Alexander M. Reiter DipTzt DrMedVet DipAVDC DipEVDC
Assistant Professor of Dentistry and Oral Surgery,
Department of Clinical Studies, School of Veterinary Medicine,
University of Pennsylvania, Philadelphia, PA 191040, USA

John G. A. Robinson BDS
Dentist to the Veterinary Profession, London, UK

Cedric Tutt BSc (Agric), BVSc (Hons) MMedVet (Med)
Cape Animal Dentistry Service, 78 Rosmead Avenue,
7708, Cape Town, South Africa

Leen Verhaert DVM DipEVDC
Trivet Veterinary Practice, Kapelstraat 52, 2540 Hove, Belgium
and Ghent University, Faculty of Veterinary Medicine,
Department of Small Animal Medicine and Clinical Biology,
Salisburylaan 133, 9820 Merelbeke, Belgium

Foreword

In 1987–88, I had the pleasure of spending time at the Dental and Veterinary Schools at the University of Liverpool while on scholarly leave from the University of Pennsylvania. There was a groundswell of enthusiasm for dentistry among a small group of British small animal practitioners at that time. During that year the British Veterinary Dental Association (BVDA) was founded and the organizational work was done that led to the publication of the original *BSAVA Manual of Small Animal Dentistry* in 1990.

In the two decades since then, dentistry has achieved its rightful place as an important part of small animal practice. The realization that the mouth is part of the body, and thus that oral health and general health are dependent on each other, is increasingly appreciated. Although rapid progress is being made, dentistry is an interesting exception to the usual development pattern for clinical specialties (in which the initial steps occur in the veterinary schools, only later spawning specialists in practice). When it comes to dentistry, in the UK as is also the case in the USA, the veterinary schools are playing catch up to enlightened practitioners. Because the standard veterinary school curriculum contains so little dentistry, post-graduate continuing professional development opportunities in dentistry are critically important. BVDA is the leading force in the UK for programs combining class-room and hands-on learning. I urge all UK-based readers of this book to join BVDA (browse to www.BVDA.co.uk for information). The *BSAVA Manual of Canine and Feline Dentistry* is the essential companion in written form.

The authors and editors of the third edition of this BSAVA Manual have built on the tradition of earlier editions by providing information tailored to the small animal general practitioner. Dentistry now has its recognized specialists, but the fundamental fact remains that all patients presented to small animal practitioners have a mouth. Every mouth should be examined every time ('LIFT THE LIP'), and the result will be very frequent recognition of oral diseases. The full breadth and depth of information on veterinary dentistry is now too large to fit into a single book – what is needed is a concise, authoritative description of what the general small animal practitioner needs to know. For example, that fractured teeth have consequences and can be treated with a good prognosis under the right circumstances - the arcane details of various endodontic and prosthodontic treatment methods are reserved for the more specialized texts and original journal publications.

BSAVA Manual of Canine and Feline Dentistry

Third edition

Editors:

Cedric Tutt
BSc (Agric), BVSc (Hons) MMedVet (Med)
Cape Animal Dentistry Service
78 Rosmead Avenue, 7708, Cape Town, South Africa

Judith Deeprose
BDS
Titchfield Dental Health, 63 Southampton Road,
Park Gate, Southampton, Hampshire, SO31 1BQ, UK

and

David Crossley
BVetMed PhD FAVD DipEVDC MRCVS
Surgical Division, Animal Medical Centre Referral Services,
511 Wilbraham Road, Chorlton, Manchester, M21 0UB, UK

Published by:

British Small Animal Veterinary Association
Woodrow House, 1 Telford Way,
Waterwells Business Park, Quedgeley,
Gloucester GL2 2AB

A Company Limited by Guarantee in England
Registered Company No. 2837793
Registered as a Charity

A catalogue record for this book is available from the British Library.

ISBN-10   0 905214 87 0
ISBN-13   978 0 905214 87 0

Typeset by: Fusion Design, Wareham, Dorset, UK.
Printed by in India by Imprint Digital.
Printed on: ECF paper made from sustainable forests.

Other titles in the BSAVA Manuals series:

For information on these and all BSAVA publications please visit our website: **www.bsava.com**

Contents

Contributors

Colin J. K. Baxter BVM&S MRCVS
Nantwich Veterinary Group, Nantwich Veterinary Hospital, Crewe
Road End, Nantwich, Cheshire, CW5 5SF, UK

Dea Bonello DVM SRV PhD DipEVDC
CVT Centro Veterinario Torinese, Lungo Dora Colletta 147, Torino,
I-10153, Italy

Anthony Caiafa BVSc BDSc MACVSc (SA Surgery and Veterinary Dentistry) MRCVS
Associate Professor in Veterinary Dentistry, University of Melbourne,
Veterinary Clinic and Hospital, Princes Highway, Werribee, Victoria
3030, Australia

David Crossley BVetMed PhD FAVD DipEVDC MRCVS
Surgical Division, Animal Medical Centre Referral Services,
511 Wilbraham Road, Chorlton, Manchester, M21 0UB, UK

Judith Deeprose BDS
Titchfield Dental Health, 63 Southampton Road, Park Gate,
Southampton, Hampshire, SO31 1BQ, UK

Thomas Eriksen DVM PhD Spec. in odont.
Associate Professor, Small Animal Hospital, Department of Small
Animal Clinical Sciences, The Royal Veterinary and Agricultural
University, 16 Dyrlaefevej-DK-1870 Frederiksberg C, Copenhagen,
Denmark

Margherita Gracis DVM DipAVDC DipEVDC
Clinca Veterinaria Milano Sud, Viale della Liberazione 26,
20068 Peschiera Borromeo, Milan, Italy

Kenneth Joubert BVSc MMedVet
Veterinary Anaesthesia, Pain Management and Critical Care
Services, PO Box 30705, Kyalami 1684, South Africa

Simone Ostermeier Tieraerztin DipEVDC MRCVS
Veterinary Dental Referral Service, Chess Veterinary Clinic,
97 Uxbridge Road, Rickmansworth, Herts, WD3 7DJ, UK

It is this core information that the BSAVA Manual covers: what conditions occur in the mouth; how to recognize and differentiate these conditions; disease progression; treatment options and prognosis; and, importantly, details of treatment for common conditions that every practice should be performing well.

The Manual is a collaborative effort of human dental and veterinary surgeons, each bringing experience from their work with small animal patients. Combine this expertise with the skills in presentation of material that the BSAVA Manual series is well known for, and the result is a book that should be ready to hand in every small animal practice.

Colin E. Harvey BVSc DipACVS DipAVDC DipEVDC FRCVS
Professor of Surgery and Dentistry
School of Veterinary Medicine
University of Pennsylvania

January 2007

Preface

Veterinary dentistry is a practical, 'hands on' part of everyday general veterinary practice that gives fulfilling results. Although a practical discipline, a thorough grounding in oral and dental anatomy and radiographic imaging of these structures helps us recognize the abnormal from the normal. Veterinary dentistry, although receiving more attention in general practice, has not achieved its potential in practice financial statements. Part of the reason for this is the feeling of ineptitude amongst some colleagues who for one or more reasons have not developed the skills required to perform these procedures.

The *BSAVA Manual of Small Animal Dentistry 2nd edition* was a comprehensive manual of small animal dentistry, including rodents and lagomorphs. With the rationalization of the BSAVA manuals to become more species-specific, the dental conditions of these animals are now dealt with within the manuals describing their husbandry, medicine and surgery.

This new edition concentrates on dental and oral conditions in dogs and cats.

The editors are grateful to the international panel of authors who have participated in this project and the new manual is a credit to their hard work and resoluteness. Although there have been some hurdles along the way, these have been overcome and the editors anticipate that this manual will build on the firm foundation provided by the previous editions.

The chapters have been set out in a logical sequence, beginning with anatomy and development and going on to clinical examination, anaesthesia and analgesia (including local and regional anaesthetic block techniques), health and safety, and the equipment required to perform veterinary dentistry adequately. From Chapter 6 more specific conditions are addressed: developmental abnormalities, infectious conditions affecting the mouth and teeth of dogs, infectious conditions affecting the feline oral cavity, physical conditions affecting the mouth and teeth, and other conditions affecting the teeth and oral cavity (including tumours). The manual is completed by a chapter on oral surgery that amongst others details the step-by-step techniques of closed and open exodontics.

The more specialized procedures of prosthodontics (including restorative dentistry and endodontics) are not covered in this manual.

Acknowledgements

The editors would like to acknowledge the support and direction of the BSAVA editorial staff, especially Nicola Lloyd, Sabrina Cleevely and Marion Jowett.

To our families who have supported us (and endured us at times) during the writing of this manual we are eternally grateful.

Cedric L. C. Tutt
Judith M. Deeprose
David A. Crossley

January 2007

Orodental anatomy and physiology

Margherita Gracis

Oral anatomy

The mouth, or oral cavity, extends from the lips to the oropharynx.

- The *oral cavity proper* is limited dorsally by the palate, laterally and rostrally by the dental arches, ventrally by the floor of the mouth, and caudally by the *isthmus of the fauces*, defined by the bilateral palatoglossal folds (Figure 1.1).
- The *oral vestibule* is the area between the lips and cheeks and the dental arches. It is relatively wide in dogs and reduced in cats.

Mucosa

The oral cavity is covered by variably pigmented mucosa.

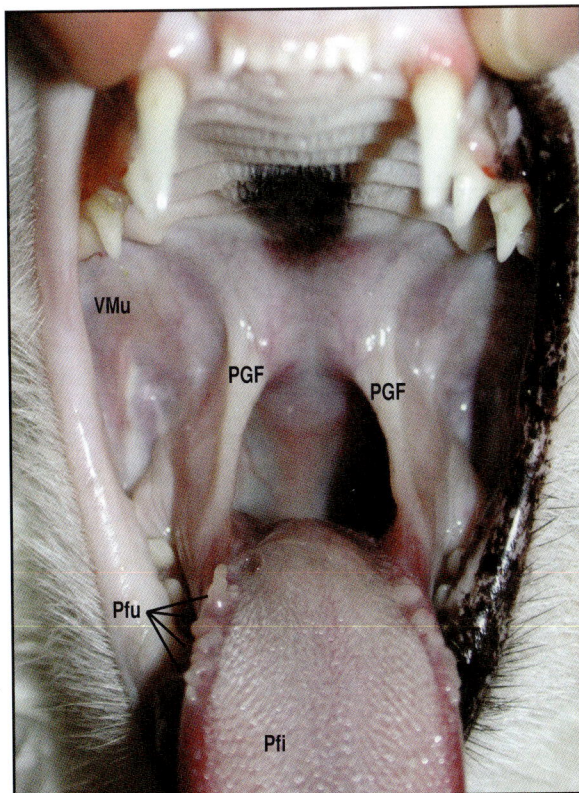

1.1 Feline oral cavity. Pfi = Lingual filiform papillae; Pfu = Lingual fungiform papillae; PGF = Palatoglossal fold; VMu = Vestibular mucosa.

- The mucosa of the oral vestibule, the cheeks, the soft palate and the floor of the mouth is composed of non-keratinized or parakeratinized stratified squamous epithelium supported by abundant connective tissue, rich in collagen fibres, which make it fairly elastic and stretchable.
- The oral mucosa lining the hard palate and the gums or gingiva, the so-called masticatory mucosa, is firmly attached to the underlying bony structures, is immovable and is mostly keratinized.

Lymphatic system

Lymphatic drainage from the face and the oral cavity is collected into mandibular, parotid, lateral and medial retropharyngeal, and superficial cervical lymph nodes. The mandibular lymph centre consists of up to five lymph nodes, easily palpable at the angle of the mandible (bilaterally), rostral to the mandibular and sublingual salivary gland. Some dogs (fewer than 10%) have a buccal or facial lymph node on the side of the face, dorsal, ventral or rostral to the angle of confluence of the facial and superior labial veins, under the zygomatic muscle. This lymph node can be unilateral or, rarely, bilateral.

Tonsils

The right and left palatine tonsils are two elongated structures located in the lateral walls of the oropharynx, caudal to the palatoglossal folds, within the tonsillar fossae, and partially covered by a mucosal fold. They have no afferent lymphatics, but drain into the medial retropharyngeal lymph nodes.

Lips and cheeks

The upper and lower lips limit the rostral opening of the mouth or oral fissure. They meet caudally at the commissures, where they continue with the cheeks. The lips and the cheeks are composed of three layers: skin, muscle and vestibular mucosa. The vestibular mucosa is continuous with the alveolar mucosa covering the jaws.

- The upper lip is grooved at the midline by the *philtrum*, which reaches the nasal plane (Figure 1.2).
- The lip carries a number of tactile hairs, the vibrissae.
- The lips may be very loose, as in dogs, or have limited mobility, as in cats, reflecting different feeding habits.

- A mucosal fold, the *labial frenulum*, attaches the lower lip to the gingival mucosa caudal to each mandibular canine tooth (Figure 1.3). Other more discrete median mucosal folds connect the upper and lower lips to the jaws, restricting labial movement.
- In cats, the maxillary labial frenulum is especially tight (Figure 1.2).

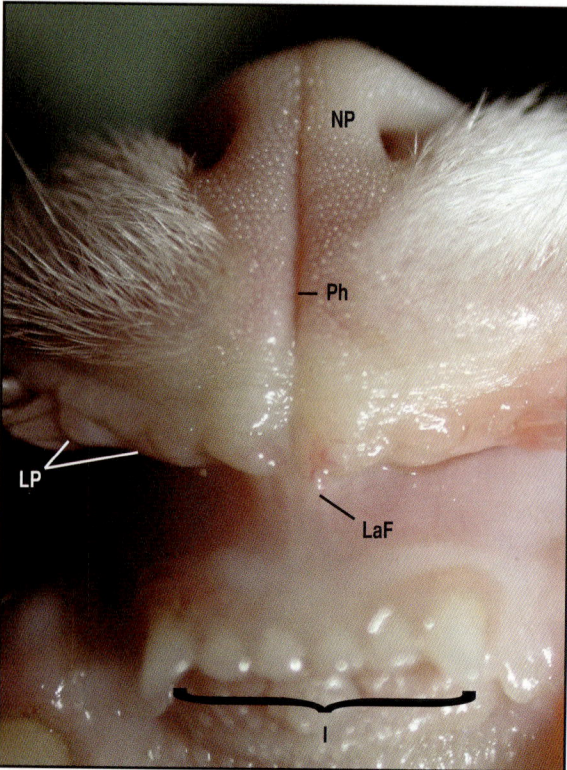

1.2 Upper lip of a cat. I = Incisor teeth; LaF = Labial frenulum; LP = Labial papillae; NP = Nasal plane; Ph = Philtrum.

- The upper lip in cats and the lower lip in dogs bear numerous large papillae for some distance on each side (Figures 1.2 and 1.3).

The muscles of the cheeks and lips include the platysma and the sphincter colli profundus, with its pars oralis (orbicularis oris muscle, incisivus superioris and inferioris muscles, maxillonasolabial muscle, buccinator muscle and mentalis muscle) and pars intermedia (zygomaticus muscle), and the levator nasolabialis muscle. They act to retract, raise and depress the lips.

Tongue

The tongue is a muscular structure that lies on the floor of the mouth, occupying the intermandibular space (see Figure 1.9). When the mouth is kept closed, the tongue normally occupies the whole oral cavity proper.

- The sensory function of the tongue is supplied by the lingual branch of the mandibular nerve, the chorda tympani of the facial nerve, and the glossopharyngeal nerve.
- The bilateral lingual arteries represent the main vascular supply to the tongue. Right and left lingual veins are located on the ventral surface of the tongue.

Muscular support

The tongue is supported by the mylohyoideus muscles that originate from the medial side of each mandibular body and meet on the midline, forming a 'sling' below it. The *root* of the tongue, which is caudal to the obvious dorsal vallate papillae and extends into the oropharynx, is attached to the hyoid apparatus through a number of muscles. From the base of the tongue, on each side, a pillar of mucosa, the *palatoglossal fold* or palatoglossal arch, extends to the soft palate, defining the caudal extent of the oral cavity (see Figure 1.1). The middle

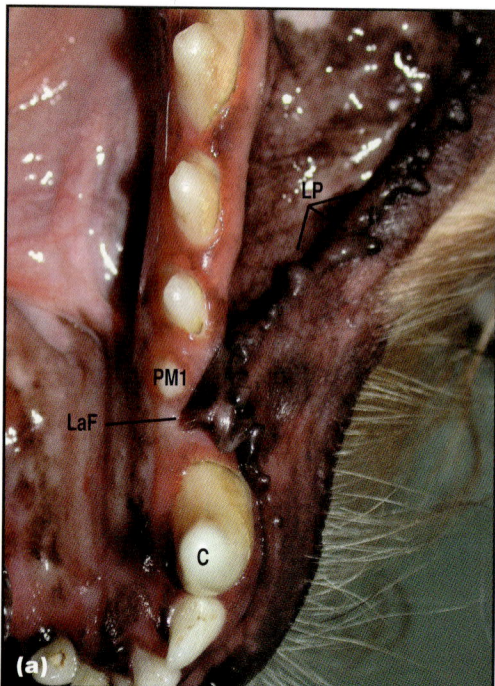

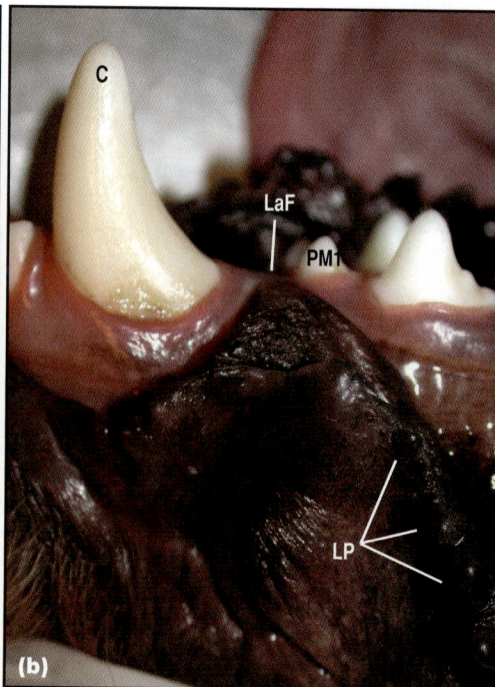

1.3 Lower lip of a dog. **(a)** Dorsal view. **(b)** Lateral view. C = Canine tooth; LaF = Labial frenulum; LP = Labial papillae; PM1 = First premolar tooth.

portion (*body*) of the tongue is attached to the medial side of the mandibles by muscular fibres, and to the floor of the mouth in the midline by a mucosal fold, the *lingual frenulum* (Figures 1.4 and 1.5). Only the rostral part (*apex*) of the tongue is free and capable of extensive movement.

The bulk of the tongue is composed of striated intrinsic and extrinsic muscles innervated by the hypoglossal nerve. Internal fibres are arranged longitudinally, perpendicularly and transversely. Extrinsic muscles include the styloglossal and hyoglossal muscles, which depress and draw the tongue caudally, and the genioglossal muscle, which depresses and protrudes the tongue.

Lyssa

In the dog, the tongue contains a single, flexible condensation a few centimetres long called the lyssa, located on the ventral surface of the apex. The lyssa is encapsulated by connective tissue and contains fat, striated muscle fibres and, occasionally, islands of cartilage. A fibrous septum departs from it and reaches the dorsal lingual surface, forming a groove on the midline that extends caudally through the whole body of the tongue (see Figure 1.4a). The function of the lyssa is still a matter of debate, but it has been postulated that it may act as a stretch receptor.

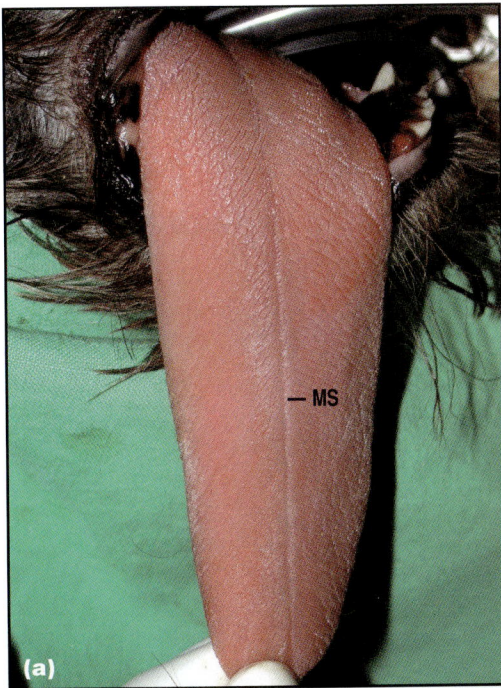

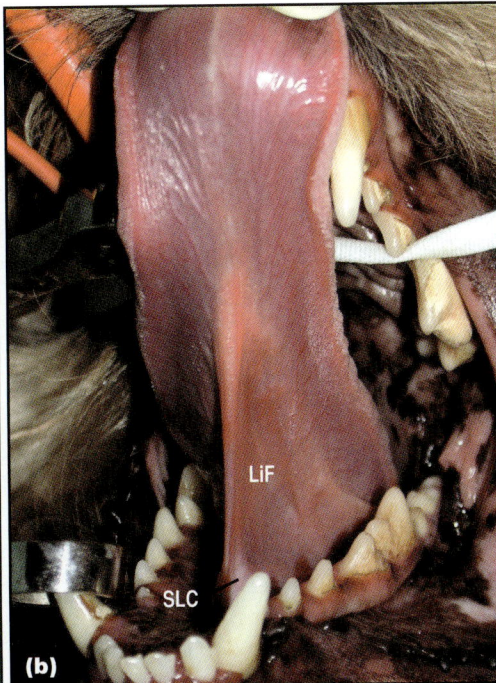

1.4

Canine tongue.
(a) Dorsal surface.
(b) Ventral surface.
LiF = Lingual frenulum;
MS = Median sulcus;
SLC = Sublingual caruncles.

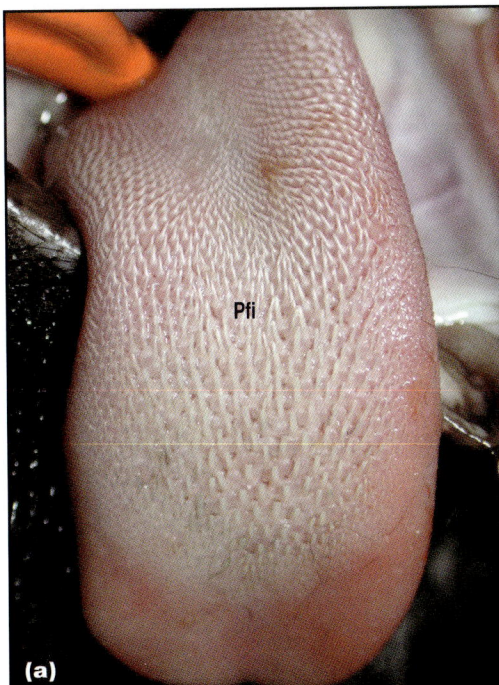

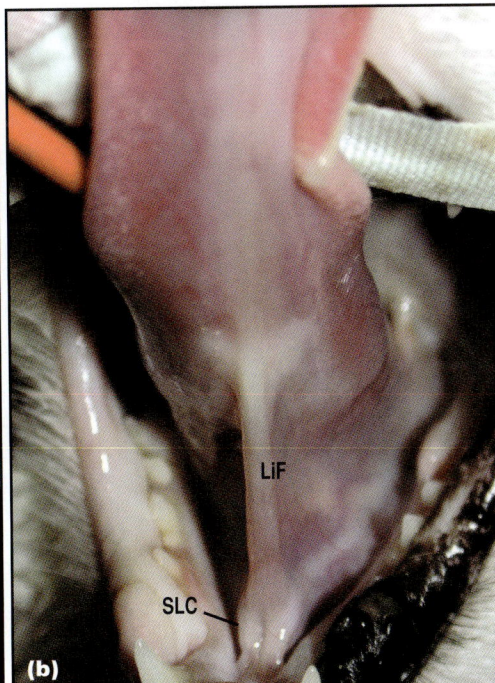

1.5

Feline tongue.
(a) Dorsal surface.
(b) Ventral surface.
LiF = Lingual frenulum;
Pfi = Lingual filiform papillae;
SLC = Sublingual caruncles.

Mucosa and papillae
The tongue is covered by stratified squamous epithelium. The ventral mucosa is rather thin and forms the lingual frenulum (see Figures 1.4 and 1.5). The mucosa on the dorsal surface is heavily keratinized and forms into papillae, namely:

- The filiform and fungiform papillae on the rostral two-thirds of the tongue
- The vallate, foliate and conical papillae on the caudal third of the tongue.

Cats also have a row of large fungiform papillae along the lateral borders of the caudal third of the tongue (see Figure 1.1). The filiform papillae are particularly well developed in cats, creating, except at the tip, a very rough surface ideal for grooming (see Figure 1.5). Fungiform, vallate and foliate papillae carry the taste buds and have gustatory functions.

Salivary glands and saliva
Salivary tissue is plentiful and broadly distributed in canine and feline oral cavities. Numerous minor glands (with multiple short ducts) are disseminated in the caudal third of the tongue, the buccal mucosa, and the mucosa of the lips and soft palate. In cats, molar salivary glands are located on the buccal (labial or buccal molar glands) and lingual (lingual molar glands) sides of the mandibular molar teeth (Figure 1.6).

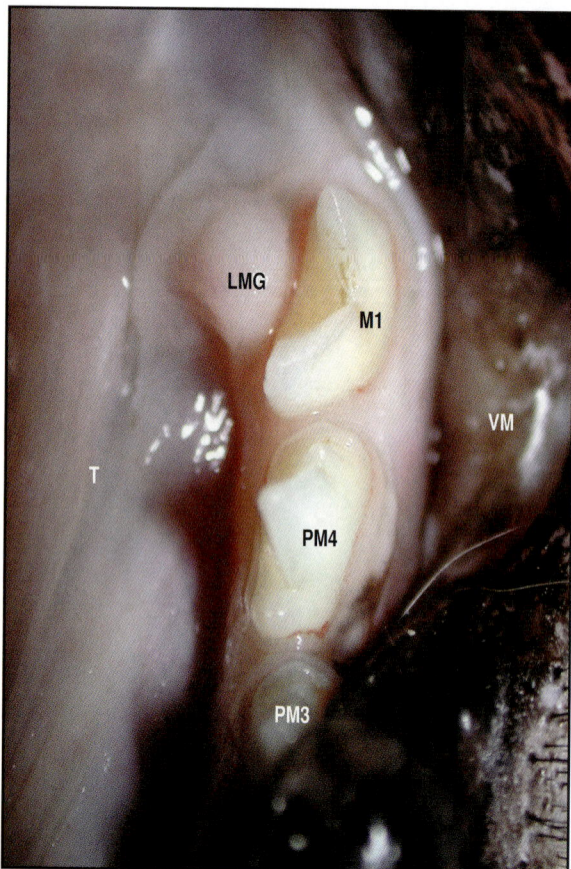

1.6 Left lingual molar gland of a cat. LMG = Lingual molar gland; M1 = First molar tooth; PM3 = Third premolar tooth; PM4 = Fourth premolar tooth; T = Tongue; VM = Vestibular mucosa.

Major salivary glands
Dogs and cats present several paired major salivary glands, namely the parotid, zygomatic, mandibular and sublingual glands. Major glands are described as having one long duct that opens in the oral cavity at a distance from the body of the gland. Because of the presence of abundant diffuse oral salivary tissue, removal or ligature of all major salivary glands has been shown not to influence saliva production in cats (Richardson, 1965).

Parotid gland: The V-shaped parotid gland lies at the base of the auricular cartilage in the retromandibular region. In dogs it may be accompanied by a number of small accessory glands. The major parotid duct, the Stenone's duct, originates from the craniomedial surface of the gland, collects the small ducts of the accessory glands variably along its length, runs lateral to the masseter muscle and opens in the upper cheek, on the buccal mucosa opposite to the maxillary fourth premolar tooth (Figure 1.7).

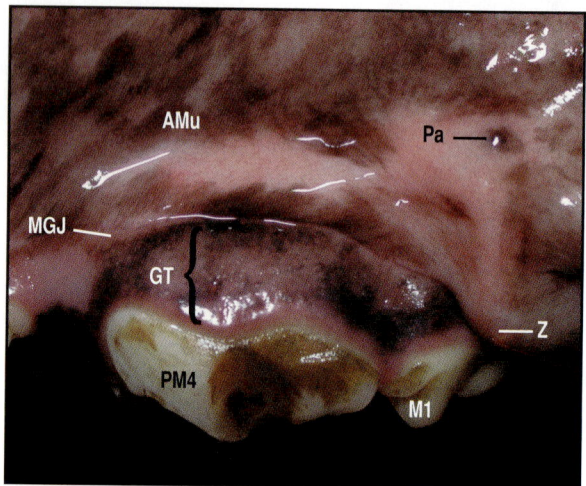

1.7 Salivary duct openings of the left parotid (Pa) and zygomatic (Z) glands in a dog. AMu = Alveolar mucosa; GT = Gingival tissue; M1 = Maxillary first molar tooth; MGJ = Mucogingival junction; PM4 = Maxillary fourth premolar tooth.

Zygomatic gland: Among domestic animals, only dogs and cats have zygomatic salivary glands. The gland lies on the floor of the orbit, in the rostral portion of the pterygopalatine fossa, ventral and medial to the zygomatic arch and dorsolateral to the last molar tooth. Its major duct, the Nuck's duct, opens in the upper cheek opposite the first molar tooth, a few millimetres rostral to a group of up to four openings of minor ducts of the same gland, and caudal to the parotid duct opening. A ridge of mucosa connects the Stenone's and Nuck's ducts' openings (see Figure 1.7).

Mandibular and sublingual glands: The mandibular salivary gland is located slightly caudal and medial to the angle of the mandible, in the region limited ventrally by the linguofacial vein, and caudally by the maxillary vein. The gland's connective tissue capsule is in common with the monostomatic portion of the sublingual gland, which is located rostrally to the mandibular gland. In dogs, and sometimes in cats, the sublingual gland also has a polystomatic portion that consists of 6–12 lobules of salivary tissue with independent short ducts that open on the sublingual mucosa beside the frenulum, next to the body of the tongue. The long mandibular gland duct, or Wharton's duct, and the duct of the monostomatic portion of the sublingual gland, the Bartolino's duct, run sublingually in the intermandibular space, and open at the sublingual papilla or caruncle, at the base of the lingual frenulum (see Figures 1.4 and 1.5). In 30% of dogs the two ducts merge before opening. If they drain independently, the sublingual duct opens dorsal to the mandibular duct (Figure 1.8).

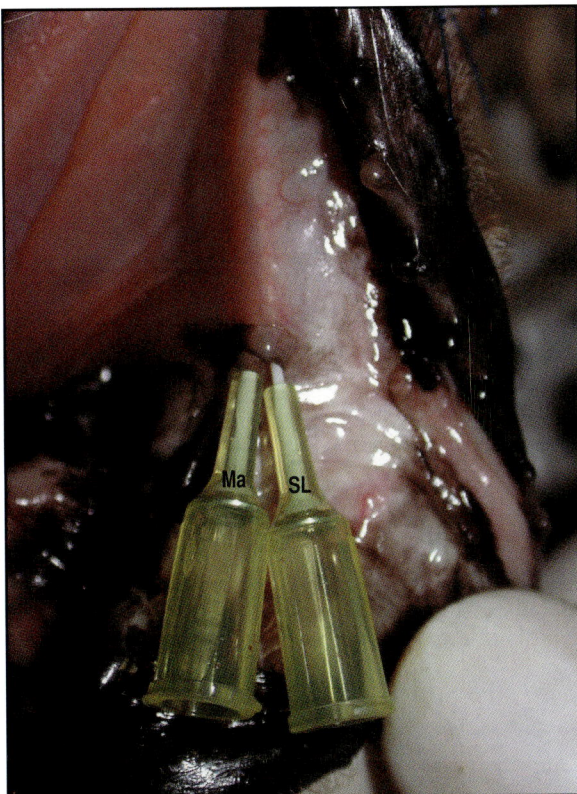

1.8 Left sublingual (SL) and mandibular (Ma) salivary ducts, catheterized with soft thin Teflon intravenous catheters. A left mandibulectomy had previously been performed on this dog.

Saliva

Salivary glands provide saliva, a secretion with a complex composition and multiple functions. Saliva can be clear and watery or mucoid and rather viscous, depending on the hydration status of the patient and the source of the sample. According to some authors, the parotid is the only gland with a pure serous salivary secretion. In contrast, all other minor and major glands produce mixed mucous and serous saliva.

In addition to lubricating the oral mucosa, saliva moistens the developing food bolus, facilitating mastication, easing its passage through the oral cavity and preparing it for deglutition. Saliva also plays an important protective role through its antimicrobial component, including enzymes, lysosomes and immunoglobulins that moderate oral colonization by bacteria.

- Besides having direct antibacterial activity, saliva secretion helps to protect the oral cavity by mechanically washing the surface of the teeth and oral mucosa, hence reducing the number of microorganisms present.
- Some salivary components (such as proteins) prevent bacterial adherence to the oral tissues by binding to the microorganisms' surface.
- Saliva possesses antifungal and antiviral activity.

However, as the composition of saliva is distinctive for each individual, the effectiveness of these mechanisms varies. Saliva also acts as a buffer, helping to maintain the normal pH of the oral cavity, which in dogs and cats is about 7.5.

Saliva production and secretion are of particular importance for thermoregulation in dogs. An increase in ambient and body temperature normally results in increased salivation.

Saliva production and secretion are regulated by the autonomic nervous system. The parasympathetic system determines a continuous basal flow of saliva that keeps the oral tissues moistened and lubricated at all times, and is vital for maintenance of oral health. Taste, visual and olfactory stimuli may cause an increase in both saliva production and secretion by sympathetic stimulation.

Jaws

Jaw development

Each of the embryonic tissues (ectoderm, mesoderm and endoderm) contribute to skull, facial and orodental development. The primitive stomodeum or oral cavity, including the epithelium of the lips, cheeks, gingiva, palate and floor of the mouth, originates from the ectoderm. The superficial ectodermal layer also contributes to salivary gland and tooth enamel formation. The ectomesenchyme, a mesoderm derivate of the neural crest cells, gives rise to the skull bones, alveolar bone, periodontal ligament fibres, cementum, dentine and pulp. The tongue is mainly of endodermal origin. The mandibles and maxillae are derived from the first branchial arch.

Maxillae: Each maxilla forms in relation to the infraorbital nerve and its anterior superior dental branch, to the outer side of the cartilaginous olfactory capsule. Maxillary development is strictly dependent on the formation of the zygomatic (or malar) and nasal septum cartilages. The palatal shelves of the right and left maxillary processes meet at the midline along the median palatine suture, and fuse rostrally with the incisive bones along two sutures that depart just caudal to the incisive papilla and run laterally to the diastema between the lateral incisor and the canine tooth (incisivomaxillary sutures) (see Figure 1.10). The incisive bones are derived from early fusion of the bilateral nasomedial processes during the embryonic stages of development. The maxillae and the incisive bones ossify by membranous ossification, characterized by direct secretion of bone matrix within connective tissues without intermediate cartilage formation. They then grow following superficial remodelling and bone apposition along the incisivomaxillary and palato-maxillary sutures (see Figure 1.10).

Mandibles: The mandibles form in relation to the inferior dental nerve, in the area of the first right and left branchial arches, as bilateral cartilaginous rods called Meckel's cartilage, or rather lateral to it. In fact, only a small portion of the Meckel's cartilage, at the level of the alveolus of the canine tooth, is incorporated in the dentary bone, the precursor of the mandible. The mandibular articular or condylar cartilage forms independently from the rest of the mandibular bone, from a secondary cartilage that fuses with the mandible during the fetal stage of development, while the most caudal part of the Meckel's cartilage becomes the malleolus of the middle ear. The condylar cartilage and the portion in the area of the canine tooth are therefore the only areas of the mandible that go through endochondral ossification (with intermediate cartilage formation), as the remaining structures ossify by membranous ossification.

The growth rate of the mandible is very rapid in the early stages of development, up until 6–8 months of age. In dogs, the rostral portion of the mandible has been shown to grow only until 50 days of age. Also, the area between the middle mental foramen and the rostral margin of the coronoid process grows only slightly in length during development. It mainly increases in height following dental eruption and alveolar process development, and because of bone apposition at the ventral border. The definitive mandibular length is therefore reached primarily by virtue of two simultaneous and opposing processes taking place at the caudal aspect of the jaw. Bone is produced at the caudal border of the vertical ramus, the condyle and the coronoid process, while bone is resorbed at the rostral borders, creating room for the molar teeth. After 6–8 months of age, when bone deposition essentially equals bone resorption, mandibular volume will not change significantly.

Craniofacial growth factors: Craniofacial growth control is multifactorial. The shape and size of the skull are genetically determined at an early fetal stage and its growth follows allometric principles: each point moves following a predetermined curve. So, if a disharmony develops, it will become evident at a critical age and follow a predictable evolvement. However, growth of the mandibles and maxillae is regulated by different genes and their development does not take place simultaneously. Each quadrant (maxillary *versus* mandibular; right *versus* left) grows independently and is individually controlled. This implies that during growth the relationship between upper and lower jaws and left and right may vary.

Furthermore, development is controlled by environmental, endocrine, traumatic, functional and other factors. Malnutrition, bacterial and viral infections, hyperthermia, chemical and teratogenic agents are only some of the factors known to alter skull growth. In addition, development and activity of the teeth and facial and oral soft tissues, such as the tongue, lips, cheeks, nasal structures and muscles of mastication,

greatly influence bone growth. Multiple studies performed in animals and humans have shown that masticatory muscle function in particular may affect craniofacial development. The caudoventral part of the mandible, the area of greatest change during jaw development and growth, is the area of attachment of the masticatory muscles and is especially subjected to this type of influence.

Jaw structure and function: maxilla

The jaws are the teeth-bearing bony structures that surround the oral cavity proper. The upper jaw, the maxilla, articulates with the incisive bone rostrally, the nasal bone dorsally, the contralateral maxillary bone and the vomer medially, and the temporal, lacrimal and zygomatic bones caudally. Normally, the incisive bone carries the incisors and the maxillary bones carry all remaining upper teeth. The maxillary alveolar process is very shallow and the roots of the teeth are actually implanted in the vertical body of the bone (Figure 1.9).

Infraorbital canal: The maxilla is perforated by the large infraorbital canal, which carries the omonymous artery, vein and nerve. The canal begins at the maxillary foramen in the pterygopalatine fossa, runs within the maxilla and opens at the infraorbital foramen on the lateral aspect of the maxilla, between the fourth and third premolar teeth (Figure 1.9a). In dogs, the infrabony portion of the canal is in strict relation to the roots of the fourth premolar tooth. It runs slightly apical and palatal to the distal root and passes in between the mesiobuccal and palatal roots. Because of its presence, particular care should be taken when performing surgical procedures in this area. In cats, the canal, which is no more than a few millimetres long, is located apical to the third premolar tooth, just below the ventral margin of the orbit (Figure 1.9c).

Hard palate: The horizontal palatine process of each maxilla articulates with the palatine process of the incisive bone, the contralateral maxillary palatine process and the ipsilateral palatine bone, forming the roof of the mouth or hard palate, which separates the oral cavity from the nasal cavities (Figure 1.10a).

- The primary palate is the incisive portion of the palate and associated soft tissues.
- The secondary palate includes the remaining hard and soft palatal structures.

Due to the embryonic origin and development of the palatal structures, congenital clefts of the primary palate typically develop along the incisivomaxillary sutures with an oblique inclination, and may be accompanied by labial defects. Secondary palate defects develop along the midline of the hard and soft palate, from the caudal margin of the palate to the incisive papilla, with variable extensions.

Rostrally, the palate is perforated by two large openings, the *palatine fissures*, through which the incisive ducts of the vomeronasal organ pass (Figure 1.10a). The incisive ducts open in the oral cavity lateral to a smooth protuberance of palatal mucosa called the

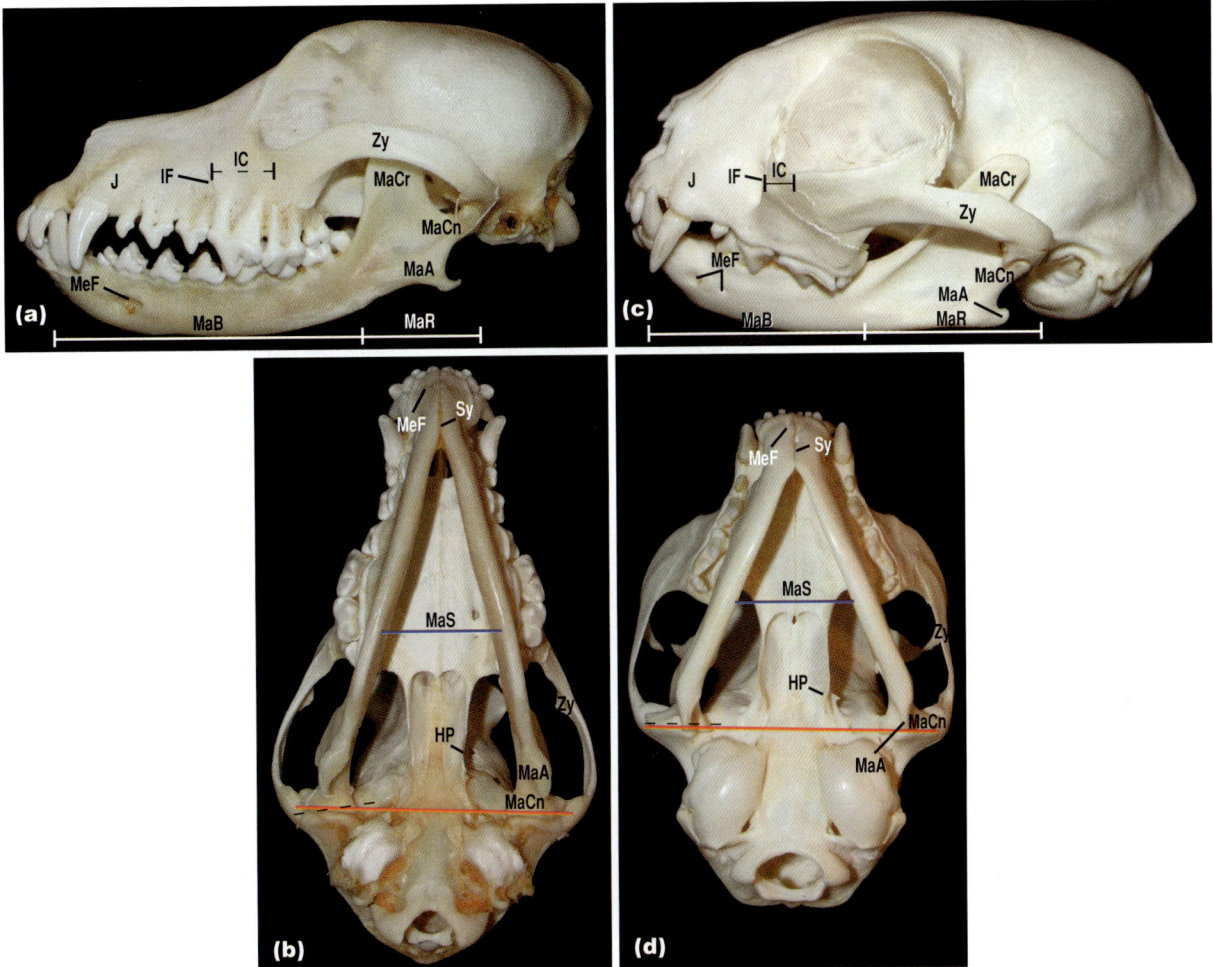

1.9 Mesocephalic skulls. **(a)** Canine left lateral. **(b)** Canine ventral. **(c)** Feline left lateral. **(d)** Feline ventral. Solid red line denotes the common axis of rotation of right and left TMJs passing through medial part of condylar processes. Broken black line (b and d) represents the long axis of condylar process. HP = Hamular process of pterygoid bone; IC = Infraorbital canal; IF = Infraorbital foramen; J = Bony jugum (canine tooth); MaA = Angular process; MaB = Mandibular body; MaCn = Condylar process; MaCr = Coronoid process; MaR = Mandibular ramus; MaS = Intermandibular space; MeF = Mental foraminae (in this canine skull the caudal and middle foraminae have merged into one opening); Sy = Mandibular symphysis; Zy = Zygomatic arch.

incisive papilla, caudal to the central incisor teeth (Figure 1.10b). The size and superficial pigmentation of the papilla varies greatly and it can be particularly evident in dogs. The hard palate is covered by thick, heavily keratinized mucosa that is firmly attached to the palatal periosteum and forms a number of transverse ridges (*rugae*), which are concave caudally (Figure 1.10b). The number of rugae is relatively consistent (7–8 in cats, 8–12 in dogs), so that in brachycephalic animals they literally fold up, creating deep depressions that often collect food particles and debris (Figure 1.10c). Cats have rows of papillae between the ridges (Figure 1.10d).

Soft palate: Caudal to the last molar teeth, the mucosa of the hard palate is continuous with the mucosa of the soft palate. The soft palate is a muscular structure covered by oral mucosa on the ventral surface and nasal mucosa on the dorsal surface. It separates the dorsal nasopharynx from the ventral oropharynx and hangs as a hammock between the hamular processes of the pterygoid bones (see Figure 1.9). Its caudal margin normally lies on the tip, or apex, of the epiglottis.

In brachycephalic animals the soft palate is often said to be long, as it covers part or all of the laryngeal inlet. However, the size of the soft palate in these individuals is simply not proportional to their pharyngeal cavity. The cause of a relatively long palate (and possibly of a 'large' tongue) is a genetic defect that is responsible for an early interruption of bony growth without affecting the oral soft tissues.

Palatine arteries and nerves: The major and minor palatine arteries are the main vascular supply to the palatal mucosa, periosteum and bone. They penetrate through the hard palate at, and caudal to the palato-maxillary suture, respectively, which usually corresponds to the level of the maxillary fourth premolar or first molar teeth (see Figure 1.10).

- The minor palatine artery mainly supplies the soft palate.
- The major palatine artery runs rostrally along the midline of each palatine process, supplying most of the soft and hard tissues of the hard palate.

7

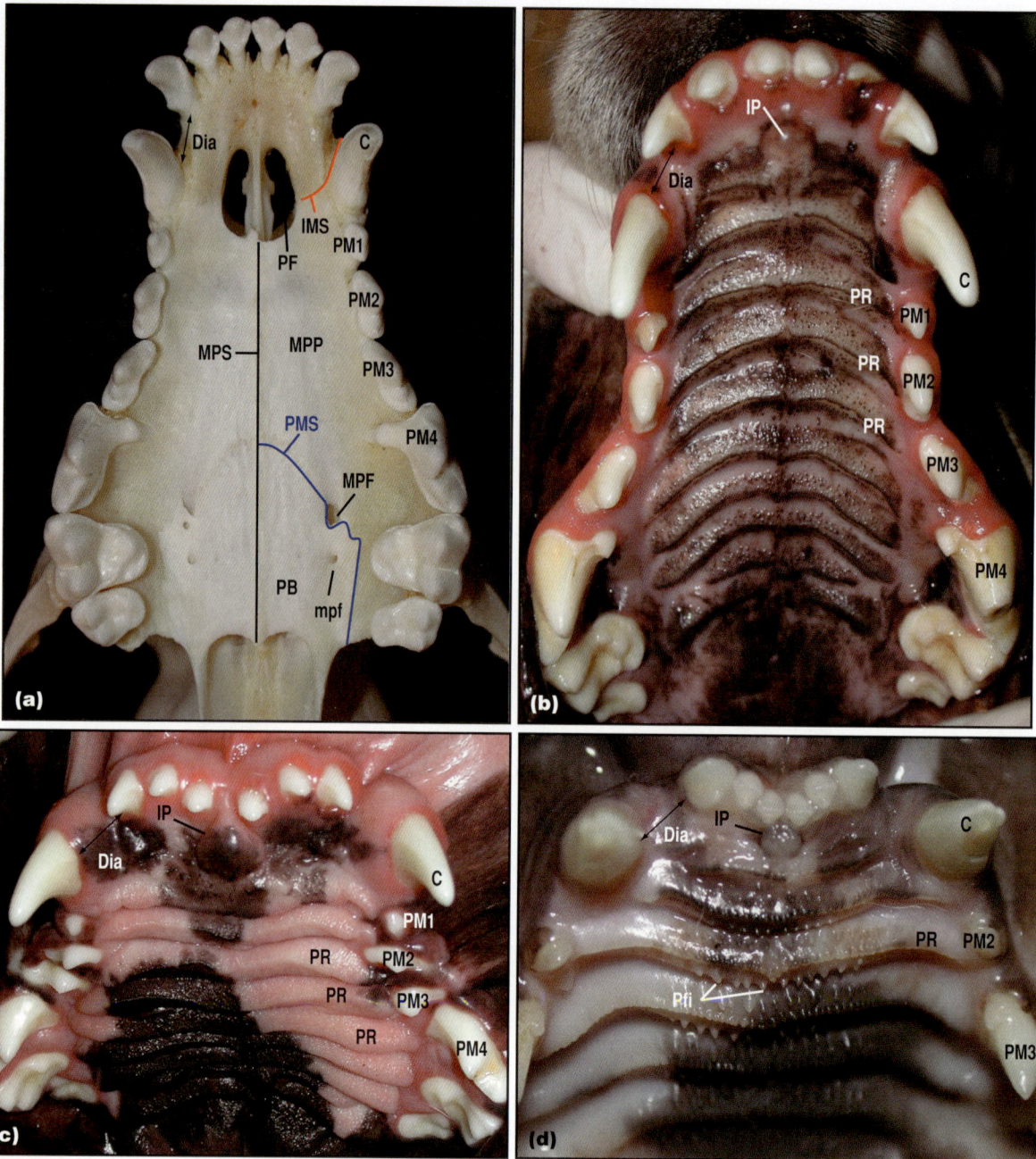

1.10 Hard palate. **(a)** Mesocephalic canine skull. **(b)** Clinical aspect in a mesocephalic dog. **(c)** Clinical aspect in a brachycephalic dog. **(d)** Clinical aspect in a brachycephalic cat. C = Canine tooth; Dia = Diastema; IMS = Incisivomaxillary suture (red line); IP = Incisive papilla; MPF = Major palatine foramen; mpf = Minor palatine foramen; MPP = Palatine process of the maxillary bone; MPS = Median palatine suture (black line); PB = Palatine bone; PF = Palatine fissure; Pfi = Filiform papillae; PM1 to PM4 = First to fourth premolar teeth; PMS = Palatomaxillary suture (blue line); PR = Palatal ridges (rugae).

Before being anastomosed with the contralateral vessel caudal to the incisor teeth, the major palatine artery gives off a branch that enters the palatine fissure to supply the nasal mucosa, and another that runs between the third incisor and canine tooth. It is then anastomosed with the lateral nasal artery. The major and minor palatine branches of the maxillary nerve follow the omonymous arteries and represent the sensory nerve supply to the hard and soft palate, while branches of the glossopharyngeal and vagus nerves supply the muscles of the soft palate.

Jaw structure and function: mandible

The lower jaw comprises the mandibles. Dogs and cats are anisognathic, i.e. they have a short, narrow lower jaw compared with the upper jaws (see Figure 1.9).

- Each mandible consists of a toothless vertical *ramus* and a horizontal *body* which carries all the lower teeth.
- Right and left mandibles meet rostrally at the *symphysis*.

Symphysis: The symphysis can develop into a true synostosis, with bony fusion of the mandibular plates, or it may persist throughout life as a synchondrosis, with a fibrocartilaginous pad and transverse connective fibres that permit some flexibility and independent movements of the right and left mandibles. However, even in animals with a flexible union, independent movements are limited by the superficial mandibular periosteum that spans the joint space and by the conformation of the temporomandibular joints (TMJs). The symphysis is vascularized by the terminal branches of the inferior alveolar arteries.

The scarcity of vascular anastomoses crossing the symphyseal space between right and left mandibles may be responsible for slowing or hindering invasion of the symphyseal region and contralateral mandible by neoplastic lesions.

Mandibular canal and foraminae: Located on the caudal medial aspect of the mandible is the entrance to the mandibular canal, the large *mandibular foramen*, midway between the last molar tooth and the angular process. The canal carries the mandibular alveolar artery, vein and nerve, and runs rostrally, paralleling the ventral border of the mandibular body. Particularly in medium size and small dog breeds, the root apices of some of the mandibular premolars and molars can reach or even cross the mandibular canal, piercing the ventral cortex (see Figure 1.17). The canal opens rostrally on the lateral aspect of the mandible through the caudal, middle and rostral *mental foraminae*, situated apical to the third and first premolar teeth and the first or second incisor tooth, respectively (see Figure 1.9). The middle mental foramen is largest, and in dogs can be palpated beneath the labial frenulum. In cats, it is at mid-height of the mandible at the diastema between the canine and the third premolar teeth.

Intermandibular space: The intermandibular space, between the right and left mandibles, is occupied by the tongue and some of the muscles of the hyoid apparatus, in particular the bilateral mylohyoid muscles, which raise the mouth floor (innervated by the mandibular branch of the trigeminal nerve), and the geniohyoid muscles, which move the hyoid apparatus cranially during swallowing (innervated by the hypoglossal nerve).

Mandibular ramus and fossa: The mandibular ramus comprises:

* The large and thin vertical *coronoid process*
* The articular or *condylar process*
* The *angular process* (see Figure 1.9).

The condylar process of the mandible articulates with the mandibular or *glenoid fossa* of the temporal bone forming the TMJ, a synovial condilatrosis (Figure 1.11). The mandibular fossa is limited caudally by the *retroarticular* (or postglenoid) *process*, and cranially by the dorsal *articular eminence* (or anteglenoid process). In dogs, the fossa is relatively flat and the articular eminence is poorly developed (Figure 1.11a). In cats, the fossa is very deep with thin but well developed cranial and caudal processes, limiting joint displacement (Figure 1.11b). A cartilaginous articular disc adheres circumferentially to the connective articular capsule, dividing the articular space into dorsal and ventral compartments. The capsule is reinforced by the *lateral temporomandibular ligament* and by a less well developed medial fibrous band. The joint is also stabilized by the powerful masticatory muscles.

The mandibular condyle of the dog is transversely elongated, with a slight dorsolateral/ventromedial inclination (see Figure 1.9). During mandibular extension, the lateral portion of the condyle slides ventrally and rostrally, stretching the lateral ligament. In the cat, the

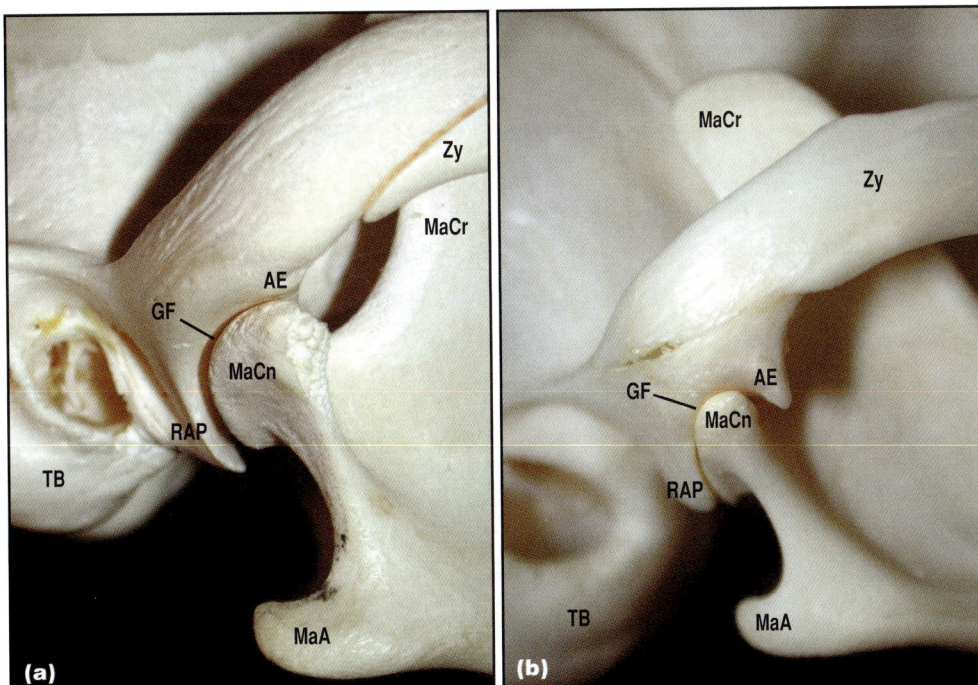

1.11

Right TMJ of **(a)** a dog and **(b)** a cat. AE = Articular eminence; GF = Glenoid fossa; MaA = Mandibular angular process; MaCn = Mandibular condylar process; MaCr = Mandibular coronoid process; RAP = Retroarticular process; TB = Tympanic bulla; Zy = Zygomatic arch.

long axes of the right and left condyles correspond to the common rotational axis, which is perpendicular to the median plane of the skull (see Figure 1.9). Consequently, in cats, the joint has very limited capability of lateral, protrusive and retrusive movement and shows, almost exclusively, hinge-like movements.

Masticatory muscles: Jaw mobility is regulated by the potent masticatory muscles, originating from the skull and attaching to the caudoventral region of the mandible.

- The *masseter* muscle extends to the lateral surface of the ramus and to the ventral and caudal borders of the mandible.
- The *temporal* muscle attaches mainly to the coronoid process.
- The *lateral pterygoid* muscle inserts on the medial surface of the condyle.
- The *medial pterygoid* muscle inserts on the medial and caudal surfaces of the angular process of the mandible, ventral to the insertion of the temporal and lateral pterygoid muscles.
- The *digastic* muscle attaches to the ventral border of the jaw.

The masseter, temporal and pterygoid muscles adduct or raise the mandible, closing the mouth. The contraction of the lateral pterygoid and deep part of the masseter also cause small lateral movements (diduction) of the lower jaw, necessary for effective mastication, especially in dogs. The digastric muscle is responsible (together with gravity) for extending or lowering the mandible, opening the mouth. The mandibular branch of the trigeminal nerve innervates all of these muscles, except the caudal belly of the digastric muscle, which is innervated by the facial nerve.

Orofacial variations

Based on craniometric evaluations, three shapes of the canine skull are recognized:

- Brachycephalic (short and wide)
- Mesocephalic (medium proportions)
- Dolichocephalic (long and narrow).

Variations occur in cats as well, but differences in size and shape are not as dramatic as in dogs. Diversity in head shape is mostly related to the size of the facial skeleton, rather than the braincase, for which measurements relative to body size remain basically consistent in all breeds.

Dental occlusion: Dental occlusion is the spatial relationship between maxillary and mandibular dental arches when the jaws are closed and in resting position. Normal or eugnathic occlusion is termed orthoclusion (Figure 1.12).

Chondrodystrophy of the chondrocranium, which causes an early interruption of growth at the base of the cranium in brachycephalic breeds, such as Bulldogs, Boxers and Pekinese, leads to the development of a disharmony or malocclusion between upper and lower dental arches defined as mesiocclusion. This condition is due to a short maxilla (maxillary brachygnathism), rather than a long mandible, and may result in extreme crowding and irregularity of the maxillary teeth (see Figure 1.10). As the mandibles preserve their growth potential, an altered contact between the rostral portion of the mandibles and the maxillae often occurs, with resultant ventral bowing of the lower jaw.

Even in brachycephalic breeds, an excessive difference in length between the mandibles and maxillae, where the mandibular incisor teeth are visible during closed-mouth examination, is considered a true defect, as it may cause a less efficacious bite.

Short mandibles (mandibular brachygnathism or distocclusion) is an unacceptable type of occlusion for any breed standard.

Oral physiology

The activities and functions of the oral structures include grooming (mainly performed by using the tongue and the incisor teeth), defence and attack by appropriately utilizing the teeth, and thermoregulation through panting and saliva production. The mouth also functions as an airway during breathing. However, the main function of the oral cavity is alimentation, with fluid ingestion, food

Teeth	Normal or eugnathic occlusion (orthoclusion)
Incisor	The mandibular first and second incisor teeth occlude on the palatal cingulum of their maxillary counterparts, with the mandibular third incisors interdigitating between the maxillary second and third incisors, creating the so-called scissors bite. An edge-to-edge occlusion, with contact between the incisal margin of the mandibular and maxillary incisor teeth, is considered acceptable by certain breed societies
Canine	The mandibular canine teeth occlude mesially to the maxillary canine teeth, equidistant from the maxillary lateral incisor and canine teeth and aligned so that there is no tooth-on-tooth contact during normal opening and closing of the mouth
Premolar	The premolar teeth interdigitate, with the maxillary premolar teeth occluding distal to their mandibular counterparts (e.g. the maxillary first premolar tooth occludes between the mandibular first and second premolar teeth). The maxillary teeth should be slightly labial to the mandibular teeth and there should not be any contact between opposite arches
Carnassial	The maxillary fourth premolar occludes on the labial side of the mesial (cat) or central (dog) cusp of the mandibular first molar tooth
Molar (dog)	The occlusal surfaces of the maxillary and mandibular molar teeth (but only the distal cusp of the mandibular first molars) come into contact

1.12 Dental occlusion in dogs and cats.

prehension and chewing, and preparation of the food bolus for swallowing. Fine coordination between the activity of the muscles of mastication, the hyoid apparatus, the tongue, the soft palate, the pharynx and the larynx is requisite for normal function, and any disturbance can significantly compromise alimentation or breathing.

Lapping

The tongue is a particularly important organ, involved in the lapping of fluids as well as prehension, preparation, translocation and swallowing of the food bolus. Fluids are licked up, transported directly between the soft palate and the base of the tongue and then swallowed.

Chewing

The chewing cycle is more complex than lapping. The tongue, lips and rostral teeth, particularly the incisors, are responsible for the initial stage of food prehension and ingestion. By sequential analysis of video footage, three distinct prehension methods for dry kibbles have been identified in cats of different skull morphology (Royal Canin Research Centre, 2002; internal data). Persians (brachycephalic breed) seemed to present a unique prehension method, defined as the lower tongue method. The lower lingual surface made the initial contact with the kibble, which was brought into the mouth after a significant number of attempts. Maine Coons (mesocephalic breed) often took the kibbles into the mouth using the dorsal lingual surface. However, Maine Coons and the dolichocephalic Siamese cats seemed to prefer the so-called labial prehension method, grasping the kibble without the help of the tongue, wedging the food between upper and lower lips and incisor teeth. Similar studies have not been performed in dogs, but it may be postulated that skull shape may influence the ability to ingest food.

Some animals chew very little or swallow their food directly. Nevertheless, normally food, once ingested, is shifted from side to side by movements of the tongue and lateral jerks of the head, and is positioned between the opposing teeth that are responsible for mastication and preparing the bolus for deglutition. Chewing is necessary to mix food with saliva, which lubricates it, and to reduce the size of the food particles to facilitate digestion by gastric enzymes once swallowed.

Voluntary muscle contraction regulates jaw movements during chewing. However, bite force is modulated by the presence of a number of specific receptors located within the alveolar bone, the muscles of mastication, the TMJ, the periodontal ligament and other dental and peridental tissues, such as the pulp, the gingiva and the alveolar mucosa. A reflex exists between the periodontal mechanoreceptors and the masticatory muscles. This reflex may cause a reduction of the bite force when an object breaks between the teeth or when opposing teeth come into contact, hence protecting teeth and supporting tissues from damaging forces. It may also increase the bite force, helping to keep food between the dental arches. Mechanical stimulation of gingival or pulpal receptors may induce an involuntary contraction of the lingual and digastric muscles, clinically observable as a twitching of the tongue and mandibular chattering. This is a relatively common occurrence during dental probing, and even if it is frequently associated with dental conditions, such as feline odontoclastic resorptive lesions, it should not always be considered an abnormal finding.

Swallowing

Once chewed, food is transported by the tongue through the fauces to accumulate as a bolus in the oropharynx. Contraction of the pharyngeal muscles and closure of the pharyngeal isthmus and laryngeal inlet allow propulsion of the bolus into the oesophagus (swallowing), avoiding aspiration into the lower respiratory tract. The bolus is brought to the lower oesophageal sphincter by sequential peristaltic contractions of the oesophageal muscles and then it passes into the stomach, where digestion begins. Swallowing occurs frequently in the conscious and sleeping animal to clear saliva and debris from the oropharynx.

Teeth

Tooth development

Odontogenesis, or tooth development, is initiated in the early embryonic development stages and continues for some time after birth. Compared with humans, in dogs and cats it is a rather rapid process. Size, shape and location are genetically and independently determined for each tooth, and tooth size is independent of mandibular and maxillary dimensions.

The biological principles and rules that regulate and influence tooth development and eruption are the same for deciduous and permanent teeth. However, it is believed that development of the permanent teeth is dependent on the normal odontogenesis of the deciduous predecessors: if a deciduous tooth is congenitally missing, the succedant tooth usually will not form.

For the tooth to develop, embryonic mesenchyme and epithelium have to interact closely.

- Initially, mesenchymal cells migrate from the neural crest into the tooth-forming region of the jaws, inducing proliferation of odontogenic epithelial cells.
- The odontogenic epithelium forms a local thickening called the *primary epithelial band*, which gives rise to the *dental lamina* in the medial nasal (premaxillary), maxillary and mandibular processes.
- During the initial stages of tooth development (*bud* and *cap stages*), cellular proliferation and migration of both epithelial and mesenchymal origin form a structure called the *tooth germ* or *organ*. In particular, the epithelium invaginates and gives rise to the *dental organ*. The ectomesenchyme condenses, partially in the *dental papilla*, which is surrounded by the dental organ, and partially in the *dental follicle*, encapsulating the dental organ and papilla.

During the succeeding stages of development (*bell* and *crown stages*), the processes of histodifferentiation and morphogenesis take place.

- The mesenchyme of the dental papilla gives rise to the *pulp* containing the *odontoblasts* that produce *dentine*.
- After the first dentine (predentine) has formed, the epithelial cells of the tooth germ (enamel organ) differentiate into *ameloblasts* that secrete enamel matrix.
- As crown enamel formation is completed, root formation commences, with differentiation of the cells of the dental follicle into *cementoblasts*, which produce *cementum*, and cells that give rise to the *periodontal ligament* and the alveolar *lamina dura*.
- Root formation is guided by a layer of epithelial cells originating from the dental organ, *Hertwig's root sheath*; these cells do not differentiate but induce histodifferentiation of the odontoblasts.
- When roots have developed about three-quarters of their length, tooth eruption occurs. As the crown penetrates through the gingival tissues, emerging into the oral cavity, the ameloblastic layer loses its nutritive supply and degenerates. For this reason, enamel cannot be repaired or replaced after tooth eruption.
- As tooth formation is completed, Hertwig's epithelial root sheath is stretched and fragmented to form a fenestrated network of cells called the *epithelial cell rests of Malassez*. The cells of Malassez persist throughout life within the periodontal ligament, retaining their odontogenic potential and being able to give rise to cystic or neoplastic lesions when stimulated.

Alterations of any specific phase of the odontogenetic process may induce specific developmental disturbances or structural defects. Tooth number and size may be altered when the induction phase (bud and cap stages of development) is disturbed, while structural changes, such as enamel and dentinal hypoplasia or dysplasia, may develop if disturbances occur during apposition and maturation (bell and maturation stages). In the case of genetic anomalies, all teeth of an individual may be affected, such as with *amelogenesis imperfecta* and *dentinogenesis imperfecta* (see Chapter 6). Environmental factors, such as trauma, metabolic, chemical or infectious agents, may affect one or more teeth.

Tooth eruption and replacement

Both dogs and cats have a *diphyodont* dentition, with deciduous and permanent sets of teeth (Figure 1.13). However, not every tooth in the mouth has a corresponding deciduous tooth. The difference between a premolar and a molar tooth is the presence of deciduous predecessors for premolars but not for molar teeth. Another exception is the first premolar tooth in dogs, which does not have a deciduous counterpart. Compared with permanent teeth, the crowns of deciduous teeth are usually smaller and whiter, because their enamel is less mineralized (Figure 1.14). In addition, deciduous teeth have relatively longer roots.

An interesting process is the so-called *molarization* of deciduous premolar teeth. Crown morphology and the number of roots of each deciduous premolar tooth is that typical of the permanent tooth positioned distal to it, rather than that of its true succeedant. For example, the maxillary deciduous third premolar tooth has three roots, like the permanent fourth premolar tooth and unlike the two-rooted permanent third premolar. Its crown shape resembles that of the permanent fourth premolar tooth, with a large mesial cusp, a shorter distal cusp and a small palatal cusp (Figure 1.14b).

Term	Definition
Diphyodont	Deciduous and permanent sets of teeth
Heterodont	Morphologically different teeth
Secodont	Teeth with sharp cutting edges
Bunodont	Teeth with rounded or conical prominent cusps
Anelodont	Limited period of growth for teeth
Brachyodont	Teeth with a short crown and relatively long root(s)

1.13 Canine and feline dentition.

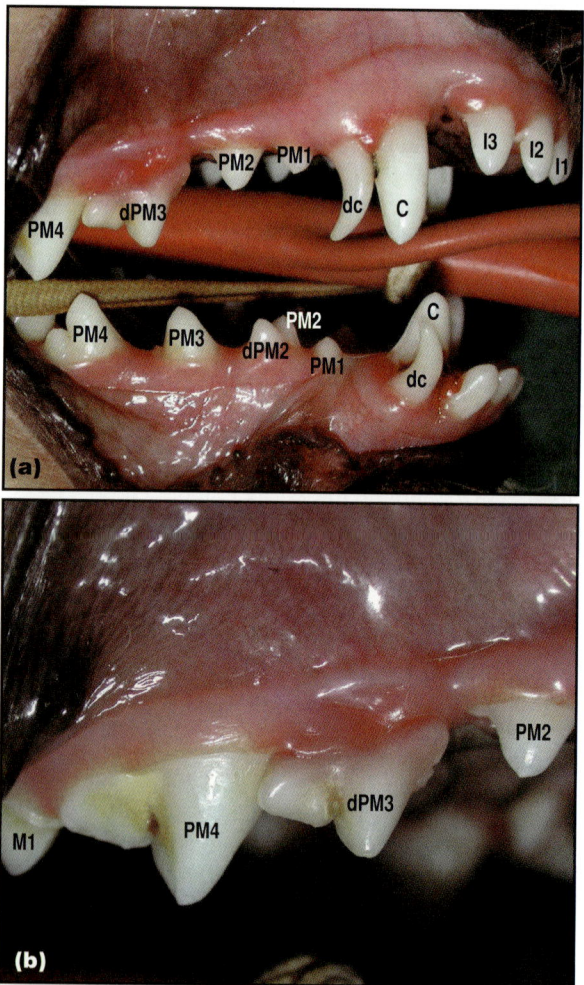

1.14 Molarization of deciduous premolar teeth. **(a)** Right side of the mouth of a dog with persistent deciduous teeth. **(b)** Detail of the maxillary right premolar teeth in the same dog as (a), showing similarity in shape of the deciduous third premolar tooth and the permanent fourth premolar tooth. C = Permanent canine tooth; dc = Deciduous canine tooth; dPM2 = Deciduous second premolar tooth; dPM3 = Deciduous third premolar tooth; I1 to I3 = Permanent first to third incisor teeth; M1 = Permanent first molar tooth; PM1 to PM4 = Permanent first to fourth premolar teeth.

Tooth eruption

Tooth eruption is defined as the process of migration of a tooth from its site of development within bone to its functional position within the oral cavity. Even if dental development begins in the fetal stage, dogs and cats are born without visible crowns, and teeth begin to erupt a few weeks after birth.

Many theories have been developed about the possible mechanisms of dental eruption of deciduous and permanent teeth but they remain poorly understood events. Eruption begins only after the dental crown has completely formed and the roots have begun to develop, showing strict chronological coordination and exhibiting precise timing in bilateral symmetry. The intraosseous phase of tooth eruption seems to depend on regulation by the embryonic dental follicle on bone metabolism on opposite sides of the tooth bud. Resorption of occlusal bone lying in the path of tooth eruption and apical apposition seem to be essential for dental eruption. Numerous studies, many performed in the dog and few in the cat, have shown that the tooth mainly plays a passive role. This theory has been supported by demonstrating that eruption is not affected by surgical destruction of the roots and periodontal ligament of developing mandibular premolars, or removal of the crown and substitution with sterile metal and silicone replicas.

Control of tooth eruption is possibly multifactorial, including genetic, environmental, infectious and traumatic factors. Some of the recognized non-genetic causes of delayed or retarded eruption in dogs and cats are radiation therapy of the skull, canine distemper virus infection, dwarfism, hypervitaminosis A, and impediment by physical trauma, supernumerary teeth, cysts and tumours.

Rotation: The definitive spatial position of an erupted tooth does not always coincide with that of the corresponding forming dental germ. Due to the small size of the growing skull, dental germs may develop with their long axis oblique or perpendicular to the dental arch. As the skull grows, the space for the teeth increases, and during eruption the teeth rotate in either a lingual/palatal or a buccal/labial direction to form, with the adjacent elements, an ordered arch. Typically, the type of rotation of the maxillary second and third premolars is such that the mesial portion of the tooth rotates buccally (B type of rotation). On the contrary, the mesial portion of the mandibular fourth premolar tooth normally rotates lingually (L rotation). However, if the mesiodistal dimension of the teeth is excessive compared with the total dental arch length, the dental germs fail to rotate, teeth erupt in the original position and tooth crowding develops, as often occurs in brachycephalic or small breed animals (see Figure 1.10c).

Exfoliation

As in eruption, exfoliation of the deciduous dentition is a relatively enigmatic process. Normally, the deciduous teeth start exfoliating and are lost before the permanent succeedant teeth begin to erupt into the oral cavity. A deciduous tooth still present in the mouth at the time of eruption of the permanent succeedant is defined as persistent (see Figure 1.14). However, the emergence of the maxillary permanent canine teeth before exfoliation of the deciduous corresponding teeth is considered normal, and the deciduous canines can persist for several days or weeks after eruption of the permanent counterpart. Eruption and root growth of the permanent teeth are normally preceded by resorption of the deciduous teeth roots, but the root of a deciduous tooth may be resorbed even when the corresponding succeedant tooth is missing. Furthermore, in the case of a missing permanent tooth it is possible that the deciduous tooth will be maintained in the oral cavity much longer than normally expected, and even for the entire life of the animal.

Dentition and eruption schedule

Dogs and cats belong taxonomically to the Order Carnivora. Based on palaeontological studies, the primitive carnivore dentition used to comprise four premolar and three molar teeth in each jaw quadrant. The *carnassial teeth* (lacerating teeth, namely the mandibular first molar and the maxillary fourth premolar teeth) are the largest teeth in all carnivores and can be used as reference to name the remaining teeth. Compared with dogs, cats are true carnivores. Probably for this reason, during evolution they have lost the bunodont molar teeth that in dogs are designed and used for chewing hard material (Figure 1.15). Dental anatomical terminology is explained in Figure 1.16.

Dogs

Deciduous dentition: In dogs, the deciduous dentition is fully erupted between the second and third months after birth, with significant breed and individual variations. There is possibly a tendency to earlier eruption in larger breeds compared with smaller breeds. The total deciduous dental formula comprises 28 teeth and is depicted as:

$$2 \ (I \ 3/3, C \ 1/1, PM \ 3/3) = 28.$$

The first deciduous teeth to erupt are usually the canine (C) teeth, followed by the incisors (I) (third, second and first in order) and the third and fourth premolars (PM). The second premolar is usually the last deciduous tooth to erupt. At three weeks of age, deciduous tooth root formation is almost completed, with apical closure occurring about six weeks after birth. In dogs, crown mineralization of deciduous teeth has been shown to begin during gestation, with mineralization of all deciduous teeth visible radiologically at the time of birth.

Permanent dentition: The first premolar and the molar (M) teeth do not have deciduous predecessors. The permanent dentition of dogs comprises 10 teeth in each maxillary quadrant and 11 teeth in each mandibular quadrant (see Figure 1.15) and is depicted as:

$$2 \ (I \ 3/3, C \ 1/1, PM \ 4/4, M \ 2/3) = 42.$$

Mineralization of the mandibular first molar tooth starts and is radiographically visible a few days before

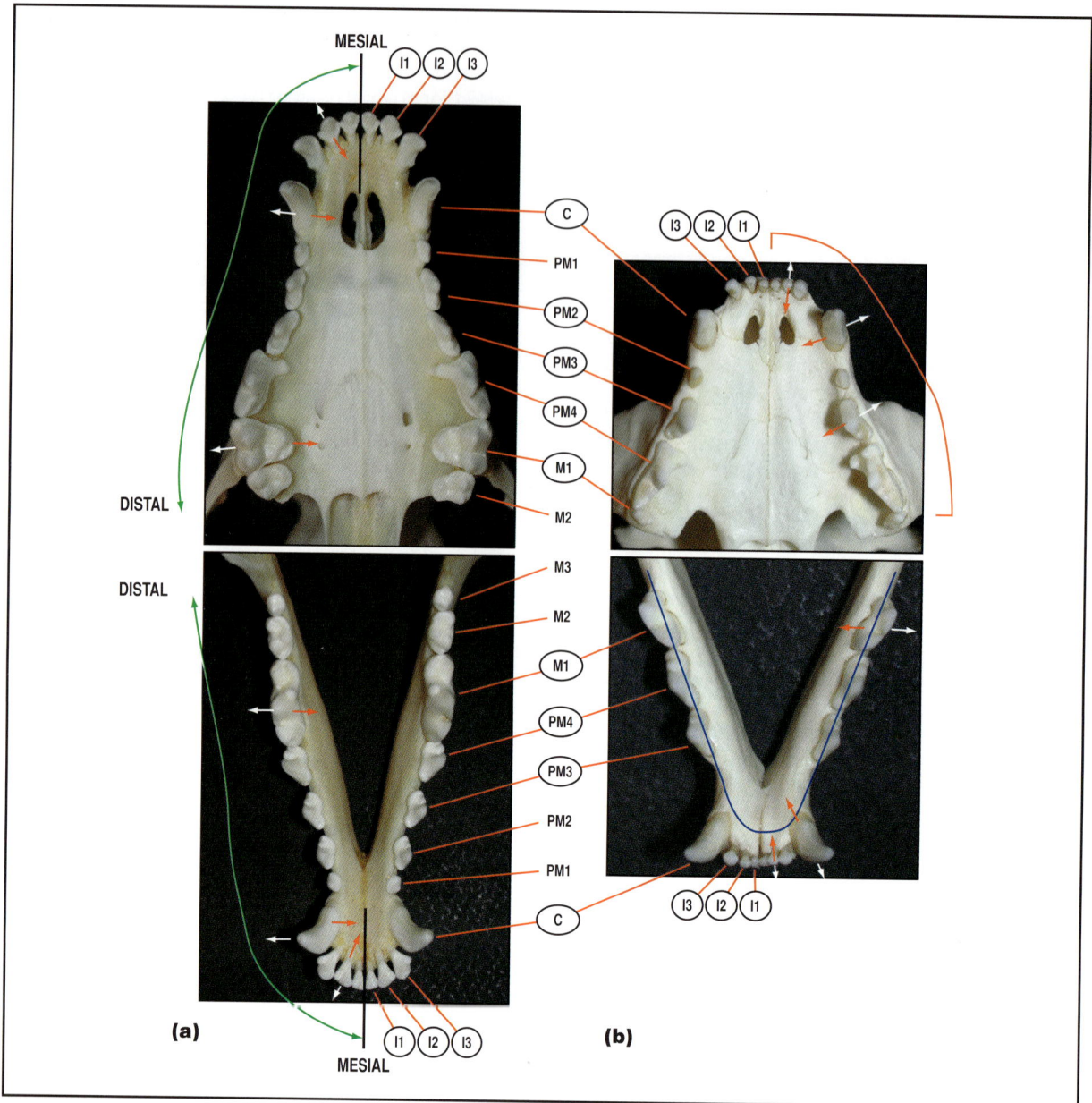

1.15 Permanent dentition of **(a)** a dog and **(b)** a cat. Note the palatal/lingual dental surface (red arrows), the labial dental surface (white arrows), the midpoint of the dental arch (black line) and the mandibular dental arch (blue line). The red line represents the left maxillary quadrant. C = Canine tooth; I = Incisor tooth; M = Molar tooth; PM = Premolar tooth.

Specific anatomical terms are used when describing dental structures. 'Cranial', 'caudal', 'dorsal' and 'ventral' can be confusing terms and should not be used.

- The teeth on the lower jaw are the **mandibular** teeth. Those on the upper jaw are referred to as the **maxillary** teeth
- Teeth are arranged in a larger maxillary and a narrower mandibular row or **arch**
- The complete dentition is divided into **quadrants**: right maxillary, left maxillary, left mandibular and right mandibular
- An area of a dental arch devoid of teeth is called a **diastema**. A large diastema exists between the maxillary third incisor and canine tooth (see Figure 1.10)
- The surface of a tooth towards the tongue or palate is defined as the **lingual** (for mandibular teeth) or **palatal** (for maxillary teeth) surface
- The portion facing the lips is the **vestibular**, buccal or labial surface
- The face of the tooth towards the midline of the dental arch (the point between the right and left first incisor teeth) is the **mesial** surface, and the opposite is the **distal** surface
- The surfaces facing adjacent teeth are defined as **interproximal** and can be either mesial or distal
- The **occlusal** surface corresponds to the masticatory surface
- The terms **apical** and **coronal** refer to directions towards the root apex or the crown of a tooth, respectively

1.16 Dental anatomical terminology.

birth. Mineralization of all other permanent teeth, and therefore presence of a complete permanent dentition, cannot be demonstrated radiologically until 3–4 months of age.

Variations in eruption schedule are common, according to breed and size of the animal, but in general the order is as follows:

- The first permanent tooth to erupt, just after the deciduous teeth, is the first premolar
- The incisor teeth (first, second and third in order) follow
- At between four and six months of age the canine teeth, the second, third and fourth premolar teeth and the molar teeth also erupt
- The last permanent tooth, generally the mandibular third molar, erupts at about 6–7 months of age.

The pattern of eruption is as follows:

- The maxillary and mandibular permanent incisor teeth erupt palatally and lingually to the deciduous predecessors
- The maxillary permanent canine teeth erupt mesially to the deciduous canines
- The mandibular permanent canines erupt lingually to their deciduous counterparts (see Figure 1.14)
- The maxillary permanent second and third premolar teeth erupt palatally to the deciduous teeth
- The maxillary permanent fourth premolar tooth erupts buccomesially to the deciduous predecessors
- The mandibular permanent premolars usually erupt lingually to the deciduous teeth.

Cats

Deciduous dentition: Eruption of the deciduous dentition of cats is completed between two and three months of age, and the dental formula is:

2 (I 3/3, C 1/1, PM 3/2) = 26.

Permanent dentition: The permanent feline dental formula (see Figure 1.15) is:

2 (I 3/3, C 1/1, PM 3/2, M 1/1) = 30.

Eruption of deciduous and permanent rostral teeth follows a similar pattern, with the incisors erupting before the canine teeth. Permanent molars usually start erupting just before the premolar teeth. Maxillary teeth may erupt slightly before the opposing mandibular teeth. Eruption of the permanent dentition is completed at about 6–7 months of age.

Dental and periodontal structures and function

Teeth are specialized structures used to prehend and prepare food for swallowing and digestion. They are also used for grooming, defence and offence.

Dogs and cats are defined as having an *anelodont* dentition, with a limited period of growth, as opposed to *elodont* teeth that grow continuously (see Figure 1.13). The teeth are of the *brachyodont* type, characterized by short crowns and relatively long roots (Figure 1.17).

Carnivores are defined as *heterodonts*, showing heterogenous dentition, with teeth morphologically different serving distinct purposes (see Figure 1.15).

- Incisors are relatively small teeth apt for cutting, with a single, long root and a short sharp crown.
- Canines are simple single-rooted teeth with a strong, long, curved conical crown used to grasp and hold, characterized by the presence of developmental grooves and shallow ridges on their crown that may allow drainage of blood while holding and killing prey. Canines are also used to lacerate flesh.
- Premolar and molar teeth have a more complicated crown morphology, with cusps, ridges and fissures that make them suitable for cutting and shearing meat and, in dogs, crushing hard materials.
- Cats have an exclusively *secodont* (cutting) post-canine dentition, with sharp dental cusps.

Despite these morphological differences, the basic structure and anatomy are identical for any tooth (see Figure 1.17). Anatomically, the neck or cervical margin of the tooth divides the crown, the portion of the tooth covered by enamel, from the root, which is deeply implanted in the alveolus.

Root

Cementum: The tooth root is covered by a layer of cementum, which is an avascular, bone-like, mineralized connective tissue composed of inorganic material (about 50%) and an organic matrix rich in collagen. Cementum is produced continuously, slightly increasing in thickness throughout life. It is normally resistant to resorption, but it can be repaired if necessary.

Root number: Teeth can have one, two or three roots, with a relatively constant number for each tooth (Figure 1.18). However, variations resulting from fusion of two roots or from the presence of an extra or supernumerary root may occur. Common examples are the maxillary third premolar tooth of both dogs and cats that often have three rather than two roots, or the feline maxillary second premolar tooth, which may have one or two roots. Roots of multi-rooted teeth may differ in size and shape (see Figure 1.17).

Root terminology:

- The area between roots of multi-rooted teeth is called the *furcation*.
- The tip of the root is called the *apex*.
- The roots are deeply implanted into their bony sockets, or *alveoli* (one alveolus per root).
- When the bone over the roots is particularly thin, such as on the maxilla, the alveolar wall may form a prominence or *jugum* that can be easily palpated under the alveolar mucosa (see Figure 1.9).

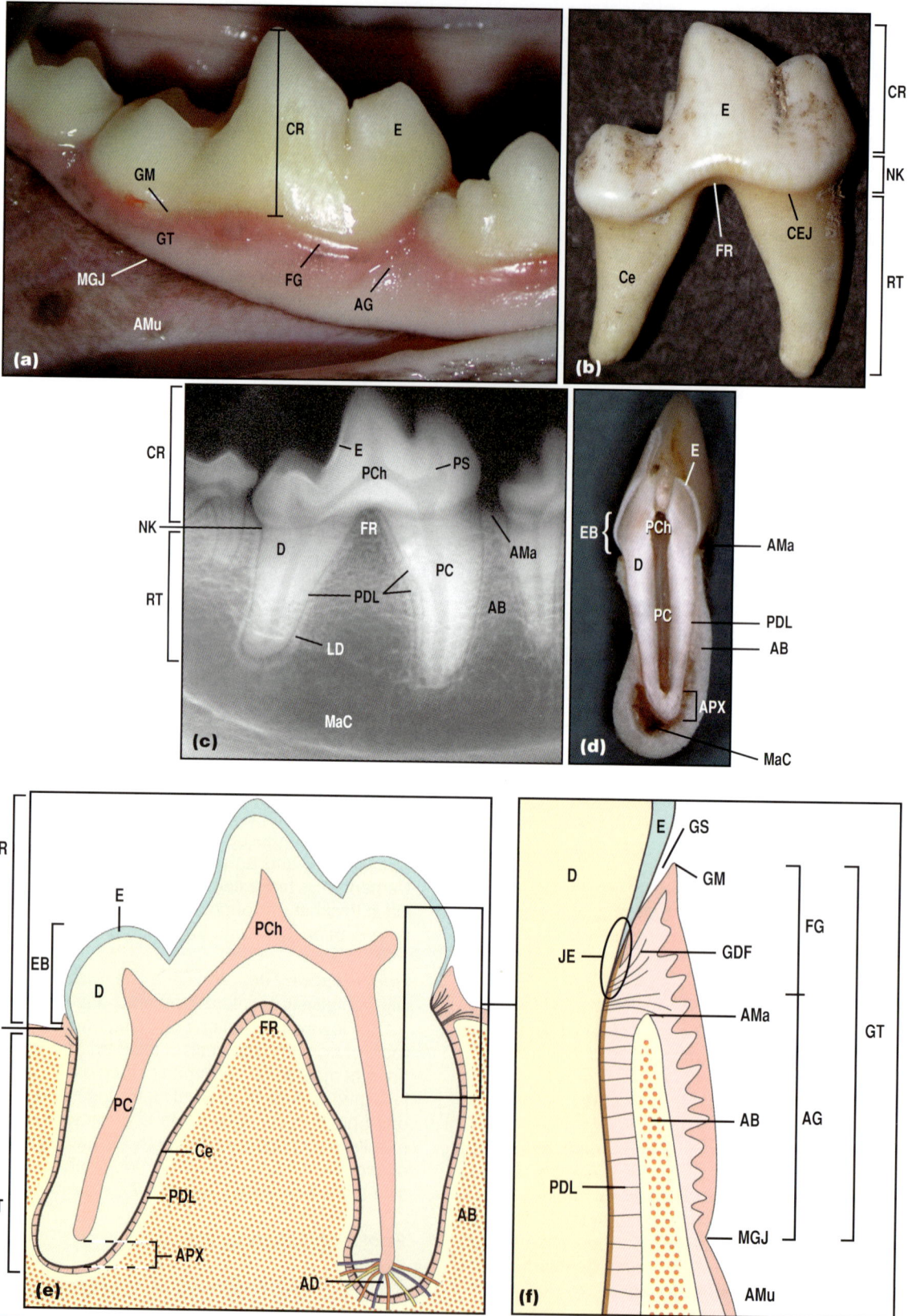

1.17 Tooth structure of the right mandibular first molar tooth of a middle-aged dog. **(a)** Clinical aspect, labial side. **(b)** Extracted tooth, labial side. **(c)** Intraoral radiographic image. **(d)** Vertical section through the mesial root. **(e)** Schematic presentation. **(f)** Detail of (e), showing periodontal structures. AB = Alveolar bone; AD = Apical delta; AG = Attached gingiva; AMa = Alveolar margin; AMu = Alveolar mucosa; APX = Apex; Ce = Cementum; CEJ = Cementoenamel junction; CR = Crown; D = Dentine; E = Enamel; EB = Tooth (enamel) bulge; FG = Free gingiva; FR = Furcation; GDF = Gingivodental fibres; GM = Gingival margin; GS = Gingival sulcus; GT = Gingival tissue; JE = Junctional epithelium; LD = Lamina dura; MaC = Mandibular canal; MGJ = Mucogingival junction; NK = Tooth neck; PC = Pulp canal; PCh = Pulp chamber; PDL = Periodontal ligament space; PS = Pulp stone; RT = Root.

Number of roots	Dog		Cat	
	Deciduous	*Permanent*	*Deciduous*	*Permanent*
One	Max/Man Is, Cs	Max/Man Is, Cs, PM1 Man M3	Max/Man Is, Cs Max PM2	Max/Man Is, Cs Max PM2
Two	Max PM2 Man PM2, PM3, PM4	Max/Man PM2, PM3 Man PM4, M1, M2	Man PM3, PM4	Man PM3, PM4, M1 Max PM3, M1
Three	Max PM3, PM4	Max PM4, M1, M2	Max PM3, PM4	Max PM4

1.18 Number of roots. Cs = Canine teeth; Is = Incisor teeth; M = Molar teeth; Man = Mandibular; Max = Maxillary; PM = Premolar teeth.

Crown and enamel

- The crown is covered by smooth *enamel*, the most highly mineralized and hardest tissue of the body, with about 96% inorganic material consisting mainly of hydroxyapatite crystals.
- The crown can have one (canine teeth) or more tubercules or *cusps*.
- The portion of the crown just coronal to the neck of the tooth enlarges to form the so-called *enamel or tooth bulge* (see Figure 1.17).

The bulge has a protective function, deflecting food particles from the gingival margin during chewing. However, its designation as the enamel bulge is inaccurate, as the bulk of the bulge comprises dentine, and the thickness of enamel is the same as adjacent areas (Crossley, 1995). Normally enamel is 0.1–0.3 mm thick in the cat and up to 0.6 mm in the dog. The area of contact between enamel and cementum is the *cementoenamel junction*, located at the neck of the tooth, where the gingiva attaches to the tooth surface.

Dentine

Enamel is very brittle and is therefore supported by dentine, which constitutes the bulk of the tooth. Dentine is a porous structure, slightly less mineralized than enamel, with an inorganic component of 70%. Up to 50,000 microscopic tubules/mm² traverse the dentinal walls from the pulp surface to the dentinoenamel and dentinocementum junctions. Each dentinal tubule is occupied by a single odontoblastic process and a small amount of gel with a rich organic component. Unusual dentinal structures, such as vasodentine (vascular inclusions) and osteodentine (intermediate cementum), have been described in the permanent teeth of cats.

Pulp system

Dentine encloses the pulp system, including the pulp chamber within the crown and the pulp canal within the root (see Figure 1.17). The pulp system contains pulp tissue, consisting of blood vessels, nerves, lymphatics, and numerous cells immersed in a collagenous matrix, such as immunocompetent cells (lymphocytes, macrophages and dendritic cells), undifferentiated mesenchymal cells, fibroblasts and specialized odontoblasts.

The pulp canal system is rather simple in dogs and cats, with one main canal for each root (see Figure 1.17). In multi-rooted teeth, the pulp chamber communicates with each pulp canal. If endodontic disease develops in teeth with more than one root, the whole pulp system will inevitably be affected. The pulp canal communicates with the external environment (the periodontal space) almost exclusively at the root apex. The apex is open, with one large canal, until 7–11 months of age, when it closes down leaving behind the so-called *apical delta*, a group of 10–20 or more microscopic ramifications that allow passage of vessels and nerves to and from the pulp canal (see Figure 1.17). Non-apical ramifications, canals that extend from the main root canal to the periodontal space anywhere along the root coronally to the apex, may be found with a relatively low prevalence in canine and feline teeth. Furcation canals have recently been shown in one-quarter of studied feline carnassial teeth.

Periodontal space

The *periodontal ligament*, together with blood vessels, nerves and lymphatics, occupies the narrow space between the tooth and the alveolar bone, the *periodontal space*. The terminal portions of its connective fibres (*Sharpey's fibres*) are embedded into cementum on one side and into alveolar bone on the other, holding the tooth in place and acting as a shock-absorber in response to masticatory stimuli (see Figure 1.17). In fact, the fibres are not arranged in a 'mat' on the tooth surface, but in interwoven and interconnected bundles that can be classified based on their functional orientation into alveolar margin, horizontal, oblique, apical and interradicular fibres.

Alveolar process

The portion of the jaw that accommodates the roots of the teeth is defined as the alveolar process and comprises cancellous or trabecular bone limited by a lingual and a labial external cortical plate covered by periosteum. The alveolar process is perforated by the dental sockets or *alveoli*. The alveolar walls are composed of a cribriform plate that provides attachment for the periodontal ligament fibres. The alveolar process forms and is maintained in relation to the teeth. If a tooth is congenitally missing, the alveolar process will not develop. If a tooth is lost or extracted, the alveolar process will gradually be resorbed. The *alveolar margin* is the coronal margin of the alveolar bone, and is normally located not more than 1 mm apical to the neck of the tooth.

Gingiva

The gingiva is that part of the oral mucosa that covers the alveolar process of the jaws and surrounds the neck of the teeth. It is a resilient tissue, able and necessary to withstand continuous masticatory trauma (see Figures 1.7 and 1.17).

Attached gingiva: The attached gingiva is tightly bound to the periosteum, and is separated from the alveolar mucosa by the *mucogingival junction* (MGJ), a line that is obviously demarcated in some dogs, but less visible in cats (see Figures 1.7 and 1.17). As the alveolar mucosa is somewhat loose, if needed it can be stretched to visualize the MGJ. On the maxillary teeth, palatally the attached gingiva blends into the palatal mucosa without a clear demarcation. The width of the attached gingiva varies greatly among individuals, and even in different areas of the same mouth. Typically, in dogs and cats the width is greatest at the maxillary canine teeth and diminishes in the incisor and pre-molar/molar regions.

Free gingiva: The free gingiva is the unattached portion of the tissue, measured from the bottom of the gingival sulcus to the coronal border of the gingiva, the *gingival margin* (see Figure 1.17). It tapers to a knife-edge at the gingival margin.

Gingival sulcus: The gingival sulcus is a shallow space between the free gingiva and the tooth. Its depth is reported in the literature to be normally less than 1 mm in the cat and less than 3 mm in the dog, but variations are common, especially taking into account the great disparity in dog breeds and sizes. Also, similarly to the attached gingiva, the sulcus depth may vary between different teeth in the same mouth.

Sulcular epithelium: The oral surface of the free gingiva is basically indistinguishable from the keratinized or parakeratinized attached gingiva. Its internal lining, the sulcular epithelium, is a thin, non-keratinized stratified squamous epithelium. The apical portion of the sulcular epithelium, the *junctional epithelium*, consists of a band of stratified non-keratinized epithelium that connects to the tooth surface by means of hemidesmosomes.

Gingival fibres: The gingival tissue is rich in connective fibres, mainly collagen, that attach the gingiva to the underlying bone and cementum, encircling the tooth in a ring-like fashion, providing rigidity to the tissue, and are continuous with the periodontal ligament fibres (see Figure 1.17). Some of these gingival fibres, the transseptal group, extend between the cementum of approximating teeth, and are considered responsible for orthodontic relapse or post-extraction tooth movement in human patients. In dogs and cats, however, the position of remaining teeth will not necessarily change following extraction of adjacent teeth. The reason is currently unknown, but it could be speculated that transseptal fibres are missing in domestic carnivores, or have a different arrangement than in humans.

Periodontium
The cementum, periodontal ligament, alveolar bone and gingiva together form the supporting tissues of the tooth or *periodontium* (see Figure 1.17).

Dental radiographic anatomy

Enamel, dentine and cementum
Enamel, dentine and cementum are highly mineralized tissues that appear radiographically opaque. Their density (Figure 1.19) is relative to their mineral content.

Radiopaque
Enamel
Alveolar bone (lamina dura)
Dentine
Alveolar bone (cancellous)
Cementum
Radiolucent
Endodontic system
Periodontal ligament space

1.19 Radiodensity of dental and periodontal structures (highest to lowest).

- *Enamel* will appear more radiopaque than the other structures. However, enamel is not always detectable, as it is normally very thin. Only when the radiographic beam passes tangential to a significant thickness of enamel, will this show as a radiopaque line.
- Because of their comparable mineral content, *cementum* and *dentine* are normally radiographically indistinguishable. In the case of a pathological increase in thickness (hypercementosis), cementum, which is normally only a few microns thick, can be seen as a slightly more radiolucent layer covering the root dentine.

Pulp system
The pulp system follows the external tooth shape and always appears radiolucent. Even in the case of pulp death, the radiodensity of the pulp canal will not change. Dystrophic pulp mineralization, or pulp stones, may be seen within the pulp chamber as discrete, round or oval radiopaque structures (see Figure 1.17). In young animals, the open apex is seen directly connected to the periodontal space, but the thin microscopic canals of the adult apical delta are not visually detectable.

Periodontal space
Healthy tooth roots are surrounded by a thin radiolucent line, the periodontal space. The size of the space should be consistent all around the root. In cases of ankylosis, the periodontal space will be obliterated. Usually, the cross-section of canine and feline teeth is round or oval. Therefore, as the X-ray beam passes tangential to the root surface, a single radiolucent line is created on the radiograph. In dogs, however, some of the roots of the mandibular premolar and molar teeth may exhibit a cashew nut-like cross-section, with a concave area

between two convex surfaces. This developmental groove adds to the physical retention properties holding the root within the alveolus and in this case the periodontal space may appear radiologically as a double radiolucent line (see Figure 1.17).

Alveolar bone and lamina dura

The radiopaque alveolar bone is cancellous bone with a variable radiographic trabecular pattern, surrounding the roots and filling the furcation area of multi-rooted teeth. Its gingival margin, the alveolar margin, should be not more than 1 mm apical to the cementoenamel junction. It appears as a radiopaque line continuous with the lamina dura, the wall of the tooth socket (the cribriform plate), and is seen around the root as a line more radiopaque than the adjacent trabecular bone (see Figure 1.17). Despite its radiodensity, the lamina

dura is not cortical bone. Its high radiopacity is due to a summatory effect of the X-ray beam passage through this thick layer of bone.

Evaluation

Rounding of the sharp angle between the alveolar margin and the lamina dura, lamina dura discontinuity and periodontal space widening are indicative of periodontal disease. The absence of the lamina dura at the apex of a root may be indicative of endodontic disease, but it can also be a normal radiological feature. Confirmation of a diagnosis of periapical pathology requires widening of the periodontal space and discontinuity of the lamina dura to be present.

When evaluating radiographic images of the teeth (Figure 1.20) and surrounding anatomical structures it is important to consider that they are two-dimensional

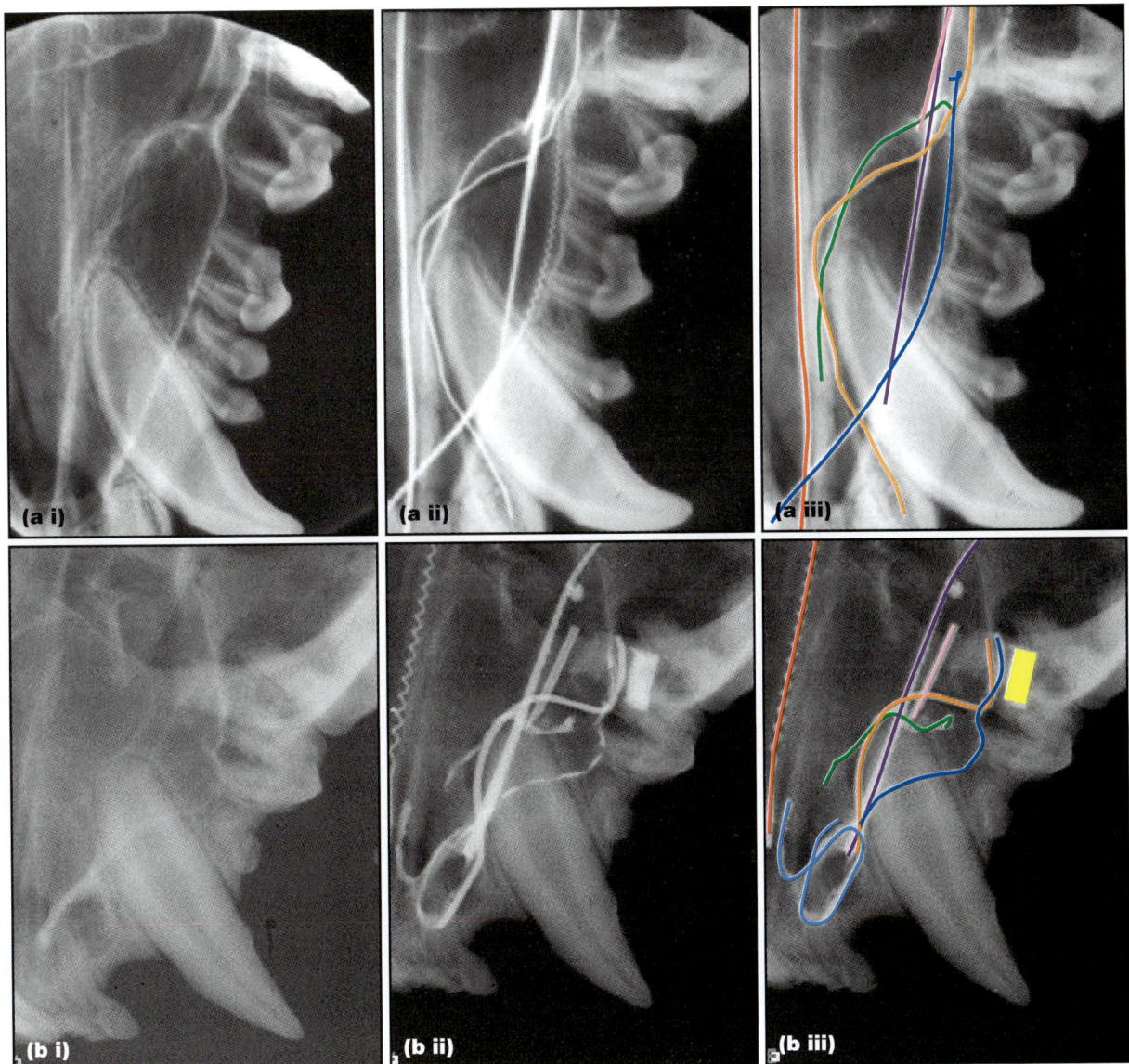

1.20 Radiographic study of the maxillary canine tooth in mesocephalic **(a)** dogs and **(b)** cats. **(i)** Survey series. **(ii)** Radiopaque markers in place. **(iii)** Coloured radiopaque markers to indicate anatomical structures visible on these images in close vicinity or superimposed on the tooth root. Blue = Palatine fissure; Green = Conchal crest; Light blue = Line of conjunction between the vertical body of the maxilla and its palatine process; Orange = Incisivomaxillary canal; Pink = Lacrimal canal; Purple = Palatine sulcus; Red = Vomer bone; Yellow = Infraorbital canal. (Reproduced and modified from Gracis and Harvey (1998) and Gracis (1999) with permission from the *Journal of Veterinary Dentistry*)

reproductions of three-dimensional objects. Differences in angulation of the X-ray beam may change the appearance of any single structure. A good example is the pulp canal of the maxillary canine tooth. As it is oval in shape, it may appear more or less wide depending upon the X-ray beam angle. Superimposition between different structures is also a common problem associated with interpretation of skull and dental radiographs. The mandibular canal and the mental foraminae may mimic periapical lucencies at the mandibular teeth roots. In mesocephalic dogs and cats the conchal crest (the attachment of the ventral nasal concha to the maxilla), the line of conjunction between the maxillary body and its palatine process, and the incisivomaxillary canal (and the lacrimal canal in cats only) have been shown to appear often superimposed on, or in close proximity to, the maxillary canine tooth on images obtained with the intraoral bisecting angle technique (see Figure 1.20). Finally, the zygomatic arch often obstructs visualization of the feline maxillary premolar and molar teeth.

Dental physiology
Following eruption, teeth do not change in size or shape, but dentine and pulp do have the ability to react to physiological and pathological stimuli.

Newly erupted teeth usually have very thin dentinal walls (made up of so-called primary dentine), a large pulp canal with abundant pulp tissue, and incomplete roots with open apices (Figure 1.21a). *Apexogenesis* (root development and apical closure) occurs within a few weeks or months following eruption. This process occurs as a result of continuous activity of the epithelial cells of Hertwig's root sheath at the tooth apex. Apical closure takes place in cats and dogs between 7 and 11 months of age, the roots of the mandibular first molar tooth being the first and the maxillary canine tooth root the last to form.

Following eruption/apexogenesis, the odontoblasts continue to produce dentine, known as *secondary dentine*. The odontoblastic layer lies on the periphery of the pulp, just below the dentine. As odontoblasts produce dentine, they move centripetally towards the centre of the canal. Therefore, the pulp canal becomes narrower with time, while the dentinal walls become thicker (Figure 1.21). Particularly in young animals, the radiographic study of root canal size can be used to determine the individual's age with more precision than using other parameters, such as tooth wear.

Vascular supply
In addition to being responsible for dentine production, the pulp has nutritive, protective and sensory functions.

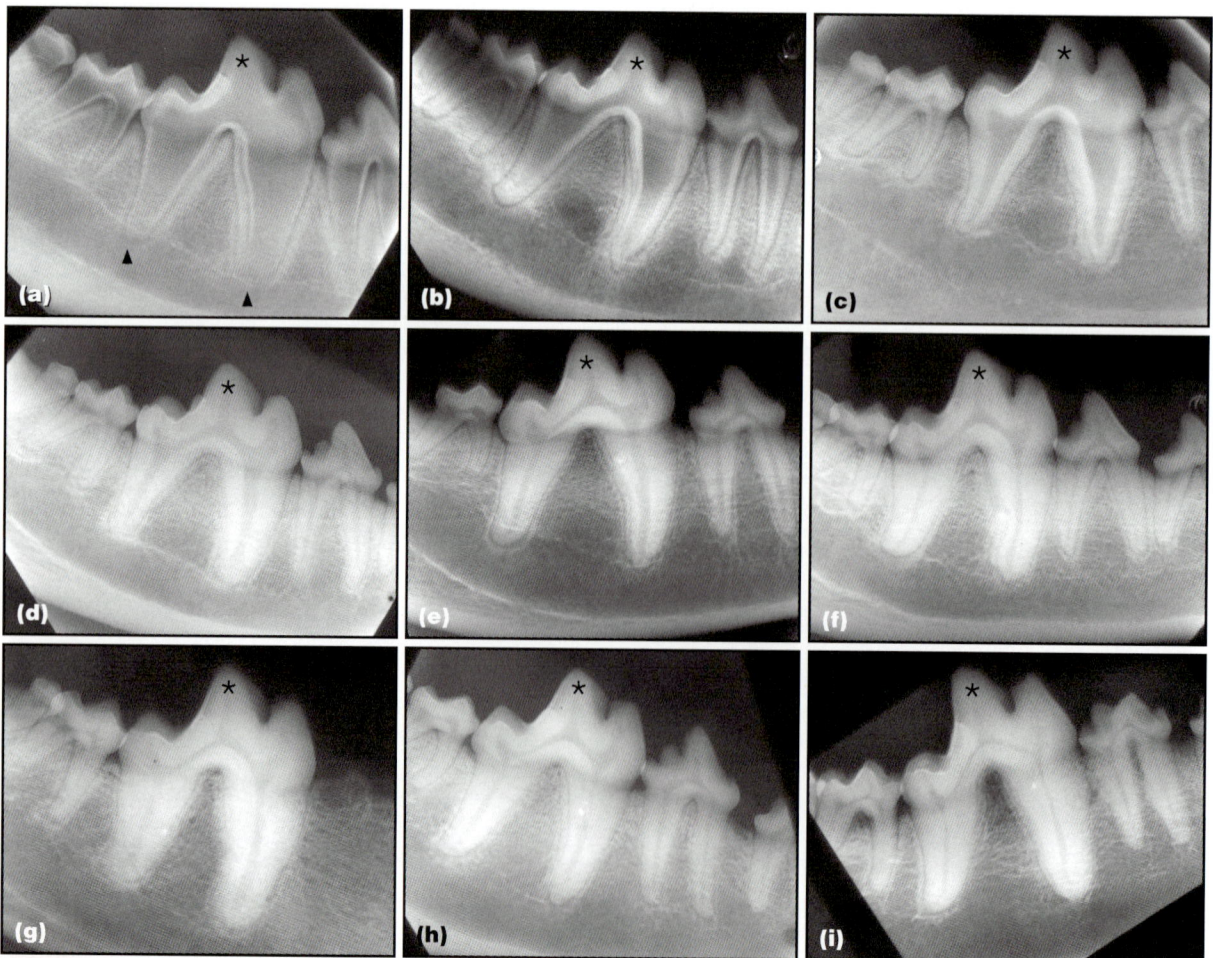

1.21 Radiographic series showing the ageing process (apexogenesis and dentine production) of the right mandibular first molar tooth (✶) of the dog. **(a)** 6 months, open apex (arrowheads). **(b)** 9 months, apical closure. Following progressive thickening of the dentinal walls and narrowing of the pulp system. **(c)** 16 months. **(d)** 2 years. **(e)** 3 years. **(f)** 4 years. **(g)** 6 years. **(h)** 8 years. **(i)** 12 years.

Nutrition to the surrounding tissues is provided by the pulp's rich vascular supply.

Mandibular artery: The vascular supply to the mandibular teeth comes from the inferior alveolar (mandibular) artery, a branch of the maxillary artery.

- The inferior alveolar artery enters the mandibular canal through the mandibular foramen, on the medial side of each mandible.
- It is accompanied by a vein and nerves and during its course gives off small vessels that penetrate the bone, reaching the apices of the roots and periodontal structures, including the alveolar bone, periodontal ligament and gingival tissues.
- The artery exits through the mental foraminae on the lateral and rostral surfaces of the mandible (see Figure 1.9), branching into the *mental arteries*, supplying the rostral part of the lower jaw and chin.

Maxillary artery: The maxillary teeth receive their blood supply from different branches of the maxillary artery.

- In the pterygopalatine fossa, just before it enters the maxillary foramen, the maxillary artery gives off the *caudal dorsal alveolar artery*.
- Small *dental branches* that leave the caudal dorsal alveolar artery reach the molar teeth.
- Within the infraorbital canal the *infraorbital artery*, the main continuation of the maxillary artery, gives off the *middle dorsal alveolar branches* to the roots of the fourth premolar tooth.
- Near the infraorbital foramen, the rostral opening of the infraorbital canal, the infraorbital artery gives off the *rostral dorsal alveolar artery* (or incisovomaxillary artery), which enters the incisivomaxillary canal.
- The *incisivomaxillary canal* and its neurovascular content run rostrally into the maxillary bone. They make a sharp turn dorsally, then run medially towards the canine tooth root apex, and continue rostrally and medially into the incisive bone, supplying the first three premolar teeth, the canine tooth and incisor teeth.
- The infraorbital artery exits the infraorbital foramen and divides into *lateral* and *dorsal nasal arteries*, supplying the muzzle.

Sensory system
Pulp tissue is rich in sensory nerve fibres entering the endodontic system through the apex in close association with arterioles, venules and lymphatics. External stimuli (e.g. variation in tooth temperature or direct injury of pulp tissues) cause sensory nerve fibres to produce a sensation of pain. In human patients, dentine exposure associated with periodontitis or aggressive tooth brushing, caries and other pathological processes may also cause perception of pain. The currently accepted theory of dentine sensitivity is the hydrodynamic hypothesis of Brännstrom, whereby noxious stimuli cause fluid movement within the dentinal tubules, which is registered by the pulpal free endings of nerves located underneath the odontoblasts and possibly by the odontoblasts themselves. Dehydration of the exposed dentinal tubule results in tension on the odontoblastic process, causing pain.

Defence mechanisms
Tooth defence mechanisms include the ability of the pulp to produce additional dentine, called tertiary or reparative dentine. *Tertiary dentine* is produced at a higher rate than secondary dentine in response to a pathological stimulus that may cause dentinal exposure, such as caries, abrasion or attrition. As its dentinal tubules are irregularly arranged and reduced in number, it reflects light differently and may appear darker than the surrounding primary or secondary yellowish dentine. Tertiary dentine is also more likely to absorb pigments and thus become discoloured.

External stimuli may also stimulate the thickening of the dentine around the tubules and obliteration of their lumens, which leads to dentinal *sclerosis*. Sclerosis may develop as an age-related physiological process with protective functions. In every case, it causes a reduction of dentine permeability. Typically, sclerotic teeth have a glossy appearance.

References and further reading

Crossley DA (1995) Tooth enamel thickness in the mature dentition of domestic dogs and cats – preliminary study. *Journal of Veterinary Dentistry* **12**, 111–113

DeBowes LJ, DeForge DH, Kesel ML and Hawkins BJ (2000) Normal canine intraoral radiographic anatomy. In: *An Atlas of Veterinary Dental Radiology*, eds DH DeForge and BH Colmery III, pp. 3–14. Iowa State University Press, Iowa

Dyce KM, Sack WO and Wensing CJG (1996) *Textbook of Veterinary Anatomy, 2nd edn.* WB Saunders, Philadelphia

Evans HE (1993) *Miller's Anatomy of the Dog, 3rd edn.* WB Saunders, Philadelphia

Getty R (1975) *Sisson and Grossman's The Anatomy of the Domestic Animals, 5th edn.* WB Saunders, Philadelphia

Gracis M (1999) Radiographic study of the maxillary canine tooth of four mesaticephalic cats. *Journal of Veterinary Dentistry* **16**, 115–128

Gracis M and Harvey CE (1998) Radiographic study of the maxillary canine tooth in mesaticephalic dogs. *Journal of Veterinary Dentistry* **15**, 73–78

Hennet P (1995) Dental anatomy and physiology of small carnivores. In: *BSAVA Manual of Small Animal Dentistry 2nd edn*, ed. DA Crossley and S Penman, pp. 93–104. BSAVA, Cheltenham

Hennet PR and Harvey CE (1992) Craniofacial development and growth in the dog. *Journal of Veterinary Dentistry* **9**, 11–18

Jayne H (**1898**) *Mammalian Anatomy. A Preparation for Human and Comparative Anatomy. Part I. The skeleton of the cat, its muscular attachment, growth and variations compared with the skeleton of man.* Lippincott, Philadelphia

Mulligan TW, Aller MS and Williams CA (1998) Normal radiographic anatomy. In: *Atlas of Canine and Feline Dental Radiography*, ed. MS Aller, pp. 68–90. Publishing Veterinary Learning Systems, Trenton

Orsini P and Hennet P (1992) Anatomy of the mouth and teeth of the cat. *Veterinary Clinics of North America: Small Animal Practice* **22**, 1265–1277

Richardson RL (1965) Effect of administering antibiotics, removing the major salivary glands, and toothbrushing on dental calculi formation in the cat. *Archives of Oral Biology* **112**, 245–253

Stockard CR and Johnson AL (1941) *The Genetic and Endocrinic Basis for Differences in Form and Behavior*. The Wistar Institute of Anatomy and Biology, Philadelphia

Ten Cate AR (1994) *Oral Histology. Development, Structure, and Function, 4th edn.* Mosby, St. Louis

2

Oral and dental diagnostics

Colin J.K. Baxter

Oral and dental pathology can be found in most animals. When oral pathology is noted by the owner, and the animal presented for consultation, the disease will often be obvious and well advanced. Only about 8% of dental cases are presented by the pet owner specifically for their oral condition. Owners are often unaware of an oral problem until signs are discovered during a full clinical examination of animals presented for either a health review or with another specific complaint.

Clinical signs and symptoms may indicate oral disease to be primary or secondary in nature. Thorough examination with the appropriate knowledge of anatomy and the correct interpretation of investigative test results leads to accurate diagnosis. This is the key to appropriate treatment planning. From a clinical perspective, diagnosis is achieved as a result of the combination of history taking, physical examination, initial oral examination, preanaesthetic diagnostic testing, full oral examination and oral diagnostic testing, i.e. radiography. The latter two components are carried out under general anaesthesia. All case details must be recorded.

History

History taking is the foundation of a complete examination. At the initial consultation, the general medical history together with a specific dental history should be obtained. The age of the animal and its lifestyle are also relevant.

The presenting complaint should be investigated. A history of the complaint should include symptoms, onset, duration, progression and whether or not any previous dental treatment has been received. The immediate history may be of major importance if, for example, the animal has been involved in an accident or received trauma to the face or head. A full history should still be taken to assist with perioperative decisions and postoperative advice, but life-saving procedures should be initiated promptly.

Clinical signs
The main clinical signs of oral disease are:

- Halitosis
- Broken or discoloured teeth
- Changes in eating behaviour
- Rubbing or pawing the face

- Drooling
- Bleeding or purulent discharge from the mouth
- Inability or unwillingness to open and close the mouth
- Change in temperament
- Facial swellings.

Halitosis
Periodontal disease (Figure 2.1) is the most common cause of halitosis and occurs as a result of the bacterial breakdown of food and other materials on the tooth surface (Figure 2.2) and in periodontal pockets. Other causes of halitosis are stomatitis, tumours, cleft palates (Figure 2.3), cleft lips (Figure 2.4), oronasal and

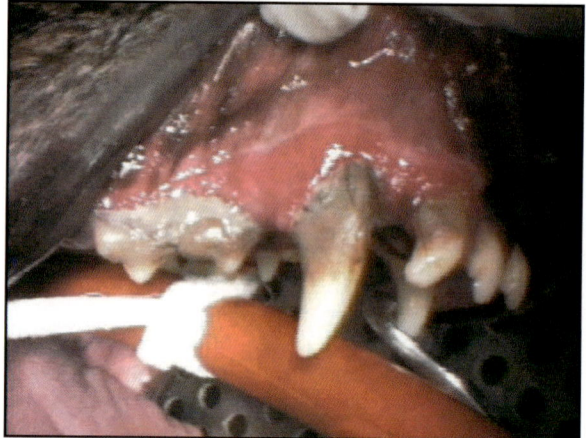

2.1 Advanced chronic periodontitis. Note the calculus on the teeth and the gingival recession.

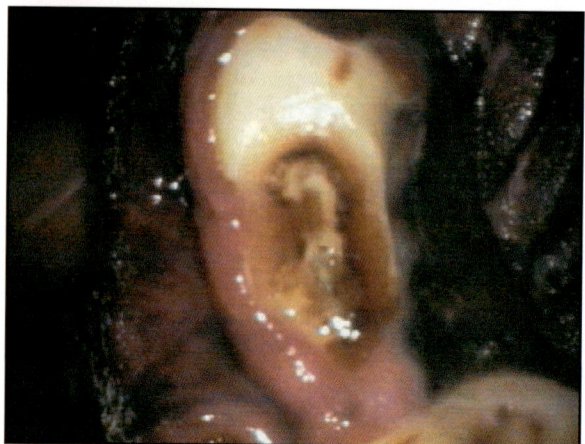

2.2 Trapped debris in a carious lesion in a dog premolar tooth (108).

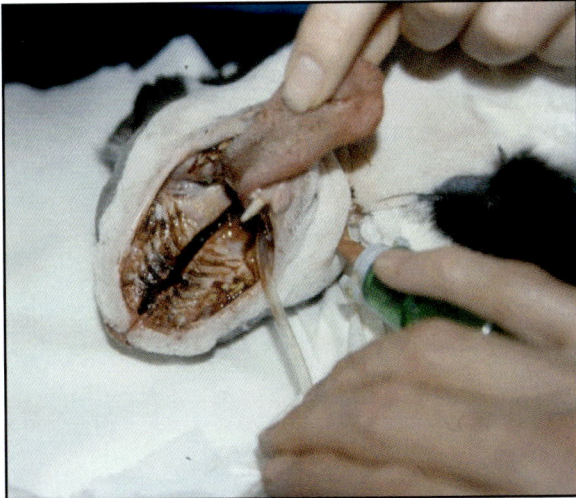

2.3 Cleft palate in a cat due to trauma.

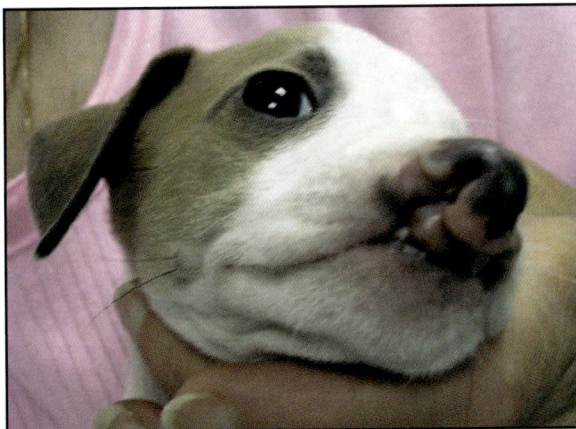

2.4 Bilateral cleft lip and cleft primary palate in a 3-month-old Italian Greyhound bitch.

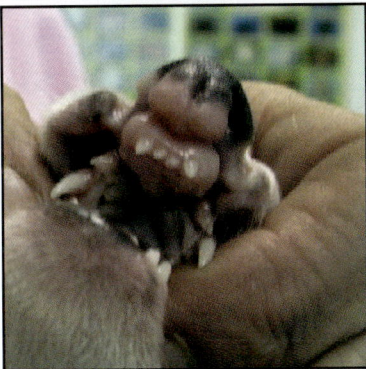

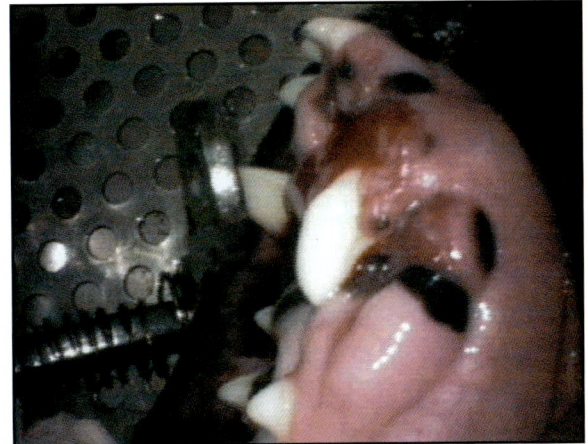

oroantral fistulae, and retained foreign bodies. Differential diagnoses include uraemia, sinusitis, gastrointestinal problems, respiratory diseases, nasal disorders, diet, lip-fold pyoderma and lesions such as abscesses or infected anal glands, being licked or chewed. Some animals consume the faeces of other animals leading to severe halitosis.

Broken or discoloured teeth
Broken and discoloured teeth as clinical signs of oral disease are discussed later in the chapter.

Changes in eating behaviour
Inappetence due to oral pathology usually only occurs in association with severe pain, mucous membrane

inflammation or ulceration. Fractured teeth, teeth affected by caries and other painful tooth-related pathology (e.g. avulsed or luxated teeth (Figure 2.5) or avulsed lip and mucosa (Figure 2.6)) may result in reluctance or hesitancy to eat, or a change in eating habits, but rarely complete inappetence.

2.5 Caudal displacement of a chronically luxated upper canine tooth in a dog.

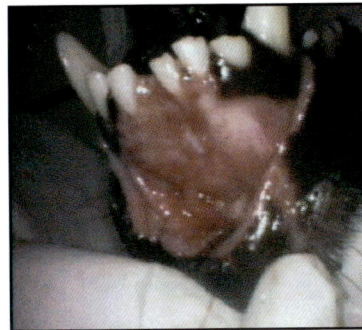

2.6 Avulsed lip and mucosa in a dog.

The animal may drop food (quidding), training aids or toys from the mouth. Food may also be shifted to one side of the mouth or a preference shown towards soft foods when periodontal or endodontic disease is present. Hesitancy in swallowing food can be due to oral inflammation, ulceration, tonsillitis or the presence of foreign bodies. In cats the most common causes of these symptoms are feline odontoclastic resorptive lesions (FORLs) (Figure 2.7) and gingivostomatitis (see Chapter 8). Breed predispositions to these conditions should be noted. In addition, the ability to smell food is very important in cats; those unable to smell for whatever reason will be reluctant to eat.

Inappetence can also be associated with general disease processes, e.g. cardiac insufficiency may result in discomfort at the time of prehension because the animal cannot eat and breathe at the same time. This may manifest itself as gulping or only taking small amounts of food at a time. All indications of systemic disease should be ruled out. The presence of a nasal or palatine mass will also result in the animal having difficulty in eating and breathing at the same time.

Rubbing or pawing the face
Pawing at, tilting, bobbing, shaking or sliding the head and mouth along the floor can be due to oral pain.

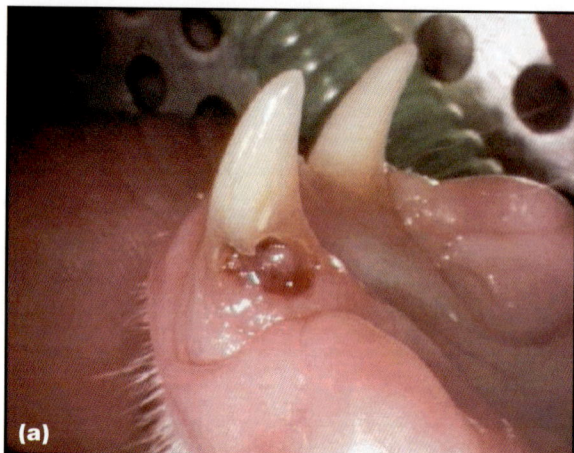

(a)

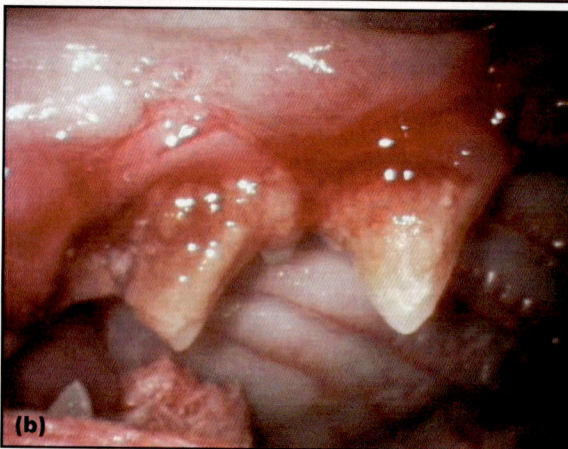

(b)

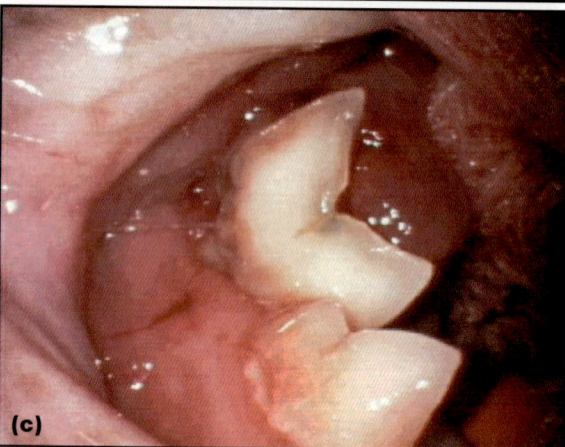

(c)

2.7   **(a)** FORL in a mandibular canine tooth.
(b) Gingivitis, stomatitis and a FORL.
(c) Gingivitis and a FORL.

Differential diagnoses include problems with the skin, lips, eyes, salivary glands and central nervous system.

Drooling

Chronic ptyalism is more commonly due to a reluctance or inability to swallow rather than increased saliva production or flow. Acute endodontic exposure, severe inflammation, ulceration or laceration of the tongue (Figure 2.8) or oral mucosa, and the presence of foreign bodies (e.g. sticks, toys and bones) are the most common causes of drooling. Foreign bodies, particularly sticks and bone fragments, can become stuck across the palate, along the dental arch

(Figure 2.9) or penetrate the mucosa longitudinally adjacent to the tongue. Systemic causes of excessive salivation include bacterial or viral infections (e.g. rabies) and toxins (e.g. organophosphates and animal toxins, such as those found on toads). Chemical irritation of the tongue can also cause ulceration and increased salivation (Figure 2.10).

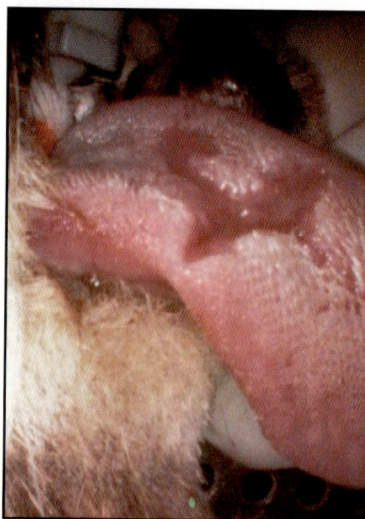

2.8   Chronic ulceration of the tongue.

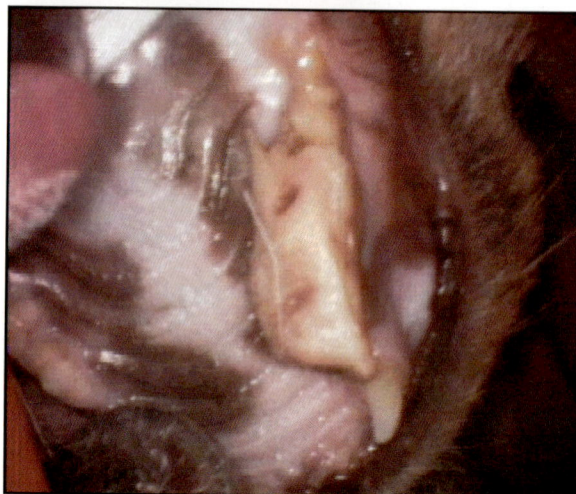

2.9   Foreign body (chicken bone) wedged along the dental arch in a cat.

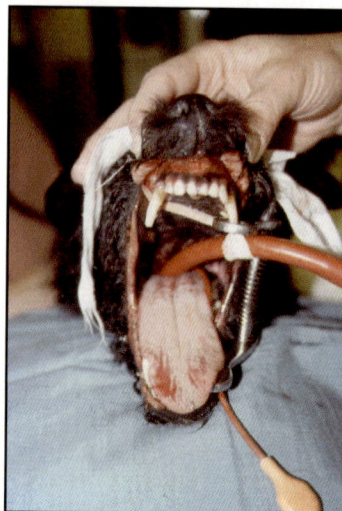

2.10   This dog had chased a small rodent and pursued it into a pile of cement dust. The resulting irritation and inflammation caused by the cement dust caused ulceration of the tongue. The dog presented with hunger, the desire to eat but the inability to ingest due to the pain and ulceration of the oral soft tissues.

Bleeding or purulent discharge from the mouth

Severe gingivitis, lacerations of the mucosa, gingiva or tongue may lead to the presence of frank blood, blood-tinged saliva or pink discoloration of the drinking water. Purulent discharges may be seen around the lips, as a nasal discharge, or on examination of the teeth. Chronic oral lacerations may lead to purulent discharge. Foreign bodies wedged within the oral cavity may present with both bleeding and a purulent discharge.

Inability or unwillingness to open or close the mouth

Clicking or popping noises and indications of acute or chronic pain associated with jaw movements are typically associated with problems with the temporomandibular joint (TMJ), coronoid process or zygomatic arch (the latter two are often associated with open jaw locking). Differential diagnoses include:

- Dental, jaw or palatal fractures
- Foreign bodies
- Salivary gland disease
- Craniomandibular osteopathy
- TMJ dysplasia
- Tumours
- Severe stomatitis
- Masticatory muscle myositis
- Mandibular neuropraxia.

Change in temperament

Pain or discomfort within the oral cavity may make the animal 'head shy' and on approaching the head a cowering or alternatively an aggressive response. may be seen. Generally dogs and cats with chronic sore mouths will not be as lively as they should be. This is often recognized in retrospect after a dental procedure has been completed.

Facial swellings

Swellings (Figure 2.11), oedema, draining sinus tracts and sores can be the result of endodontic, periodontal or salivary gland disease. Differential diagnoses include insect and snake bites, allergic reactions, tumours, haematomas and emphysema.

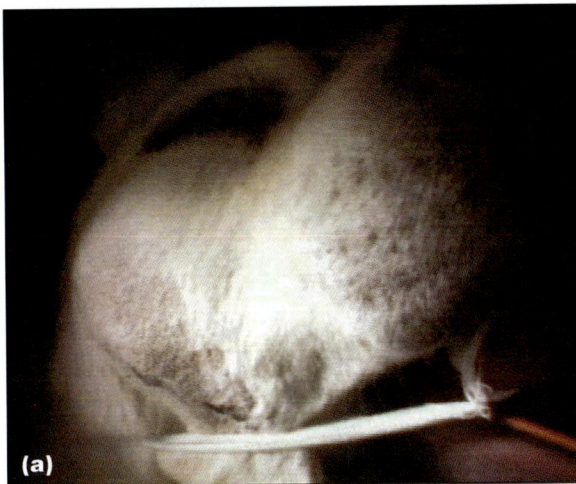

2.11 **(a and b)** Malar abscess in two dogs. Note the sinus tract below the left eye (continues). ▶

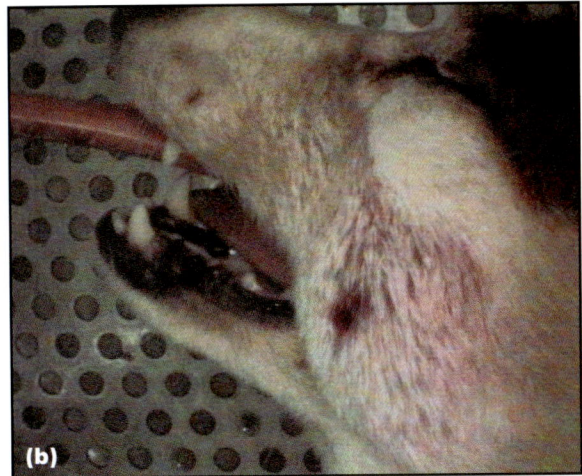

2.11 (continued) Malar abscess in two dogs. Note the sinus tract below the left eye.

Other

Additional oral clinical signs, secondary to systemic conditions, may also be found and include pallor, congestion, cyanosis, icterus (Figure 2.12), petechiae and echymoses, ulceration and malodour.

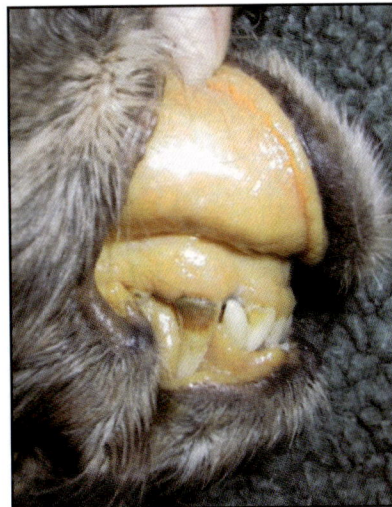

2.12 Severe chronic icterus in a dog with liver failure.

General and medical history

A more general dental history should investigate factors that may result in dental problems and be used to advise the client on the prevention of further dental problems.

Damaging habits include chew toys that are too hard, cage or chain biting, stone chewing (perhaps as a result of boredom or lack of appropriate chew toys), the animal carrying abrasive objects in its mouth, and excessive grooming. These habits may result in excessive attrition, abrasion (Figure 2.13) and fracture of the teeth (Figure 2.14).

Relevant dietary habits include the usual diet, treats or table scraps (which may contain fermentable carbohydrates and therefore predispose to caries) and nutritional supplements. Dental home care is a relevant part of the history in terms of what the client is willing and able to achieve to maintain oral health.

A full medical history should be obtained to determine conditions that may affect the anaesthetic protocol, affect the cause, predisposition, progress or prognosis of the dental condition, or mean that adjunct therapy to dental treatment is required.

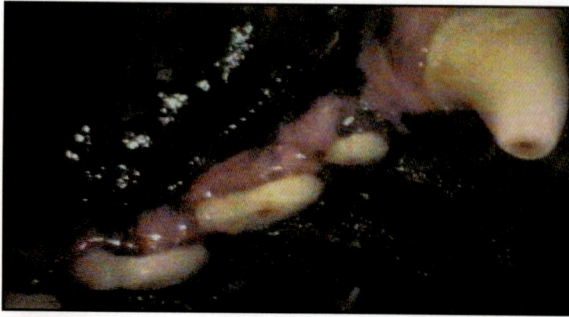

2.13 Chronic abrasion as a result of stone chewing.

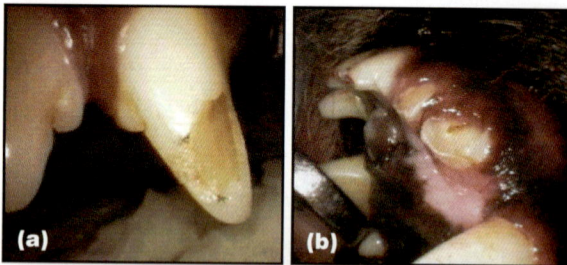

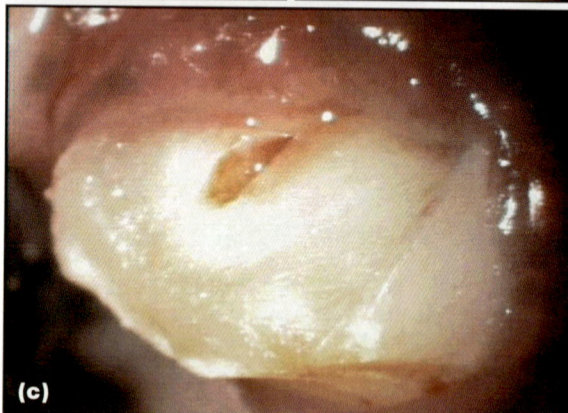

2.14 **(a)** Enamel chipped off an upper incisor (203) in a dog. **(b)** Fractured upper incisor teeth in a dog. **(c)** Close-up of a lateral incisor, showing chronic exposure of the pulp chamber.

General physical and extraoral examination

The entire animal should be observed but special attention paid to the respiratory and cardiovascular systems as these in particular will affect the anaesthetic protocol required for a full oral examination and dental treatment.

The face, head and jaws should be examined, with reference to:

- Swellings
- Lips
- Lymph nodes
- Salivary glands
- Asymmetry of the face or head
- TMJs
- Eyes.

Swellings can indicate neoplasia, cellulitis or abscesses. Cellulitis or abscess formation can be as a result of foreign bodies, fight wounds, periodontal disease or periapical disorders. Sinus tracts with or without discharge may be present.

The lips may show ulcerative lesions, neoplasia, wounds, cheilitis, lip-fold pyodermas and other localized infections.

The lymph nodes should always be palpated for enlargements or indications of pain as a result of oral infection or lymphatic neoplasia. It should be noted whether any enlargements are unilateral or bilateral. Other peripheral lymph nodes should also be examined to rule out the presence of a systemic rather than a localized condition.

The salivary glands may be enlarged or atrophied as a result of neoplasia, infection or duct obstruction.

Asymmetry of the face or head can be seen in hereditary or congenital conditions, inflammatory disease, neoplasia, dislocations, fractures and nerve damage. Muscle wastage may indicate poor muscle usage as a result of the reduced activity of the relevant part of the face. Muscle wastage can be either unilateral or bilateral. Unequal growth of paired facial bones can result in asymmetry and may cause bite or occlusion abnormalities, e.g. cross bite (Figure 2.15) or wry bite.

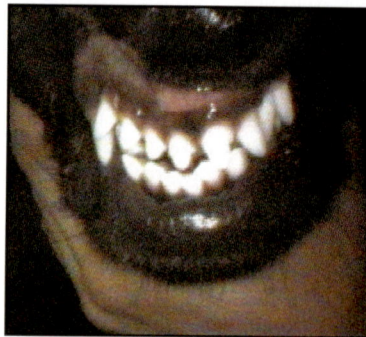

2.15 Mandibular prognathism in a dog with cross bite.

TMJ examination may reveal crepitus, limitation of opening, deviation on opening or closing, and is especially relevant if there is a history of head trauma. Open-mouth disorders are usually a result of trauma to the TMJ, maxillary or mandibular fracture, nerve damage or disease. Some breeds are predisposed to open-mouth locking, e.g. Red Setters. Closed-mouth disorders include dislocation of the TMJ, locking of the teeth and jaw by a foreign body, and craniomandibular osteopathy as seen in West Highland White, Scottish and Cairn Terriers.

The eyes should be examined for the presence of orbital or retrobulbar abscesses, neoplasia or the presence of enlarged zygomatic salivary glands, as these can result in unilateral exophthalmos.

Initial oral examination

The oral examination of a conscious animal is limited and dependent on the animal's temperament, but it will provide significant information, reduce the number of differential diagnostic possibilities and help to formulate an initial treatment plan. This plan should then be discussed with the owner and informed consent to the treatment options and costs obtained. The owner must be aware that the final treatment plan can only be formulated once a full dental examination has been carried out under general anaesthesia. The consent form should indicate this and cover any possible treatment requirements. A contact telephone number for use whilst the treatment is being carried out is essential to enable discussion of the treatment plan after the full examination if necessary.

Only visual inspection and a gentle approach are used at the initial examination, which should be carried out in a quiet, well lit room. Larger dogs may be more comfortable being examined sitting on the floor rather than on the examination table. The help of an experienced assistant can be invaluable should the animal require gentle restraint. Gentle retraction of the lips allows examination of the vestibular surfaces of the teeth and gingiva and the exposed mucosa. Examination of the bite or occlusion can also be performed at this stage. Progression to an open-mouth examination can then occur.

Dogs

To open a dog's mouth:

1. Place one hand over the muzzle and place the index finger and thumb on either side under the lips behind the upper canine teeth.
2. Place the other hand under the chin and insert a finger and thumb over the lower lip and on to the alveolar ridge in the second premolar region.
3. Lift the upper hand to extend the head dorsally and open the mouth.

Care must be taken not to squeeze the dog's cheeks against the teeth or pull the facial hair to force the animal to open its mouth. Special care should be taken in trauma cases.

Cats

To open a cat's mouth:

1. Place one hand across the top of the head in front of the ears and place the thumb and index finger just behind the commissures of the lips.
2. Pull the lips gently backwards and slightly upwards and then hold firmly just below the zygomatic arch.
3. Tilt the head dorsally and press down on the lower incisors with the index finger of the other hand.
4. Push the ring or middle finger into the intermandibular space, raising the tongue to enable sublingual examination.

For both dogs and cats the mucous membranes should be examined for colour, moistness, ulceration, lacerations and swellings. The gingiva should be examined for colour, inflammation, hyperplasia, recession, bleeding and the presence of swellings. The teeth can be inspected for occlusion, avulsions, fractures, discoloration, plaque, calculus, caries, developmental defects and abnormal shape. It may be possible to examine the palate for swellings, defects and foreign bodies. The tongue may be visualized and its general appearance noted. The mobility and the presence of lesions on the tongue surface, in the body of the tongue or underneath the tongue should be noted, for example, the presence of ranulae (Figures 2.16 and 2.17). Halitosis, bleeding, epistaxis and rhinitis should also be noted. However, it must be reiterated that a full oral examination can only be performed with the patient under general anaesthesia.

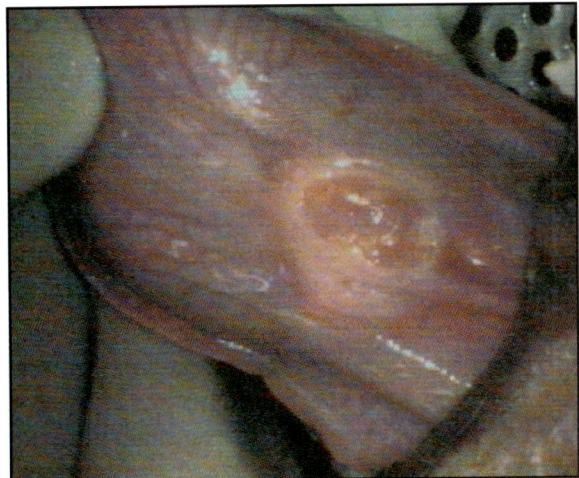

2.16 Sublingual ulceration due to squamous cell carcinoma in a dog.

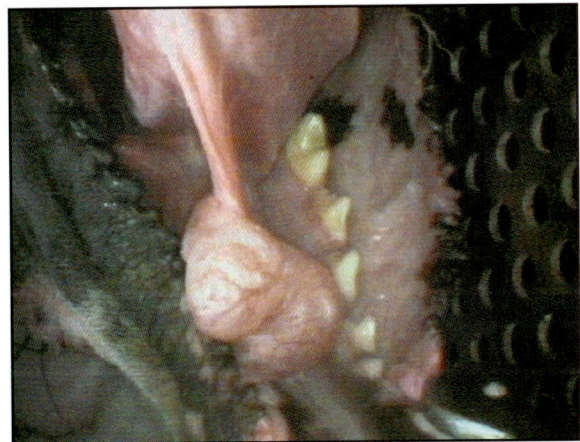

2.17 Sublingual ranula in a dog.

Preanaesthetic diagnostic tests

Preanaesthetic diagnostic tests are often indicated after the general medical and initial oral examinations. They should be performed and the results collated and evaluated before the induction of general anaesthesia.

- Blood tests, including screening tests (preanaesthetic or geriatric) and specific tests (feline immunodeficiency virus (FIV), feline leukaemia virus (FeLV), feline coronavirus (FCoV), feline herpes virus (FHV), *Chlamydia*, feline calcivirus (FCV).

- Special tests may be indicated for some cardiovascular or respiratory diseases, e.g. electrocardiogram (ECG), cardiac ultrasonography and blood pressure. In some cases specialist opinion should be sought before proceeding.
- Radiographs are indicated in most dental cases but are usually best performed with the full dental examination when the patient is anaesthetized.
- Microscopic examination. Cytological examination of a swab or scrape sample can give a diagnosis in some cases, e.g. *Candida* or *Aspergillus* infection. Biopsy samples are required to differentiate between inflammatory, hyperplastic and neoplastic lesions. Immunofluorescent techniques are employed in the diagnosis of immune-mediated disorders.

Full oral examination

A definitive oral examination is only possible under general anaesthesia. Information is obtained from oral (soft tissue), periodontal (structures supporting the teeth) and dental examinations. The information obtained must be recorded in a systematic way.

Case records

A permanent record must be made of the relevant medical and dental history, diagnostic data and details of all treatment carried out. They should include written or electronic clinical records, a dental chart and radiographs, together with digital or other photographic records. Plaster cast models of the dentition are an accurate way of recording tooth position; this is especially relevant in orthodontic cases.

Case records are important from legal as well as clinical aspects. They facilitate reference at a later date for review or follow-up and allow accurate comparisons of the progression, stabilization or resolution of a specific disease process to be made over a period of time. They can also be useful by providing a database for reference when determining disease incidence. All clinical records or charts must identify the client and patient, the findings at examination and the treatment carried out. This may represent several stages of the same procedure and the records need to be able to be updated periodically.

Dental charting is the process of diagrammatically recording the health status of the oral cavity and the teeth in particular (see Chapter 5). Many different types of dental chart are available and operator preference will determine the one used. All charts must make provision for the recording of detail required by the operator. This may be quite basic information, e.g. pocket depth, missing dentition or the presence of fractured teeth, or more complicated information where more detail is required, e.g. gingival recession, pseudo-pockets, fracture description, gingivitis and calculus indices. Specific dental charts are available for orthodontic assessments. The best type of chart allows information to be recorded without becoming too crowded. Commonly used abbreviations and the use

of an index on the chart enable details to be universally understood.

It is important during charting to be able to refer to a specific tooth. There are many tooth-naming and coding systems in current use, all with advantages and disadvantages. A universal system has evolved for animal dentitions that is interchangeable between species. In humans a two digit system for recording each tooth allows both the quadrant and the individual tooth to be recorded. In animals, however, there are often more than nine teeth in a quadrant so the system described was adapted by adopting a three digit system. This system (described by Professor Triadan from Switzerland) had its limitations when used for species, such as cats, that have naturally missing teeth. The numbering system has been modified to record the gap resulting from missing teeth and is known as the modified Triadan system.

The modified Triadan system is regarded as the standard for identifying teeth and should be used wherever possible. It is universally recognized, easy to write and record. A three digit number is allocated to each tooth in each quadrant of the mouth. The first digit denotes the quadrant of the mouth and whether the tooth is part of the permanent or deciduous dentition.

Permanent dentition:

- 1 = upper right quadrant
- 2 = upper left quadrant
- 3 = lower left quadrant
- 4 = lower right quadrant.

Deciduous dentition:

- 5 = upper right quadrant
- 6 = upper left quadrant
- 7 = lower left quadrant
- 8 = lower right quadrant.

The second and third digits together denote the tooth. In dogs the teeth are numbered consecutively from the dental arch midline to the caudal end of each quadrant. In cats with a reduced compliment of teeth (i.e. rostral premolars and caudal molars absent) some numbers are skipped in the premolar region and omitted in the molar region, therefore, incisors start at 01, canine teeth are always 04 and the first molar is 09. This system enables the numbering of other teeth to be determined, even in unfamiliar species.

Soft tissue examination

Once general anaesthesia has been induced, the oropharynx is inspected prior to the insertion of an endotracheal (ET) tube. The lips, cheeks, tongue, sublingual area and palate are then fully examined and any abnormality noted.

Mucosal ulceration as a result of trauma, infection, systemic disease or autoimmune disorder should be recorded. Salivary gland disorders, e.g. sialolithiasis, ranula, salivary cele and tumours, should be looked for during soft tissue examination of the mouth.

The oropharynx should also be examined for neoplasia, gingival hyperplasia and localized reactive or inflammatory change. Examination for intraoral osseous lesions, including osteoporosis, fractures, exostoses and neoplasms, should also be performed.

Prior to an in-depth oral cavity examination under general anaesthesia, the patient should have a cuffed ET tube placed together with a throat pack. The throat pack should be changed as required during the anaesthetic period to avoid fluid saturation. At the end of the procedure the back of the throat and the mouth should be checked to ensure there is no liquid, mucus or foreign material remaining that could be inhaled during the recovery period.

Before examination, the use of a chlorhexidine solution to rinse the mouth will reduce the bacterial load in the oral cavity. The operator should wear gloves, eye protection and a facemask during all operative procedures, including the examination (see Chapter 4).

Dental examination

A dental examination needs to be carried out in a systematic way. A starting point should be chosen (e.g. the upper right central incisor, 101) and a full and thorough examination of that tooth unit together with its periodontium carried out. A dental probe will facilitate the examination and a periodontal probe is essential for assessing periodontal pocket depth (see Chapters 5 and 7). Each tooth in that quadrant should then be examined unit by unit starting from the dental arch midline and moving caudally. The process should then be repeated for all remaining quadrants, starting in each case from the midline and moving caudally. In this manner, none of the teeth are omitted.

It is easier to examine the tooth surface when it is dry; this may be facilitated by the use of a three-in-one syringe. Disclosing solution may be used on the teeth to highlight the presence of plaque. Various indices can be used to record the level of plaque, gingivitis and calculus for each tooth. These enable a repeatable record of the progression, stabilization or improvement of these parameters to be kept. The root below the gingival attachment and its supporting alveolar bone can only be examined radiographically.

The following are assessed during a dental examination:

- Number of teeth (see Figures 2.18 and 2.19)
- Tooth appearance, including developmental defects, tooth fractures, colour and destructive processes. Any previous restorations should also be evaluated and noted

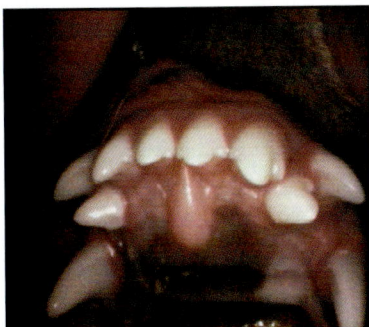

2.18 An oral examination may reveal abnormalities in the number of teeth present. Note the extra (supernumerary) bilateral upper incisors in this dog.

- Gingiva, including contour and inflammation, recession and hyperplasia
- Periodontal pocket depth and loss of periodontal attachment
- Presence, distribution and quantity of calculus
- Tooth mobility
- Tooth position and jaw shape.

Number of teeth

Retained deciduous teeth should be recorded (Figures 2.19 and 2.20). Any missing teeth should be noted. Teeth may be missing as a result of exfoliation, extraction, uneruption or may be congenitally absent. Teeth may be unerupted as a result of impaction or an ectopic position. Unerupted teeth may or may not have associated pathology. If a persistent deciduous tooth is noted without the concurrent eruption of its permanent successor, radiography is required to determine

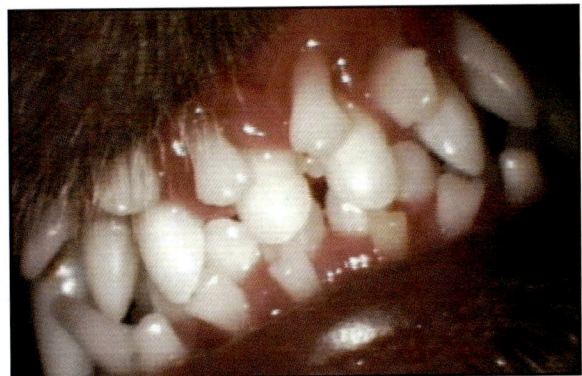

2.19 Persistent deciduous teeth in a male neutered 10-month-old German Spitz-Klein.

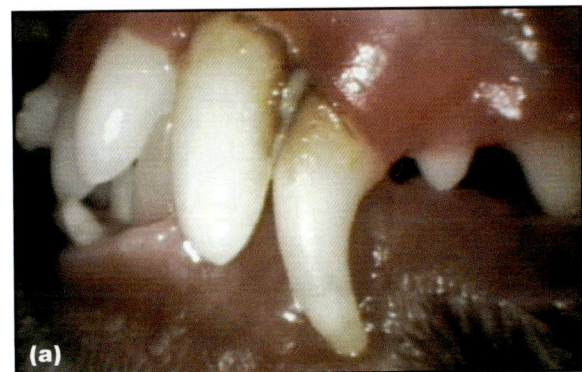

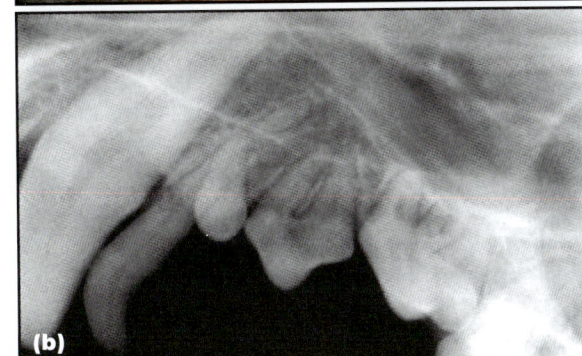

2.20 **(a)** Trapped debris, gingivitis and periodontitis associated with a persistent maxillary canine tooth in a dog. **(b)** Radiograph showing persistent deciduous maxillary canine tooth in a dog. Note the length of the root.

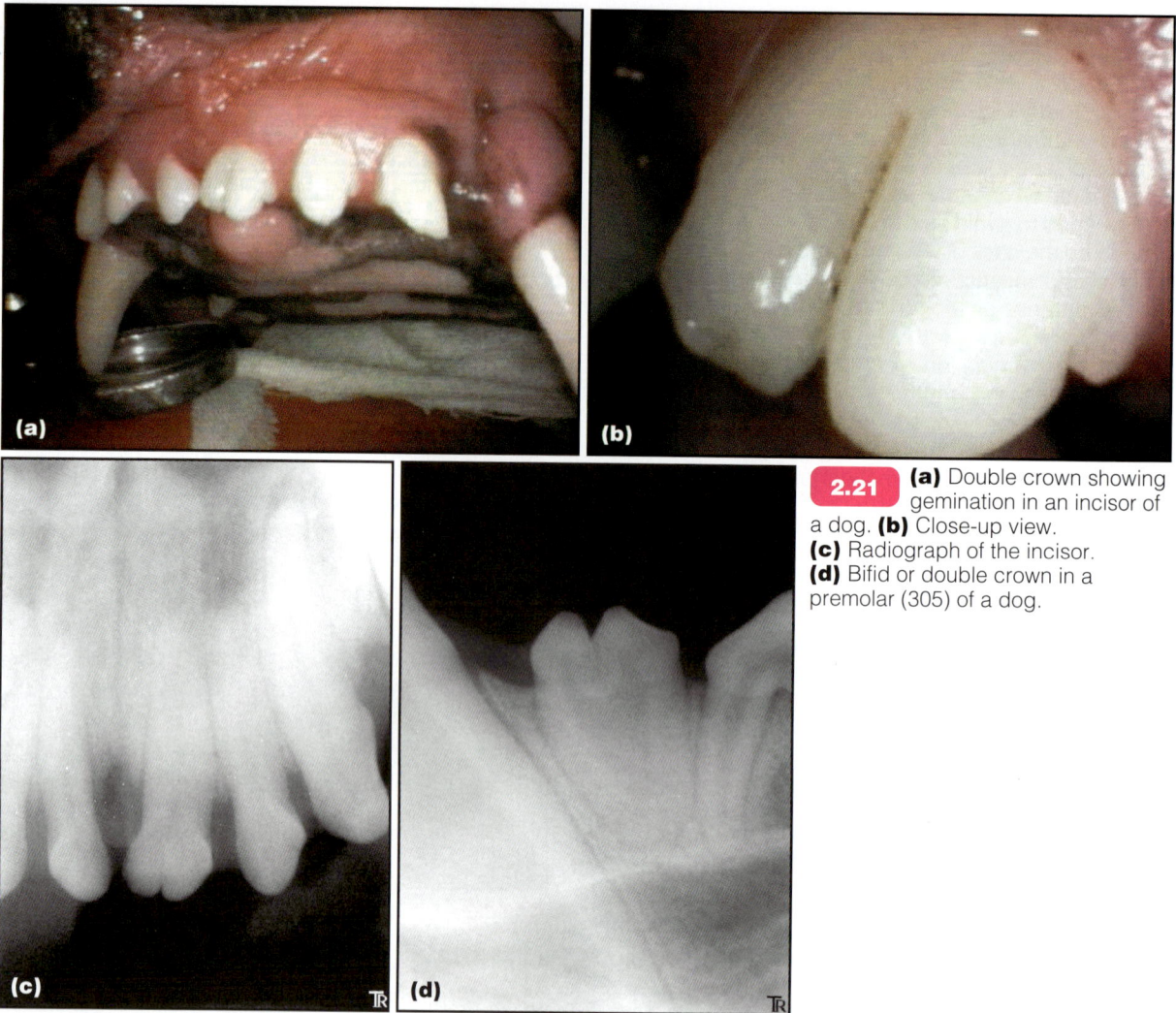

2.21 **(a)** Double crown showing gemination in an incisor of a dog. **(b)** Close-up view. **(c)** Radiograph of the incisor. **(d)** Bifid or double crown in a premolar (305) of a dog.

the cause of non-eruption of the permanent tooth, thereby, forming the basis of the optimal treatment plan.

Supernumerary teeth are not uncommon (see Figure 2.18). When persistent deciduous or supernumerary teeth predispose to periodontal disease as a result of crowding (see Figure 2.20) or when they are involved in a traumatic occlusion, they need to be extracted. Two teeth should not occupy the same location.

Tooth appearance

Developmental defects: Developmental defects, i.e. geminated or fused teeth, should be noted as well as any defects in enamel formation, e.g. enamel hypoplasia, dysplasia and rarely aplasia (see Chapter 6).

Severe systemic illness and pyrexia (such as that caused by canine distemper virus infection during tooth development) will result in all of the teeth that develop at that time exhibiting a disruption of formation. Typically, multiple teeth are affected in a bilaterally symmetrical pattern (see Figure 2.24). A single tooth exhibiting a developmental defect will probably have suffered a local disturbance during tooth formation, e.g. trauma or infection of the deciduous predecessor, but may also be due to a hereditary disorder. Missing,

supernumerary, bifid (Figure 2.21) and other misshapen teeth may all have a genetic origin.

Tooth fractures: Tooth fractures should be noted and classified as either crown, with or without pulpal involvement, or root fractures. If one tooth is fractured, it is likely that other teeth are also damaged (see Figures 2.14b, 2.22 and 2.23).

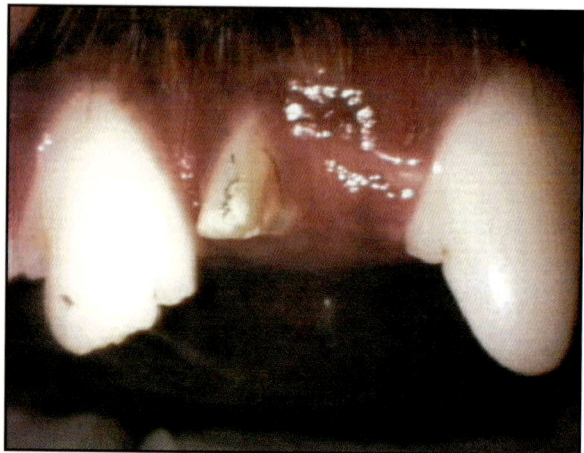

2.22 Fractured upper incisor in a dog. Note also the chipped enamel on the adjacent tooth.

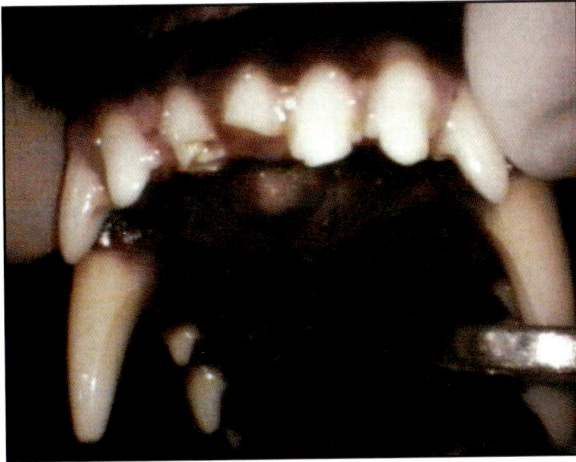

2.23 Fractured teeth in a 3-year-old male Flat Coated Retreiver. Note the supernumery incisor, a common finding in this breed.

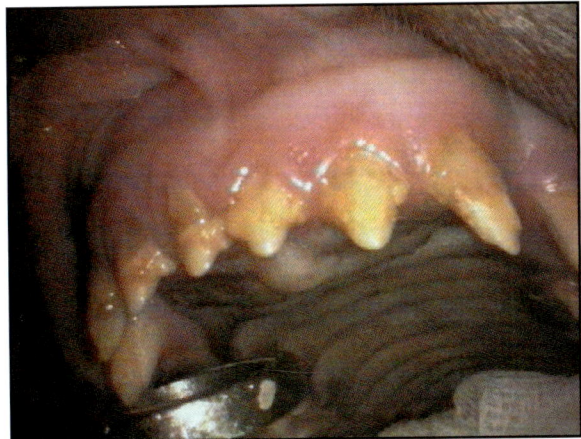

2.24 Poor mineralization or formation of enamel (dysplasia) resulting in discoloration of teeth, in a young adult dog.

The vitality and viability of all traumatized teeth needs to be assessed. Where pulpal involvement is not apparent, pulpal necrosis will only be evident as crown discoloration and periradicular radiographic changes. Radiographic changes as a result of periapical pathology take a minimum of ten days to become apparent. Pulpal necrosis, where there has been obvious pulpal involvement, will present as a black spot which does not bleed on probing. Exploration of an exposed pulp cavity with an endodontic file may elicit the presence of smelly necrotic debris. An exposed vital pulp will be seen as pink or red soft tissue at the exposure site. It will bleed on probing.

A tooth that is mobile after trauma may have a root fracture or be subluxated. Radiographic examination is required to determine the diagnosis.

Discoloration: Tooth discoloration can be either localized extrinsic staining, which can be removed, or intrinsic staining, where it is incorporated within the enamel. Intrinsic staining can occur during periods of enamel demineralization, when the relatively softer enamel surface permits absorption of stains. When it remineralizes, the stain is locked into the now relatively harder enamel. Intrinsic stains can range in colour from light brown to almost black.

Plaque deposits can be seen when they are heavy, but slight deposits may require staining with a disclosing solution to render them visible.

Generalized tooth discoloration can be as a result of the use of some systemic agents during the tooth development stage, e.g. tetracycline will result in a grey/blue band of discoloration, the location of which is dependent on the stage of development the tooth was at when the tetracycline was administered (Figure 2.24).

A necrotic pulp will cause the tooth to appear darker, or grey, in colour. Pigments released from haemoglobin breakdown within the pulp cavity leach into the dentine, resulting in a grey discoloration that often darkens with time. Severe pulpal bruising, recent pulpal haemorrhage or internal resorption will result in a tooth that appears pink or purple.

Destructive processes: Caries (Figure 2.25), resorptive lesions, attrition, erosion and abrasion all result in the destruction of hard tooth tissue (see Chapter 9). Rostral dental attrition can be as a result of excessive grooming (Figure 2.26). Habits, such as stone chewing and carrying abrasive objects in the mouth, can result in worn premolar teeth. Abnormal tooth contact as a result of malocclusion can result in wear facets. Cage biting typically results in wear facets on the distal surfaces of canine teeth.

Caries is most commonly seen in the central pit of upper first molars and in lower first molars in dogs (see Chapter 7) (Figure 2.25). However, pits, fissures and

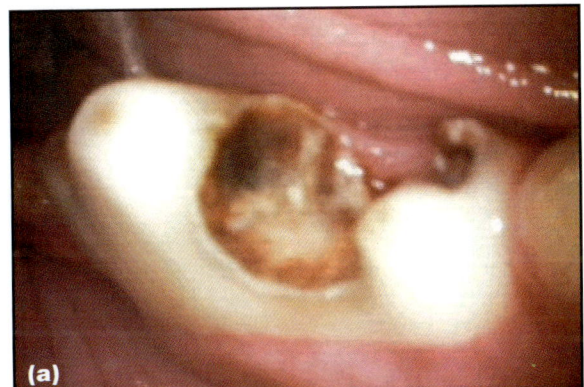

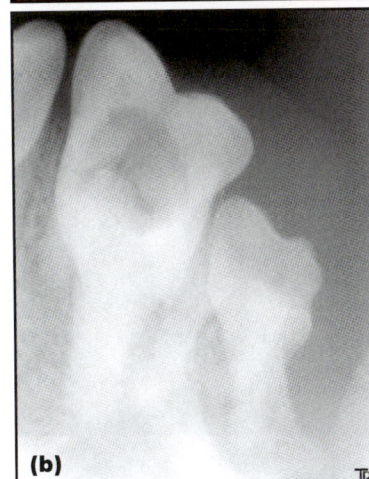

2.25
(a) Caries affecting a dog's mandibular molar. **(b)** Radiograph of a dog's maxillary molar with caries.

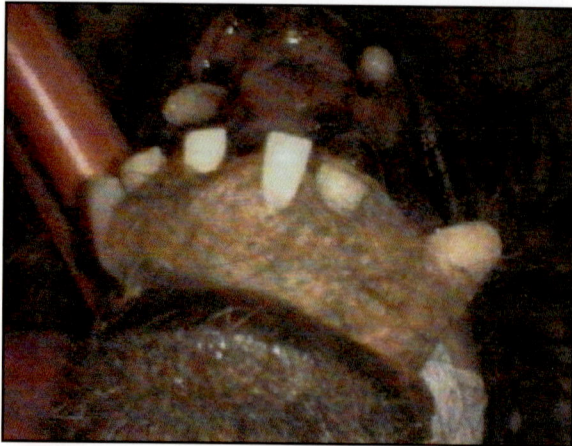

2.26 Hair matted around the incisor teeth due to excessive grooming in a dog.

tooth areas that contact the adjacent teeth should also be examined for carious lesions. Smooth surface caries have also been described in dogs.

Restorations: Any existing restorations should be examined for marginal defects and deterioration.

Gingiva

Gingivitis (inflammation of the gingiva): Gingivitis is the initial reversible reaction by the gingiva to infection and trauma. It can range from mild, with some oedema

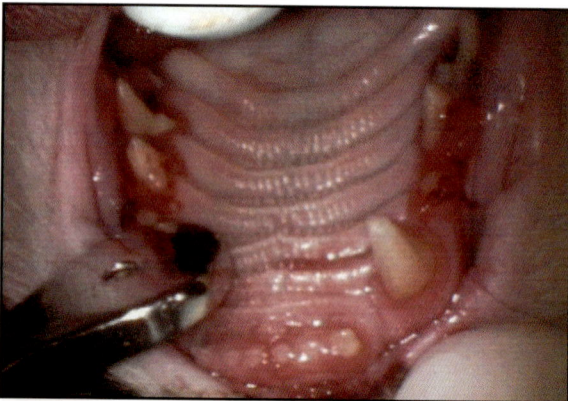

2.27 Gingivitis in a cat.

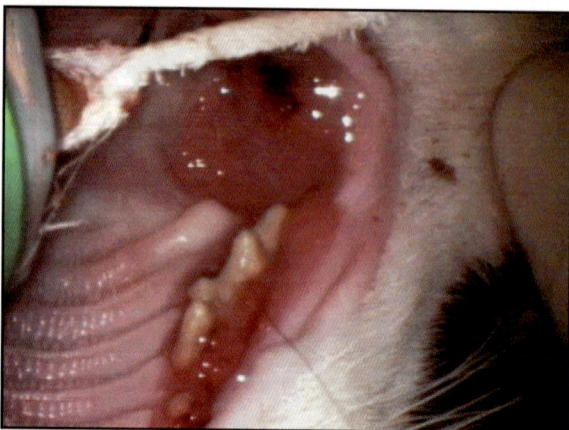

2.28 Severe gingivitis and stomatitis in a cat.

of the gingiva, to a severe inflammatory reaction accompanied by haemorrhage (Figures 2.27 and 2.28). Gingival bleeding is gauged by gently running a periodontal probe around the gingival sulcus.

A gingivitis index is used to allocate a gingivitis score to each tooth. Since the degree of inflammation may vary around one tooth the worst score is recorded (see Chapters 7 and 8). A suggested gingivitis index for veterinary dentistry is given in Figure 2.29.

Index	Description
0	Clinically healthy
1	Mild inflammation, slight redness or oedema. No bleeding on probing
2	Moderate inflammation, redness, oedema and glazing. Bleeding on probing
3	Severe inflammation, extensive redness, oedema and possible ulceration. Profuse bleeding on probing, tendency to spontaneously bleed

2.29 Example of a gingivitis index used in veterinary dentistry.

Gingival contour: Assessment of the gingival contour is important as it can influence the treatment choice and prognosis of periodontal disease. The position of the gingival margin should be drawn on the dental chart. Gingival hyperplasia will result in an increased probing depth and should be recorded (pseudo-pocket). Marginal recession should also be recorded as this can predispose to root and furcation exposure (Figures 2.30 and 2.31).

An area of inflamed, hyperplastic gingiva in a cat may be masking an early FORL and should be investigated further. Hair (and other foreign material) impacted within the gingival sulcus will increase the rate of periodontal destruction.

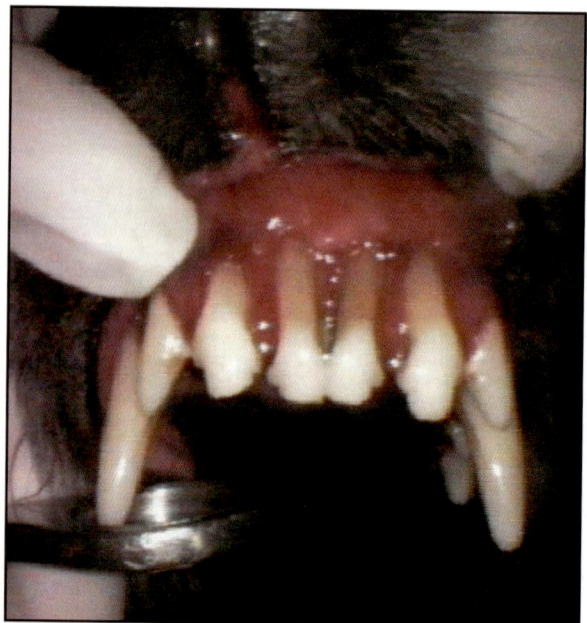

2.30 Gingival recession affecting the upper incisor teeth of a dog.

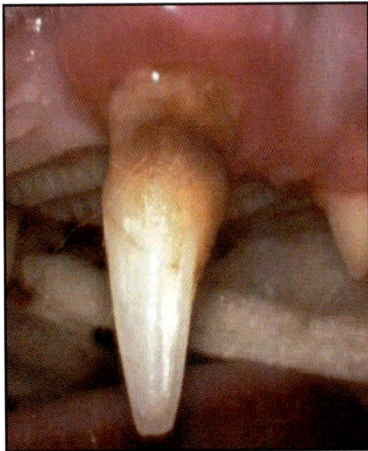

Gingival recession affecting a maxillary canine tooth of a cat.

Epulis: This is the term used to describe a proliferative mass on the gingiva and is not a diagnosis (see Chapter 10). Various lesions manifest themselves as epulides and can be reactive or neoplastic in nature, for example, localized fibrous hyperplasia, pyogenic granuloma, peripheral ameloblastoma and squamous cell carcinoma. Definitive diagnosis relies on histopathological examination of the tissue.

Periodontal examination

A periodontal examination will highlight the presence, location and extent of periodontal disease and differentiate between gingivitis and periodontitis.

Periodontal pocket depth measurement is carried out around the entire circumference of the tooth and is defined as the distance from the free gingival margin to the base of the periodontal pocket, where the junctional epithelium (JE) forms an attachment to the tooth. It is measured by means of a periodontal probe and where pocketing exists, four or six readings are taken around each tooth. In dogs with clinically healthy gingiva a sulcus depth of 1–3 mm is considered normal. The sulcus depth in cats with clinically healthy gingiva is 0.5–1 mm. Variation in pocket depth and any areas of localized deep pocketing should be noted on the dental chart. It may be necessary to remove heavy deposits of plaque and calculus on certain teeth before an accurate periodontal assessment can be performed (Figure 2.32).

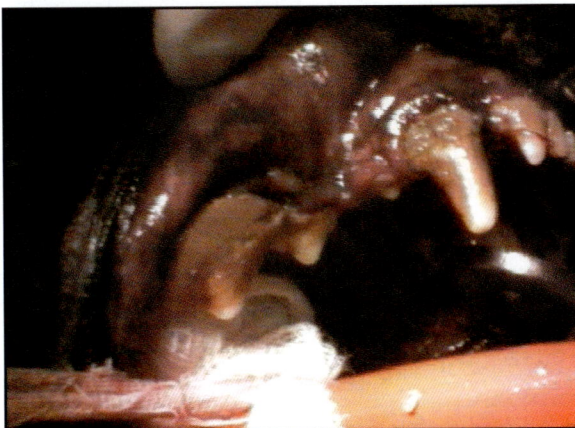

Heavy deposits of calculus on the dental arch of a dog. These need to be removed before a complete periodontal examination can be made.

However, the measurement of pocket depth alone is an unreliable indicator of periodontal destruction as the gingival margin does not always maintain its original position.

In animals with a healthy periodontium, previously unaffected by periodontitis, the gingival margin is positioned above the cementoenamel junction (CEJ) and the JE is attached to the enamel surface of the tooth, extending from the base of the gingival sulcus to where the periodontal ligament starts at the CEJ. As periodontal disease progresses the JE retreats apically following destruction of the periodontal ligament. If the gingival margin recedes at the same rate there will be little or no pocket formation. However, if the gingiva remains at its normal level, or if there is gingival hyperplasia, there will be pocket or pseudo-pocket formation.

By recording the level of the gingival margin relative to the CEJ in conjunction with actual pocket depth measurements, the true loss of periodontal attachment can be measured. The loss of periodontal attachment together with the pocket depth is important to assess the treatment of choice and the prognosis for the tooth. The use of radiography to evaluate the extent and type of bony destruction is mandatory. If periodontitis affects a multi-rooted tooth, the bone between the roots may be destroyed. The degree of bone loss in the furcation area is measured in the horizontal plane with a periodontal probe and recorded on the dental chart using the grading system described in Figure 2.33.

Grade	Description
0	No furcation involvement
1	The furcation can be palpated using a probe, but there is minimal horizontal destruction
2	The furcation is partially exposed but a probe does not go completely through the furcation. One aspect of the interradicular bone is intact
3	Full furcation involvement. Complete loss of interradicular bone such that a probe is able to pass through the furcation from buccal to lingual/palatal

An example of the grading system used to describe the degree of bone loss in the furcation area of multi-rooted teeth.

Calculus

The presence, distribution and quantity of subgingival calculus can often be detected whilst measuring pocket depth with the periodontal probe. The presence of supragingival calculus can be observed on visual examination of the tooth. Calculus deposits are most commonly noted on the dental chart as being slight, moderate or heavy; however, there is also a calculus index used in veterinary dentistry (Figure 2.34).

There is little correlation between the amount of calculus present and the severity of periodontal destruction. Sometimes removal of heavy, radiodense calculus deposits from the teeth prior to radiography is required to prevent superimposition of calculus over relevant dental or pathological structures.

Index	Description
0	No calculus
1	Supragingival calculus
2	Either moderate deposits of both supragingival and subgingival calculus or subgingival calculus only
3	Heavy deposits of both supragingival and subgingival calculus

2.34   Example of the index used to describe calculus deposits.

Root surface irregularities: These are more readily detected by running the tip of a sharp explorer over the root surface within the pocket. The long axis of the probe should be kept almost parallel to the root surface.

Tooth mobility

Periodontal disease, which results in loss of periodontal attachment and bone support, will lead to an increase in tooth mobility. However, tooth mobility may also be as a result of widening of the periodontal ligament space following prolonged lateral forces on a tooth, e.g. gnawing habit or orthodontic treatment.

Tooth luxation, root fractures and alveolar bone fractures will also result in increased tooth mobility. The lower central incisors of the cat and dog often appear loose due to movement in the fibrous mandibular symphyseal joint. Proper evaluation of tooth mobility requires radiographic examination.

Tooth mobility is assessed in the horizontal plane using the blunt end of, for example, a mirror handle. Fingers should not be used as the yield of the tissues at the tip of the fingers can give a misleading impression of tooth mobility. Tooth mobility is graded according to the grading system described in Figure 2.35.

Multi-rooted teeth are graded more severely than single-rooted teeth, and horizontal mobility >1 mm in a multi-rooted tooth is classified as Grade 3 mobility even though vertical movement may be absent.

Grade	Description
0	No mobility
1	Horizontal movement of <1 mm
2	Horizontal movement of >1 mm
3	Vertical as well as horizontal movement

2.35   Grading system used to grade tooth mobility.

Tooth position and jaw shape

Teeth may be rotated, abnormally positioned (Figure 2.36) or angulated (Figure 2.37), over or under erupted. Jaw shape, width and length discrepancies will affect relative tooth positions (Figure 2.38). Crowding (Figure 2.39), occlusal problems or soft tissue trauma can result from an abnormal tooth position or jaw shape (Figure 2.40).

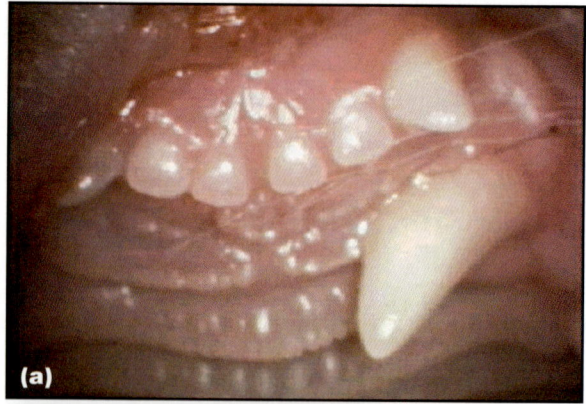

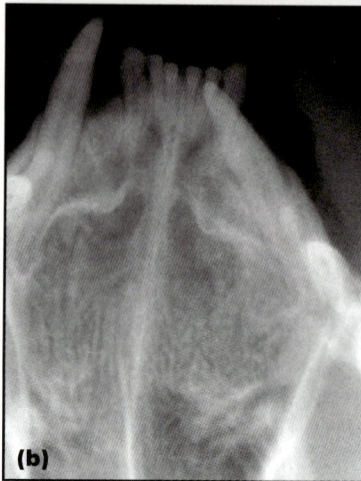

2.36
(a) Abnormal position of 204 (upper left canine) in a cat.
(b) Radiograph of the same tooth.

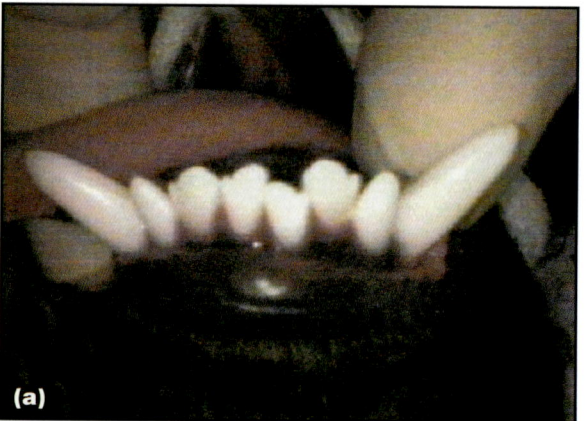

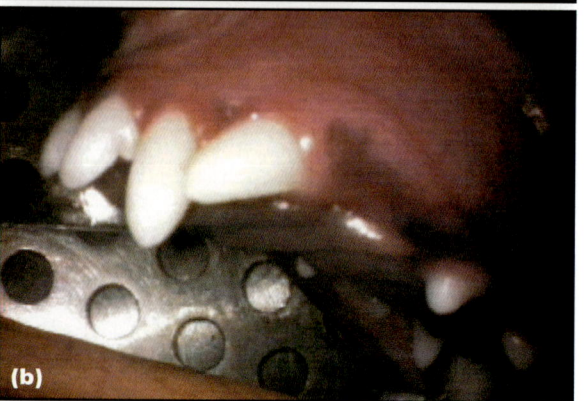

2.37   **(a)** Mandibular canine teeth in a dog. Note the exaggerated sloping/deviating angle.
(b) Rostral displacement of tooth 204 in a dog. This is also known as a 'lance' or 'spear' canine tooth.

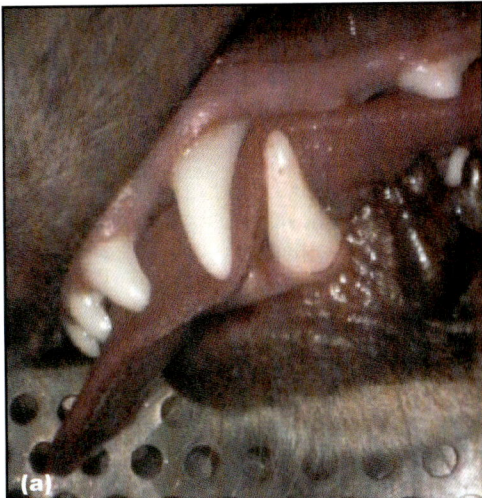

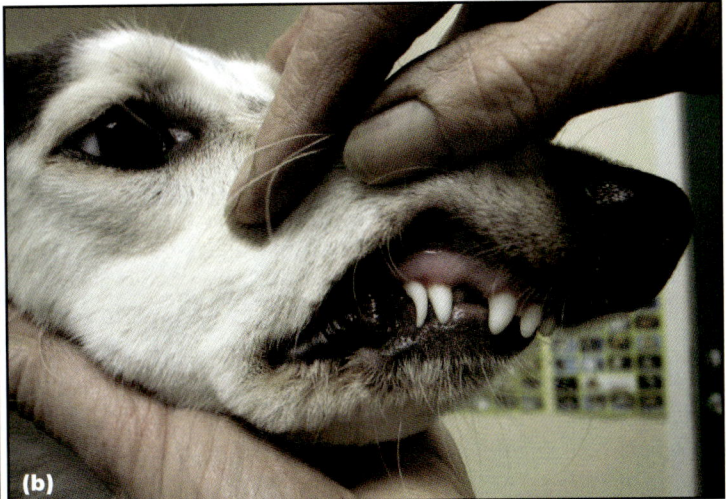

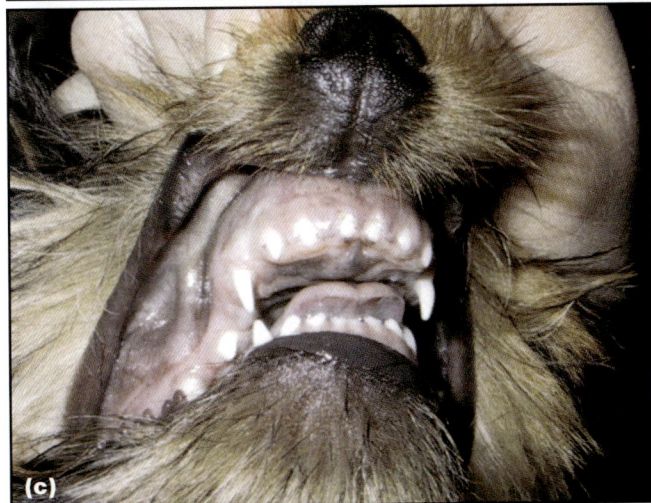

2.38 **(a)** Reverse position of upper and lower canine teeth in a dog with mandibular brachygnathism. **(b)** Mandibular brachygnathism in a young Whippet with a persistent 504 (upper right deciduous canine) tooth. **(c)** Mandibular brachygnathism in a terrier showing reverse occlusion of the canine teeth.

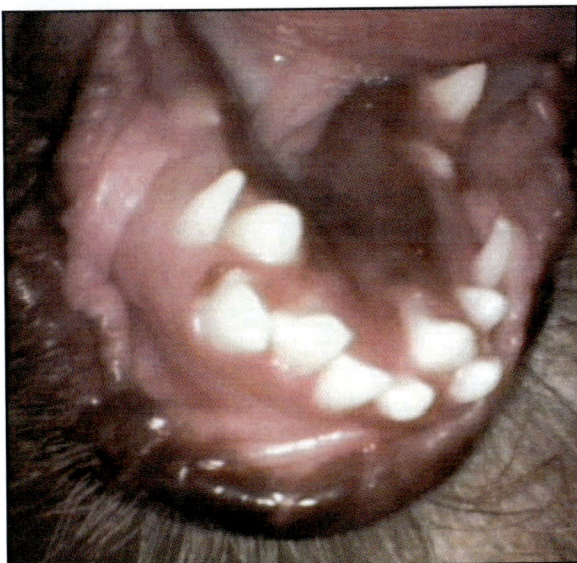

2.39 Overcrowding of incisors in a dog. Note persistent 704 and 804 causing lingual deviation of lower canines 304 and 404.

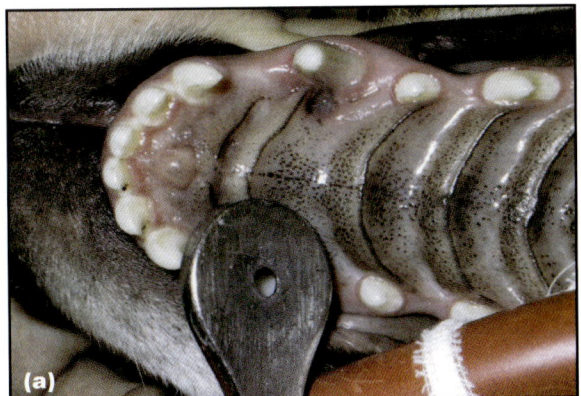

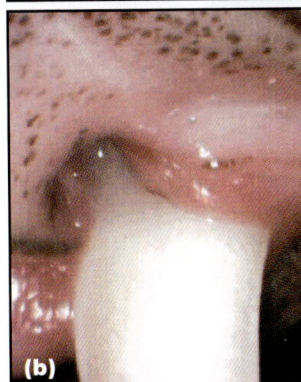

2.40

(a) Linguoversion or lingual displacement of lower canines causing palatal trauma medial to 204 and creating a 'pocket' of several millimetres depth. **(b)** Upper canine (104) of dog showing the point of impact of a lower canine palatally, causing trauma to gingival margin.

Dental impressions and the resultant study models are required for an accurate assessment of orthodontic problems.

Review examinations

Any clinical examination only reveals the situation at that time. Subsequent changes may occur with time and a diagnosis may require revision as sequelae occur. Each condition and each patient should be evaluated with reference to the interval of follow-up or review examinations.

Oral and dental imaging

Radiography is a fundamental part of veterinary dentistry, assisting in the diagnosis, treatment and monitoring of oral disease as well as being an integral part of the patient record. A knowledge of the radiographic appearance of normal anatomy enables the clinician to determine whether an abnormality exists, including variations in development (e.g. missing teeth and acquired diseases) that affect the bone and tooth structure (e.g. hyperparathyroidism secondary to renal dysplasia (rubber jaw) (Figure 2.41), osteomyelitis (Figure 2.42) and neoplasia).

The tooth root and most of the periodontium can only be visualized by means of radiographs, therefore, a complete clinical examination must include radiography. Radiography can provide information to aid in the diagnosis of some lesions and assist in treatment planning for patients with, for example, periodontitis, FORLs, caries, endodontic lesions, fractures (Figure 2.43) and neoplasia where the extent of lesions can be more accurately assessed.

Periodontitis: radiographs provide information on the amount and pattern of bone loss, and can assist in the assessment of furcation involvement. A series of radiographs taken at suitable time intervals can be used to assess the stabilization or progression of periodontal disease and the efficacy of treatment provided.

Extractions: preoperative radiographs are mandatory before any extraction to assess root size and shape, impacted and ankylosed teeth. Any abnormality in the supporting bone will also become apparent. Postoperative radiographs will show any remaining root remnants (Figure 2.44) and aid location of root tips which have been forced into the nasal cavity, mandibular canal or facial soft tissues (Figure 2.45).

Fractures: radiographs enable detection and accurate assessment of tooth root and alveolar fractures.

Necrotic pulp: a discoloured tooth or one with a fractured crown, extensive caries or that has been subject to trauma may have a necrotic pulp. The presence of a periapical/periradicular radiolucency can indicate pulpal pathology.

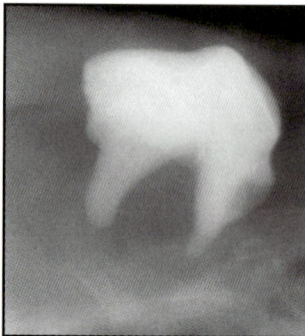

2.41 Tooth of a dog with secondary hyperparathyroidism. Note calculus deposits on the tooth and poor mineralization of the bone surrounding this tooth; this condition is known as 'rubber jaw'.

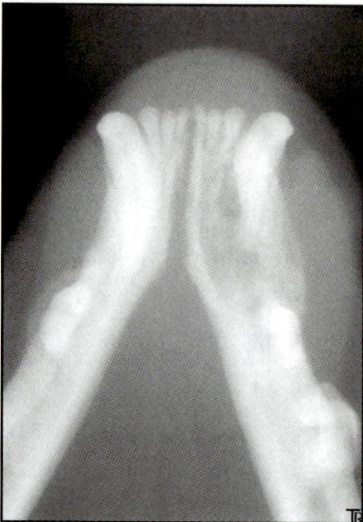

2.42 Radiograph of a 5-year-old neutered female Domestic Shorthair cat, showing osteomyelitis around the root of the mandibular canine.

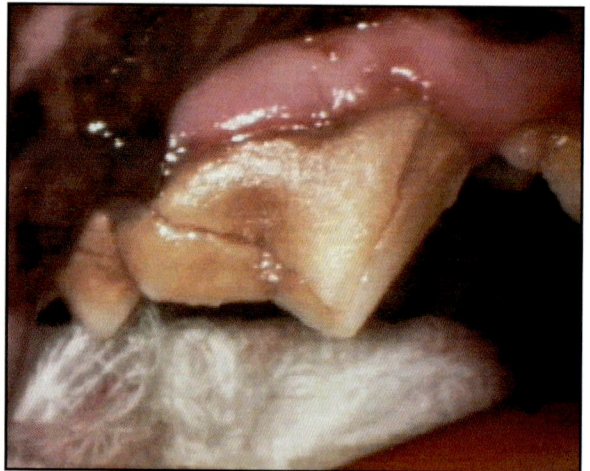

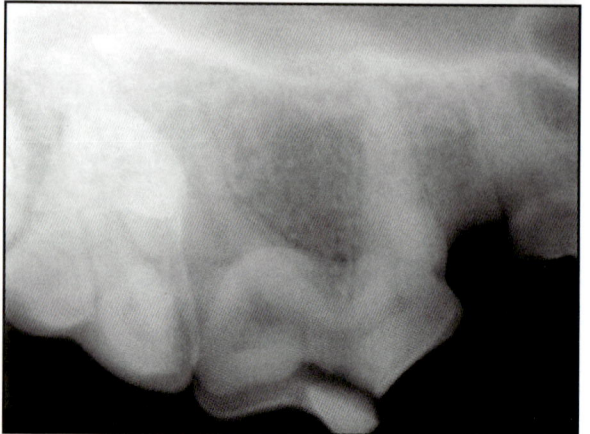

2.43 Slab fracture of upper right fourth premolar (108) in a dog.

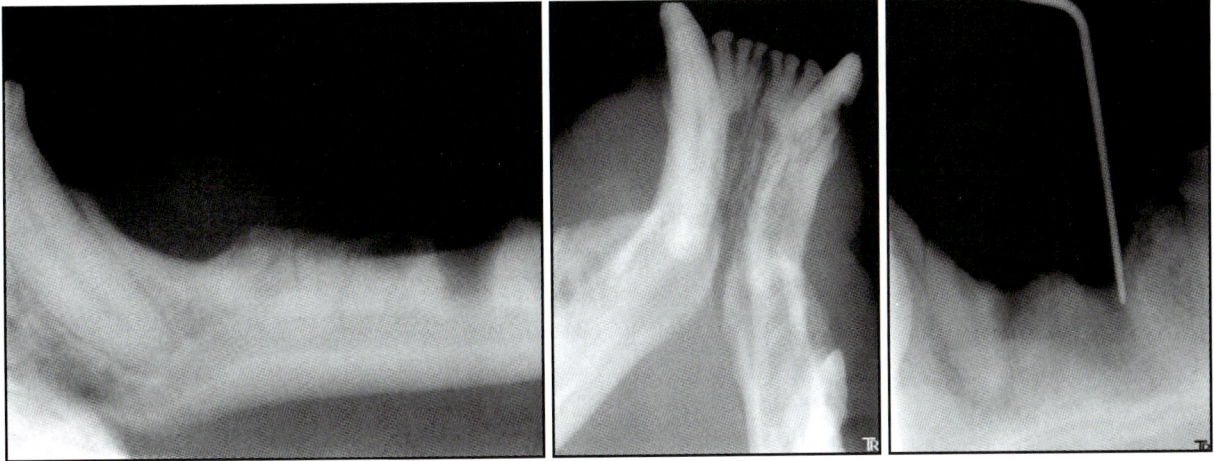

2.44 Root remnants in various positions within the mandible of feline patients.

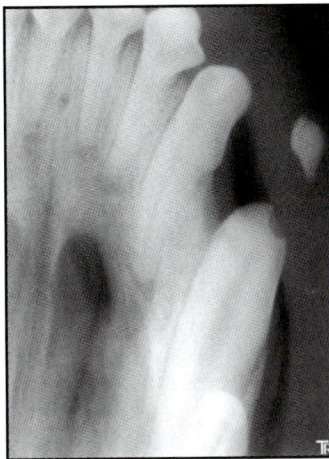

2.45 Fractured tip of a canine tooth wedged in the lip mucosa; it is not detectable without radiography.

Resorptive lesions: radiographs detect root surface resorptive lesions (both internal and external). Once one resorptive lesion is found then all the teeth in that animal should be radiographed for signs of resorptive lesions.

Missing teeth: clinically missing teeth may be absent or unerupted. Teeth that are unerupted may be impacted or ectopic and may have associated pathology. Radiography will assist in the evaluation of these teeth.

Endodontic treatment: multiple radiographs are taken throughout the endodontic procedure to evaluate the suitability of a particular tooth for endodontic treatment, to confirm the working length for instrumentation and to check obturation of the final root filling. Follow-up radiographs taken at suitable time intervals will monitor the success of the treatment by indicating a resolution of the periapical/periradicular radiolucency.

Oral abnormalities: radiographs can also assist in the investigation of other oral abnormalities, e.g. discharging sinuses, neoplasms and cysts.

Radiographs are necessary to formulate a diagnosis, aid treatment planning, enable effective treatment to be carried out, to assess the immediate outcome of treatment and to monitor the long-term success of that treatment. A good radiograph will be an accurate representation of the size and shape of the subject being examined, show the subject clearly, with good definition and contrast, avoiding superimposition of adjacent structures and enable clear interpretation of the image. In the field of veterinary dentistry this is best achieved by means of intraoral radiographic techniques.

Equipment and materials

The reader is also referred to Chapter 5 where the equipment and materials for dental radiography are also described. A summary of the equipment required is as follows:

- Dental X-ray machine
- Dental X-ray film
- Dental X-ray film processing (manual or automated).

Dental X-ray machine

A standard medical veterinary unit can be used for dental radiography, including intraoral techniques, but a dental X-ray machine has the following advantages:

- It can be wall mounted close to the treatment site, reducing patient movement once anaesthetized. Free standing units are also available
- It has a manoeuvrable head that allows accurate positioning with minimal adjustment of the patient position
- It has an optimal film–focal distance, enabling reduced exposure settings. Most dental X-ray units have a fixed kV and mA and use electronic timers to adjust the exposure time.

Dental X-ray units have guideline exposures for different sized patients and for different teeth. A series of trial exposures should be taken on different sized animals and for different teeth (preferably on cadavers) to make up an exposure chart prior to undertaking dental radiography on patients.

Dental X-ray film

Dental X-ray film is single emulsion, non-screen and high definition. The film is contained in a moisture resistant, light-proof, flexible paper or plastic envelope, which also contains a protective black paper sheet and a lead foil sheet to absorb radiation passing through the film.

Human dental X-ray films are available in numerous sizes; the three most commonly used in veterinary dentistry are:

- Occlusal (5.5 cm x 7 cm)
- Adult periapical (3 cm x 4 cm)
- Paediatric periapical (2 cm x 3.5 cm).

Dental film is commonly available in two speeds: D (ultra) and E (ekta). E-speed film is twice as fast as D-speed film and therefore requires less exposure time, but this is at the expense of the quality of the image. D-speed film is most commonly used in veterinary dental practice.

Mono-processing or self-developing films are also available in adult periapical size. They are processed by means of a single developer and fixer solution contained within a pouch attached to the film package and therefore no darkroom facilities are required. The film must be thoroughly rinsed after the package is opened but the final image is of comparable quality to other dental film. These films should be fixed again prior to storage or they will deteriorate.

All dental films have a small raised 'dot' on one side. This embossed dot should face the X-ray beam when the exposure takes place; it is the side without the lead foil and should also face the viewer when the film is orientated for evaluation. If the film is exposed through the back of the envelope the lead sheet will absorb a lot of the X-rays, resulting in an underexposed radiograph with the pattern of the lead sheet imposed upon it.

Dental X-ray film processing

Dental film is processed in a light-proof system. Most normal semi-automated systems for standard X-ray films will not cope with the small sized dental film. A dental film processing system is required, which may be automated or manual, using a three or four bath system in a darkroom or light-proof box. 'Rapid' developer and fixer solutions can be used to reduce developing and fixing times. Films must be handled carefully during processing to avoid scratching, and thoroughly fixed so that the image quality is retained during storage. Complete rinsing of the final fixing solution from the film must occur to avoid fixation stains.

Once dry, the radiographs should be examined on a backlit dental viewing box, preferably with magnifying facilities, and then carefully stored and linked to patient records, if possible in cardboard or plastic holders.

Extraoral radiography

Extraoral radiographs are sometimes required to investigate, for example, the TMJ. Views of the TMJ and of larger areas of the head can be achieved with fixed head X-ray machines. Veterinary surgeons may also have access to computed tomography (CT) or magnetic resonance imaging (MRI) through specialist referral practices, although cost can prohibit their general use.

Digital radiography

Digital radiography is the latest advancement in dental imaging and is rapidly being adopted by the dental profession. Digital imaging incorporates computer technology in the capture, display, enhancement and storage of radiographic images and offers some distinct advantages over film. Essentially there are two types of digital imaging systems:

- Direct digital
- Indirect digital.

Direct digital radiography: This technique is based around solid-state sensor technology. There are two types of sensor: the charge coupled device (CCD) and the complementary metal oxide semiconductor-active pixel sensor (CMOS-APS). This type of digital imaging system provides immediate, real-time image acquisition. Once the sensors are exposed to X-ray energy, the image is electronically processed and displayed on the computer ready for evaluation. This process typically takes less than one second.

Indirect digital radiography: This technique employs a variant of the film system. It relies on photostimulable phosphor (PSP) plates. These PSP plates, when exposed to X-rays, retain a latent image. The image is procured from the PSP plates by processing it through a special laser scanner. Once the image is scanned it is transferred automatically to the computer, typically taking less than one minute. Although slower than direct digital radiography it is still faster than the wet film system.

The milliampere seconds (mAs) of the exposure, in either digital method, is dramatically reduced by up to 90% when compared with traditional radiography. On dental X-ray machines with fixed kV and mA this means a reduction in exposure time. Once an image is captured it can be enhanced by altering the density and contrast; magnification and coloration of specific areas is also achievable. All this allows the clinician to achieve maximum diagnostic quality and a high level of interpretation from the radiographic images.

Film and digital imaging are not significantly different in their ability to record dental disease states. Digital imaging does have distinct advantages over film in terms of diagnostic quality, reduction of radiation doses, elimination of processing chemicals, instant or real-time image production and display. Reduced operative times, image enhancement and convenient storage are also advantageous. However, there are some drawbacks, e.g. infection control. Sensors cannot be sterilized, other than by cold sterilization, and care needs to be taken to prepare, cover and ensure the cross-infection barrier is not broken during patient imaging procedures.

Digital systems lend themselves to having photographic programmes incorporated. This can be a useful tool for the clinician's case record and the client can receive photographic records of the treatment carried out.

Techniques for intraoral radiography

The correct film, exposure, development and fixing of the radiograph are all essential for a clear image. Correct patient and beam positioning is critical to achieve a diagnostically valuable radiograph.

The use of intraoral radiography techniques, namely the parallel and bisecting-angle techniques, enable radiographic films to be produced without superimposition of the contralateral side. Film size is selected such that wherever possible the film is large enough to include the entire area to be examined but without the need to bend the film. This minimizes the risk of distortion of the image. For further information see *BSAVA Manual of Canine and Feline Musculoskeletal Imaging.*

Parallel technique

The parallel technique requires the film to be placed parallel to the long axis of the tooth or structure to be radiographed. To prevent magnification and distortion, the film should be as close as possible to the tooth and the radiographic beam positioned perpendicular to the tooth and film. In the dog this technique is used most frequently for the mandibular cheek teeth: the patient is placed in lateral recumbency with the area to be examined uppermost. The film is then positioned lingual to the premolar or molar teeth to be examined. Care must be taken to ensure the lower border of the film is placed as close as possible to the ventral border of the mandible. The film is then held in position by means of special film holders or by packing, such as screwed up paper towels or foam wedges and blocks.

The parallel technique will produce a true image of the subject being examined but the shape of the oral cavity only permits this technique to be used for the mandibular premolar and molar region caudal to and including the second premolar tooth. In other areas of the oral cavity, parallel film placement is not possible due to the adjacent anatomy, e.g. the film cannot be placed parallel to an upper fourth premolar due to the vault of the palate. Radiographic examination of all other teeth, therefore, requires the use of the bisecting-angle technique.

Bisecting-angle technique

With the bisecting-angle technique the film is placed at the smallest possible angle to the subject (i.e. as close to parallel to the subject as possible) and held in position. Care should be taken to avoid bending the film.

- If the X-ray beam is directed perpendicular to the film, a foreshortened image will be obtained.
- If the X-ray beam is directed perpendicular to the tooth, then the resultant image will be elongated.

To avoid these discrepancies, an imaginary line is drawn half way between the long axis of the tooth and the plane of the film; this is known as the bisecting line (Figure 2.46). The X-ray beam is directed perpendicular to this imaginary line, and the resultant image closely approximates the real situation. This technique requires the ability to visualize the long axis of the tooth and its root(s); spatulas, fingers or instrument handles can help to visualize these planes outside the mouth.

Occasionally, two or more views of an area can help to visualize fractures or to eliminate the presence of an artefact. The canine teeth can be viewed lateromedially or rostrocaudally, depending on the reason for examination. In general, the lateral view is better for maxillary canines whilst the rostrocaudal view is better for man-

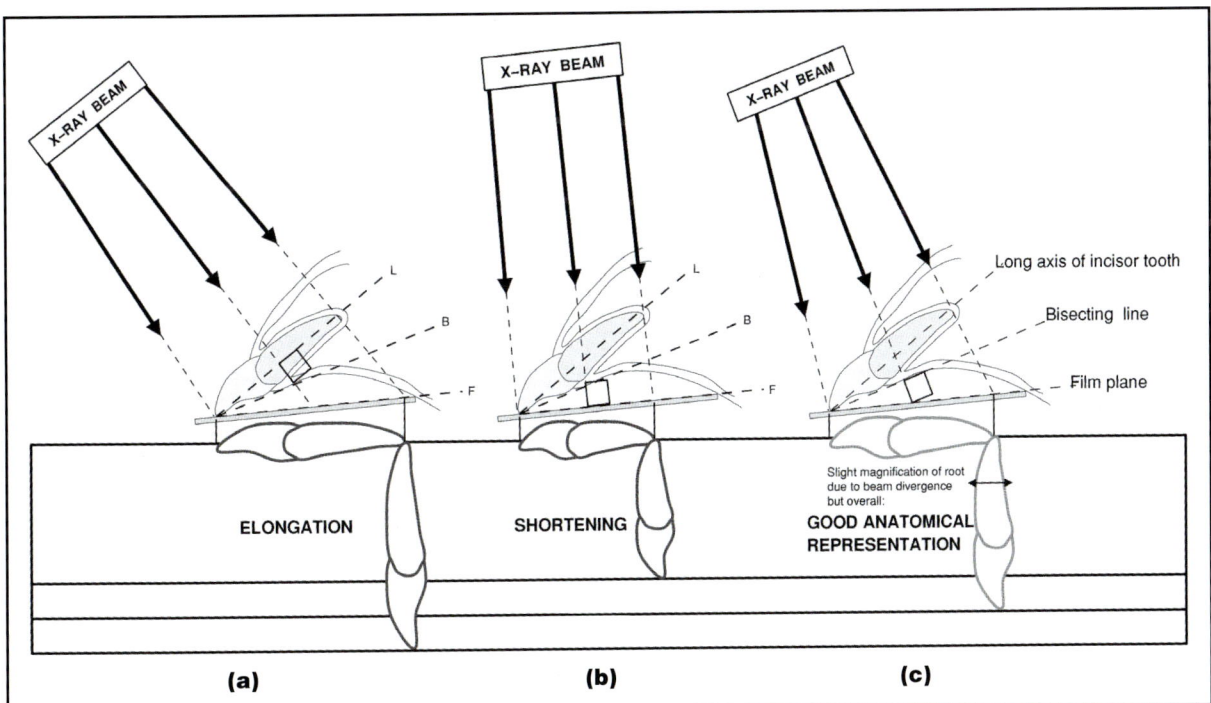

2.46 **(a)** Incident beam perpendicular to tooth: elongation of image. **(b)** Incident beam perpendicular to film: foreshortening of image. **(c)** Incident beam perpendicular to bisecting line: life-size image.

dibular canines. Feline maxillary premolar and molar views are difficult to achieve without superimposition of the zygomatic arch. Tilting the head of the cat upwards to make the dental arch parallel to the table can help to avoid this problem. Superimposition of the mesio-buccal and mesiopalatal roots of the upper fourth premolar tooth in both dogs and cats is also a problem. Often more than one view of the subject, slightly changing the angle of the incident beam rostrally or caudally is required to visualize both roots separately.

Techniques for extraoral radiography

Extraoral views are not ideal for dental examinations, mainly due to the superimposition of the contralateral side, which obscures the image and can result in distortion of the image due to its incorrect angulation.

In some instances useful extraoral radiographs of premolar and molar teeth can be obtained. The radiographic film is placed on the table and the animal placed in dorsolateral recumbency with the side under investigation closer to the film. The mouth is held wide open using a radiolucent device, e.g. plastic needle cap. By tilting the head and opening the mouth, the incident beam should only pass through the soft tissues of the contralateral side. The bisecting-angle technique is required when aiming the incident beam, in order to reduce distortion of the resultant image.

Parallax effect

Radiographic films are two dimensional and cannot give information on the relative depths of different structures. Determining the spatial location of an object can be vital when locating a foreign body or an unerupted, ectopic tooth. By taking two intraoral views of the same area, altering the beam position around the axis of the object between exposures, two images will be obtained. When the object appears to move in the same direction as the change in X-ray beam, it is lingually positioned, i.e. closer to the film. When the object appears to move in the opposite direction to the change in X-ray beam, it is buccally positioned, i.e. farther away from the film. This technique can also be used to separate and identify two overlying roots. This is known as the parallax effect and can be remembered with the help of the mnemonic 'SLOB':

- S = same (direction)
- L = lingual
- O = opposite
- B = buccal.

Viewing and interpretation

After X-ray films have been exposed, developed, fixed and dried they can be mounted and viewed. Systematic viewing procedures should be followed to ensure that the maximum amount of information is obtained from each radiograph. Ideally radiographs should be examined on a viewing box with minimal peripheral light and with the aid of magnification.

Radiographic interpretation involves identification of the structures on the radiograph, differentiation between normal and abnormal appearances, and the diagnosis of pathology. Contour, detail, variation in density and any structure displacement should be noted. Radiographic examination of the contralateral side can be useful comparatively. In some instances a series of radiographs taken over a period of time are required to assess whether pathology is in an active, static or regressive phase.

The radiographic features of normal dental structures are detailed in Chapter 1. The radiographic features of various pathological processes are covered in Chapters 7, 8, 9 and 10.

Client education

Excellence in veterinary dentistry requires directed enthusiasm and understanding of dental and oral conditions. This enthusiasm can help to motivate a client to maintain the oral health of their animal and prevent the future occurrence of any preventable pathology.

Positive marketing of the benefits of oral health for animals will bring rewards, both for the animal through improved oral health and general well-being, and for the veterinary practice. Clients can receive dental charts or records detailing the work carried out on their animals together with photographs of the treatment stages. These, together with leaflets describing home care and dietary advice relevant to the mouth, can help to reinforce the important message of oral health care for animals.

Specialist nurse clinics can be vitally important in showing the client how to care for, and maintain the health of their animal's mouth. Ideally, oral hygiene techniques should be demonstrated on the client's animal or on a practice pet to demonstrate how animals will tolerate oral hygiene procedures. These nurse led clinics can enhance client compliance and create a favourable bond between the client and the veterinary practice. Review appointments can be scheduled to monitor progress, offer corrective advice and most importantly encouragement.

References and further reading

Bezuidenhout AJ (2003) Applied Oral Anatomy and Histology. In: *Textbook of Small Animal Surgery 3rd edn*, ed. D Slatter, pp. 2630–2637. WB Saunders, Philadelphia

Gorrel C (2004) Oral examination and recording. In: *Veterinary Dentistry for the General Practitioner*, ed. C Gorrel, pp. 47–56. WB Saunders, Philadelphia

Holmstrom SE (1995) Canine Oral Diagnosis. In: *BSAVA Manual of Small Animal Dentistry, 2nd edn*, ed. D Crossley and S Penman, pp. 114–128. BSAVA Publications, Cheltenham

Mulligan T, Aller M and Williams CA (1998) *Atlas of Canine and Feline Dental Radiography*. Veterinary Learning Systems

Robinson J and Gorrel C (1995) Oral Examination and Radiography. In: *BSAVA Manual of Small Animal Dentistry, 2nd edn*, ed. D Crossley and S Penman, pp. 35–49. BSAVA Publications, Cheltenham

Shipp AD and Fahrenkrug P (1992) Eruption and dentition. In: *Practitioners Guide to Veterinary Dentistry*. Dr Shipps Laboratories

Verstraete FJM (1999) *Self assessment colour review of small animal dentistry*. Manson Publishing, London

Verstraete FJM (2003) Oral Pathology. In: *Textbook of Small Animal Surgery*, ed. D Slatter pp. 2638–2651. WB Saunders, Philadelphia

Wiggs RB and Lobprise HB (1997) *Veterinary Dentistry*. Lippincott Williams and Wilkins, Philadelphia

3

Anaesthesia and analgesia

Kenneth Joubert and Cedric Tutt

To be completed successfully, almost all dentistry work requires very deep sedation or anaesthesia. Sedation is not safer than general anaesthesia, as many of the fundamental practices of safe anaesthesia are often ignored (e.g. patent airway, monitoring).

In most hospitals one or two standard anaesthetic protocols are used for routine surgery on healthy patients. The standard protocol must be evaluated for its suitability to the individual patient, and changes made when necessary for patient safety.

The patient's physical status is not the only factor that determines the anaesthetic protocol to be used. Other factors that may affect the decision include:

- Availability of facilities and equipment (some anaesthetic techniques require the use of specialized equipment)
- Familiarity with the agents
- Nature of the procedure requiring anaesthesia
- Special patient circumstances
- Specific disease processes present or medications that the patient may be receiving
- Cost
- Urgency
- Critically injured animals requiring rapid induction of anaesthesia to initiate emergency therapy.

The anaesthetic period is broken down into preanaesthetic, anaesthetic and recovery periods. During the entire time the anaesthetist is responsible for the safety and well-being of the patient.

In the preanaesthetic period, two important procedures need to occur. The first is an evaluation of the patient and the second is the preparation of the patient for anaesthesia.

Patient evaluation

Patients vary in age, temperament, physical appearance, health status and with regard to the surgical procedure to be carried out. Given this diversity, it is unrealistic to assume that the same anaesthetic technique will apply to all patients and that all patients will respond in exactly the same way. It is very important to gather as much information as possible before the anaesthetic episode in order to plan an appropriate anaesthetic protocol.

The patient's admittance form must include the owner's name, address and telephone numbers to facilitate contact if necessary. The signalment and description of the patient should be included so that the patient can be identified, together with the procedure to be performed. An identification tag showing the owner's name, the patient's name or a description of the patient and the procedure to be performed should be placed on the patient. It is the anaesthetist's responsibility to ensure that the correct procedure is performed on the correct patient. The patient should be weighed on a suitable scale and the weight recorded on both the admission form and on the identification tag.

Geriatric patients are those that are considered to have lived at least 75% of their expected life span. Large-breed dogs are usually considered to be geriatric when an age of 8 years is achieved, while small-breed geriatric dogs are older. An increase in organ dysfunction (e.g. kidney, liver, heart) is seen with increased age. Older patients are also associated with an increase in neoplasia and cardiac disease. During the preanaesthetic evaluation particular attention should be paid to evaluation of these organ systems.

History

The current medical status of the patient needs to be established and should include information about known medical problems and concurrent medication. This should be reviewed and provision made for the continuation of vital medication (for example, insulin for diabetic patients or angiotensin converting enzyme (ACE) inhibitors for patients with heart disease).

Specific questions with regard to alternative and complementary therapy should be asked. People do not always consider these to be relevant and may not declare them when asked about medication. There are several known drug interactions and complications that may arise as a result of herbal remedies (Ang-Kee et al., 2001; Abede, 2002; Hodges and Kam, 2002; Tessier and Bash, 2003).

Other questions should be aimed at the general well-being of the animal. This may include questions about appetite, coughing, sneezing, scratching, vomiting, listlessness, diarrhoea, polyuria, polydipsia, ocular discharges, behavioural abnormalities, musculoskeletal problems and central nervous system abnormalities. Exercise intolerance is an important indicator of cardiovascular and pulmonary status. All recent treatments should be recorded, including vaccination status, worming, dipping (or other ectoparasite control measures taken) and any other routine treatments.

It is customary at this point to obtain a signed release authorizing the anaesthesia and surgery. The risks and complications associated with the procedure and anaesthetic should be fully explained to the owner.

Clinical examination

A full clinical examination should be performed, preceded by observation of the patient at rest from a distance. The basic clinical examination includes temperature, pulse and respiration.

The patient should then be examined from the tip of the nose to the end of the tail. This includes examination of the oral and pharyngeal cavities and ears, palpation of all the peripheral lymph nodes, abdomen and limbs, auscultation of the heart and lungs and examination of the skin. Overall body condition should be noted. A brief neurological examination should be conducted, including the eyes and ocular reflexes. All abnormalities must be recorded and all the systems examined should be noted in the records.

A blood smear can be made and examined for blood components (e.g. thrombocytes, monocytes, lymphocytes, neutrophils) and for blood-borne parasites. A urine sample (dipstick, specific gravity and sediment) and faecal sample (faecal float, wet preparation and smear) should be examined.

Any abnormalities or suspected abnormalities should be followed up with appropriate tests and procedures. These may include haematology, serum chemistry, radiography, electrocardiography, coagulation tests and blood gas analysis.

Following the clinical examination, the anaesthetic risks should be determined and recorded. The American Society of Anesthesiologists' (ASA) risk classification system is the most widely accepted. In the case of an emergency procedure an 'E' is usually added to the risk classification (Figure 3.1).

Status	Condition	Clinical situation
I	Normal healthy patient	Ovariohysterectomy, hip dysplasia radiographs, castration, declaw
II	Mild systemic disease; able to compensate	Neonate, geriatric, obesity, fracture without shock, mild diabetes
III	Moderate systemic disease; clinical signs	Anaemia, anorexia, moderate dehydration, low grade kidney or heart disease
IV	Systemic disease; life-threatening	Severe dehydration, shock, anaemia, uraemia, fever, uncompensated heart disease
V	Moribund, less than 24 h survival	Advanced heart, liver, lung, kidney, or endocrine disease, profound shock, major head injury, trauma
E	Emergency	

3.1 ASA risk classification.

Most dentistry is elective and should therefore be postponed until after any relevant medical condition has been treated or stabilized. Timing of the dental procedure should take into account the general medical condition of the patient.

Preparation of the patient for anaesthesia

During the preanaesthetic period the patient should receive appropriate nursing care, food should be witheld for the appropriate period, intravenous catheterization and fluid administration, resuscitation (if required), premedication and any other procedures requested by the veterinary surgeon.

Fasting

Animals that are anaesthetized without prior fasting may regurgitate or vomit during anaesthesia or in the recovery period. Stomach contents may be aspirated and this is followed by pulmonary complications (i.e. aspiration pneumonia). The pH of the aspirate is important in determining the outcome. Aspiration of gastric contents with a pH <2 results in severe pneumonia.

- In general, for adult animals food is withheld for 12 hours (minimum 4–6 hours) and water is allowed up to 2 hours before anaesthesia.
- Neonates (puppies and kittens) are particularly prone to hypoglycaemia and fasting for 12 hours may be detrimental to them. Neonates and infants are generally allowed clear liquid up to 2 hours before anaesthesia; milk and solids are usually taken away 6–8 hours prior to anaesthesia.
- Patients with renal and gastrointestinal disease may dehydrate rapidly if water is withheld for a short period of time. These patients should be placed on intravenous fluids when water is withheld.
- Critically ill and geriatric patients require particular attention when fasting is considered. These patients are very often in a negative nitrogen balance and may have dramatic fluid shifts due to altered renal and gastrointestinal function.
- Despite withholding food, some patients will still vomit or regurgitate.

Intravenous catheterization

Intravenous catheterization is essential for anaesthesia. A catheter should be placed for the following reasons:

- Allows for the safe use of anaesthetic agents that are irritant if injected perivascularly (e.g. thiobarbiturates)
- Allows for the administration of multiple drugs intravenously (e.g. diazepam and fentanyl for induction)

- Allows for the administration of emergency drugs rapidly without the need to find intravenous access (e.g. adrenaline)
- Allows for the administration of crystalloid fluids, colloids and blood during anaesthesia (e.g. Ringer's lactate, Balsol, hetastarch, blood). This also allows for the maintenance of an open intravenous line
- Allows for the maintenance of anaesthesia with injectable anaesthetics (e.g. propofol)
- Allows for the continuous administration of drugs during anaesthesia (e.g. dobutamine).

A hypodermic needle can be used for a once-off administration of an agent but is not advisable, due to the high risk of complications and the ease with which intravenous access is lost. The risks associated with intravenous catheterization are low.

The flow rate through a catheter is directly proportional to the diameter of the catheter and hence the largest-bore catheter that can be placed into the vein should be used. This is important if a crisis should arise and the rapid administration of fluid is required. Aseptic catheter placement should be performed.

Needles and catheters must be placed to their full length into the vein, avoiding nearby joints and other movable parts. This helps to prevent accidental damage to the vein and deposition of the anaesthetic agents subcutaneously.

Fluid therapy

The primary aim of fluid therapy is to maintain preload for the optimal delivery of oxygen and tissue perfusion. The normal body consists of 60% (55–75%) water on a mass basis. Of this, 30–40% is intracellular, 30% extracellular, 20% interstitial and 5% in plasma. Total blood volume is 8–10% of body mass. Water is normally distributed between these compartments following Starling's Law, osmosis and diffusion. Most anaesthetic agents result in some degree of vasodilation, hypotension and a relative hypovolaemia. The clinical signs of normal and inadequate perfusion are listed in Figure 3.2.

Parameter	Normal	Inadequate
Urine output	2 ml/kg/h	<2 ml/kg/h
Mental status	Alert	Depressed
Capillary refill time	1–2 seconds	>2 seconds
Mucous membrane colour	Pink, moist	Dry and dark
Temperature	Warm extremities	Cold extremities
Pulse rate	Normal	Fast and weak
Acid–base status	Normal	Acidotic
Lactate levels	Normal	High
Mixed venous saturation	Normal	High or low
Central venous pressure	Normal	High or low

3.2 Clinical signs of normal and inadequate perfusion.

Figure 3.3 may be used as a guide to giving fluids perioperatively. Care must be taken to ensure that a sufficient volume of fluid is administered. The rate of fluid administration should be calculated taking the following into consideration:

- *Maintenance requirements (80–100 ml/kg/day).* The maintenance amount includes normal urine production of 2 ml/kg/hour. This should be adjusted accordingly if the patient is oliguric. In anuric patients the normal urine production must be subtracted. Maintenance fluid requirements without including urine production are approximately 20 ml/kg/day
- *Fluid deficits (% dehydration x body mass).* Dehydrated patients require additional fluid to correct this imbalance. A 10% dehydrated patient would require approximately 10% of its body mass in fluid to correct this deficit. This may be given over a short period (± 2 hours) or over 6 hours. It is advisable to correct as much of this imbalance as possible before induction of anaesthesia
- *Ongoing losses.* Ongoing losses to the gastrointestinal tract through diarrhoea or vomiting may amount to several litres of fluid per day in a large dog. The volume of stool or vomitus produced can be used as a guide to increase the volume of fluids given
- *Third-space losses.* These are difficult to quantify as no fluid leaves the body; the fluid in the intravascular space is redistributed to other organs in the body and generally results in oedema of these organ systems. Diarrhoea is sometimes considered as a third-space loss
- *Haemorrhage.* Intraoperative blood loss can be measured through assessment of blood on the swabs and the amount of blood accumulated in the suction system. This fluid loss must be replaced. Some patients may lose their entire circulating volume of blood during a procedure, while others will lose only a negligible amount. It is recommended that if a patient loses more than 20% of their circulating volume, or if their haematocrit (Ht) falls below 20%, they should receive a transfusion
- *Loss to the environment.* Evaporation from exposed surface areas can be high in hot dry operating theatres. Most operating theatres are air-conditioned, resulting in low relative humidity. Theatre lights create heat, resulting in increased evaporation. This loss is difficult to calculate but an additional 2–6 ml/kg/hour can be allowed for it

Type of surgery	Fluid rate required
Minimally invasive	6 ml/kg/h
Moderately invasive	8 ml/kg/h
Severely invasive	10 ml/kg/h

3.3 Intraoperative fluid requirements.

- *Increased intravascular space.* An increase in intravascular space may occur due to vasodilation as a result of the anaesthetic agents used. This 'loss' needs to be replaced urgently.

The ultimate volume of fluid given is determined by adding the above losses together. This may result in a continually changing fluid rate. Fluid rates may initially be high to correct a deficit (e.g. dehydration, third-space losses). Haemorrhage can occur at any stage and would require a sudden increase in fluid adminis-tration. Particular attention should be paid when administering fluid to patients with cardiac disease (usually volume overloaded) and renal failure (oliguric – reduced urine production; polyuric – increased urine production).

- Resuscitation fluids are generally used to replace fluid losses due to haemorrhage, dehydration and vasodilation.
- Diarrhoea and vomition may result in electrolyte disturbances with the result that additional sodium, potassium or bicarbonate may be required.
- A patient may require more than one infusion to replace all their losses.
- Replacement of blood loss with crystalloid fluids is done at 3–5 times the volume of blood lost.
- Signs of over-hydration include ocular and nasal discharges, chemosis (swelling and oedema of the conjunctiva), increased lung sounds, cyanosis, increased respiratory rate and dyspnoea.
- The choice of fluids varies depending on the status of the patient and the procedure.
- Colloids are beneficial in patients with endothelial dysfunction to maintain oncotic pressure.
- Blood should be given to anaemic patients and when blood loss is greater than 20% of the circulating volume.

Precautions for rapid fluid administration include the following:

- Maximum fluid administration rate in dogs is 90 ml/kg/hour (1 blood volume/hour)
- In cats, maximum fluid administration rate is 45–60 ml/kg/hour (1 blood volume/hour)
- Monitor cardiopulmonary status carefully
- Monitor Ht and total plasma protein (TPP) levels: maintain Ht > 20% and TPP > 4 g/dl
- Direct blood loss can be replaced rapidly (over a couple of minutes) if required to support cardiovascular function.

Oxygen, the airway and endotracheal intubation

Oxygen
Patients presenting with respiratory compromise (lung oedema, pulmonary contusions or pneumonia) and debilitated patients benefit from receiving oxygen prior to anaesthetic induction. This improves blood oxygen status and allows for a safer induction to be performed.

The induction of anaesthesia in a cyanotic patient is associated with increased morbidity.

Airway and endotracheal (ET) tubes
One of the essential functions of an anaesthetist is to ensure the maintenance of a patent airway. The nature of dentistry inevitably compromises the airway and certain oral procedures are hindered by orotracheal intubation.

Cuffed tubes: Either cuffed or uncuffed tubes can be used to protect the airway. The function of the cuff is to ensure a seal between the trachea and the tube, preventing the leakage of air around the ET tube and preventing foreign bodies from entering the trachea. A cuffed ET tube offers the following advantages:

- It ensures a patent airway
- Airtight cuff prevents leakage of anaesthetic gases
- It reduces the risk of aspiration of blood, saliva, vomitus and other material into the lungs
- It prevents the dilution of anaesthetic gases with room air during inhalation
- It reduces environmental pollution
- It minimizes dead space (if inserted correctly)
- Positive pressure ventilation can be performed.

Tube material: ET tubes are made of either rubber (red), silicone (clear) or plastic (clear).

- *Rubber tubes* are relatively inexpensive but their use is associated with several problems: the rubber surface may absorb disinfectants, anaesthetic agents or other solutions; the tubes crack with time and these cracks form a protected environment for the colonization and growth of microorganisms; the tube may also leak through these cracks; rubber tubes usually contain a low-volume high-pressure cuff, which is more likely to cause tracheal damage.
- *Silicone tubes* have the advantage of being smooth, flexible and non-porous and are less irritating than the other tubes. They have high-volume low-pressure cuffs, which are less likely to induce tracheal damage.
- *Plastic tubes* are usually one-use disposable tubes that have high-volume, low-pressure cuffs.

Tube diameter: ET tubes come in different sizes determined by the internal diameter of the tube. Some tubes are reinforced with a metal spiral to prevent obstruction when the tube is bent. Uncuffed ET tubes usually have a smaller external diameter than cuffed tubes of the same internal diameter. The inverse squared law applies to the radius of the tube and resistance. This means that, for very small tubes, a small increase in radius results in a significant reduc-tion in resistance. All patients (particularly those that are small) should have the largest ET tube possible placed to ensure that airway resistance remains low.

Intubation: Intubation of patients after induction of anaesthesia is standard practice, especially if the procedure is expected to last longer than 30 minutes. The technique for the insertion of an ET tube is simple. Dogs are intubated in a light plane of anaesthesia while cats are intubated in a deep plane of anaesthesia. In cats, the vocal chords can be sprayed with a topical local anaesthetic to reduce the risk of laryngospasms. Prior to placement the ET tube should be lightly lubricated, using a water-soluble lubricant, to prevent damage to the respiratory epithelium lining the trachea.

A laryngoscope may be used to aid in the visualization of the larynx. The position of the ET tube needs to be confirmed by palpation of the trachea: the tube should end just in front of the thoracic inlet. It is then secured in place with gauze or string. The tube should be trimmed to the level of the incisors to reduce dead space. In order to assess whether or not the tube is in the trachea, the following criteria may be used:

- The reservoir bag will inflate and deflate as the patient breathes
- The mouth can be opened and the larynx visualized to see the tube passing between the vocal chords
- A cough may be heard on manipulation of the tube or on insertion in lightly anaesthetized patients
- During expiration the patient's breath can be felt at the end of the ET tube. This can also be demonstrated by the movement of cotton wool or gauze as inspired and expired air flows through the opening of the tube
- Vocalization is impossible if the tube is inserted correctly.

Cuff inflation: The technique for inflating the cuff is to apply a normal ventilatory pressure of 20 cm H_2O to the reservoir bag at the same time as inflating the cuff. The cuff is inflated until the gas stops escaping past the cuff. If a large volume of air is required to inflate the cuff, a larger tube should be used instead. The pilot balloon indicates that the cuff is inflated. Over-inflation of the cuff can lead to tracheal necrosis and stenosis and in severe cases tracheal rupture.

Aspiration and micro-aspiration: During dentistry, the mouth is contaminated with water, calculus, bacteria and blood. The primary technique for protecting the airway is the placement of an ET tube. A cuffed tube usually provides a good seal to prevent the aspiration of large particulate matter but unfortunately does not protect the airway from micro-aspiration and the passage of fluid.

The narrowest part of the upper airway is between the vocal chords, while the broadest part is immediately behind the vocal chords. Fluid and small particulate matter can pass between the vocal chords and the ET tube. This fluid then accumulates between the vocal chords and the cuff of the ET tube. When the cuff is deflated and the tube removed, aspiration can occur. In addition, movement of the ET tube during ventilation can allow for the slow movement of fluid between the cuff and the tracheal wall in a process known as micro-aspiration.

For these two reasons, a cuffed ET tube does not guarantee against aspiration. The throat should be packed with swabs or pharyngeal packs after endotracheal intubation, to prevent particulate matter (e.g. calculus, blood clots) from entering the upper airway. However, fluid can still accumulate. Raising the thoracic inlet above the mouth allows fluid to drain away by gravity and is invaluable in protecting the airway. At the end of the procedure, the pharynx should be inspected and any accumulated fluid and particulate matter should be removed by suction before the ET tube cuff is deflated and removed.

Tube hygiene: After use, the ET tube should be placed in a solution of bicarbonate of soda to loosen the saliva and mucus build-up on the tube before it is cleaned with a suitable disinfectant.

Difficulty in intubating patients

Temporomandibular joint (TMJ) disease can prevent the mouth from opening, making intubation almost impossible. A number of techniques exist to enable successful intubation of these patients.

Tubes can be placed blindly but this requires experience and a certain amount of luck for successful intubation. Blind techniques can be facilitated by external manipulation of the larynx, alignment of the upper airway and trachea into a straight line and by listening at the end of the tube for respiratory sounds.

If a small gap is present, a stylet can be used. A light source or laryngoscope is useful to assist with visualization of structures in the pharynx. The stylet is advanced into the trachea and used to guide the ET tube into the trachea using a 'railroad' technique. If this fails, an endoscope can be used to find the airway and advanced into the trachea before 'railroading' the ET tube in.

Alternatives to endotracheal intubation

Jaw fracture alignment and intraoral surgery are often facilitated by not having an ET tube in the mouth. Nasotracheal intubation is unfortunately not possible in most canine and feline patients. Alternatives are pharyngostomy or tracheostomy.

Pharyngostomy: Pharyngostomy intubation is a simple technique to perform. Following induction of anaesthesia and the placement of a standard ET tube, the hair coat caudal to the mandible is clipped and aseptically prepared. A gloved hand is used to palpate the hyoid apparatus from within the pharynx. Curved artery forceps are placed immediately caudal to the hyoid apparatus and pressure is applied on the forceps to force the tip laterally to tent the skin on the lateral aspect of the neck. A scalpel is used to incise the skin and blunt dissection is used to exteriorize the forceps. The tip of a guarded ET tube (reinforced by a steel spiral within the wall) is placed between the jaws of the forceps and pulled through the pharynx and out of the mouth. The forceps can then be used to guide the guarded ET tube into the trachea once the normal ET tube is removed. At the end of the procedure the tube is removed and the skin defect is allowed to heal by second intention.

Tracheostomy: If pharyngostomy fails, or if the airway is expected to be compromised after surgery, a tracheostomy can be performed. For the tracheostomy technique, refer to standard surgical texts.

Premedication

The purpose of premedication (drugs administered to a patient before anaesthesia, as either a single agent or a combination of drugs) is to improve the quality of anaesthesia. Sedation not only enhances patient comfort but also simplifies the task of anaesthesia. Not all patients require sedation; debilitated, sick and old patients may experience excessive central nervous system depression after the administration of a tranquillizer or sedative.

Acepromazine maleate

Acepromazine maleate (ACP) is a commonly used tranquillizer. It has a ceiling tranquillizing effect and increasing the dose beyond this point results in an increase in side effects. The most common side effect is hypotension due to vasodilation. ACP is not always effective in aggressive animals, which may become more aggressive due to a loss of fear (Collard, 1958; Meyer, 1997). ACP has an anti-arrhythmic effect by desensitizing the myocardium to catecholamines. At clinically used doses the effects on respiration are minimal.

ACP is contraindicated in debilitated or sick patients, hypovolaemic and hypotensive patients, epileptics, hepatically compromised patients and aggressive dogs. It should be avoided in brachycephalic breeds, as relaxation of the upper airways can result in a critical narrowing and an obstruction with dyspnoea. ACP can also cause a dose-independent atrioventricular block in these breeds.

Benzodiazepines

Benzodiazepines are known as sedative hypnotics, but in dogs the sedative and hypnotic effects appear to be absent. At clinical doses these drugs have minimal effects on the cardiovascular system. Slight respiratory depression does occur due to down-regulation of carbon dioxide perception.

Benzodiazepines are good muscle relaxants but they are seldom used on their own and are very often combined with opioids to improve their sedative action. They are safe in most compromised patients.

Alpha$_2$ adrenergic agents

Alpha$_2$ adrenergic agonists are potent sedatives in dogs and cats. They decrease anaesthetic requirements by 50–90%, which is important to remember in order to prevent a relative anaesthetic overdose. After intravenous administration an initial dramatic rise in blood pressure occurs, followed by a reflex bradycardia and a drop in cardiac output. Centrally, a drop in sympathetic tone occurs, resulting in a further drop in cardiac output, which may decrease by up to 60%. These drugs are responsible for respiratory depression through a reduction in respiratory frequency and tidal volume. Marked hypoxaemia is seen in patients following administration of these drugs. The use of alpha$_2$ agonists should be limited to healthy patients.

Opioids, NSAIDs and analgesics

Opioids, non-steroidal anti-inflammatory drugs (NSAIDs) and analgesics are usually administered in the preoperative period to improve analgesia in a process known as pre-emptive analgesia. Pre-emptive analgesia improves pain control in the postoperative period. These drugs are discussed in more detail in the section on analgesia.

Anticholinergics

Anticholinergic drugs are used to control secretions and prevent vagal inhibition. They have several effects on the lungs, including a reduction of bronchial secretion, a decrease in mucociliary apparatus clearance and an increase in dead space as a result of bronchodilation. These effects may predispose certain patients to hypoxia.

Vagal inhibition of the heart results in bradycardia. Such vagal inhibition may occur as a result of drugs (xylazine and opioids) and surgery, procedures or manipulations of the eyes (oculocardiac reflex) and larynx. Anticholinergics have been shown to attenuate these responses.

Anticholinergics are also used to treat bradycardia. An initial slowing of the heart is seen after the administration of anticholinergics but this is followed by an acceleration of heart rate. The increase in heart rate may predispose the patient to cardiac arrhythmia. Tachycardia increases myocardial energy demands and may be fatal.

Hypothermia

Hypothermia can be a complication of prolonged dental procedures and has a major influence on mortality rate (Beal *et al.*, 2000; Oncken *et al.*, 2001; Tyburski *et al.*, 2001). Patients with a core temperature of 34°C or less had a mortality rate of 40%, compared with patients with core temperature greater than 34°C who had a mortality rate of 7% (Kongsayreepong *et al.*, 2003). Hypothermia causes a left shift of the oxygen dissociation curve, resulting in impaired oxygen delivery, increased lactic acidosis with hypovolaemia, inhibition of the pulmonary hypoxic reflex, shunting of blood and coagulopathy (Oncken *et al.*, 2001). The coagulopathy is the result of reduced enzyme function, enhanced plasma fibrinolytic activity and reduced platelet aggregation. The bleeding and prothrombin times are particularly prolonged. Metabolism decreases by 8% for each degree Celsius below normal (Oncken *et al.*, 2001). Hypothermic patients therefore have reduced anaesthetic requirements, which should be taken into consideration to avoid an overdose of anaesthetic agents.

Hypothermia should be prevented by the use of insulation between the patient and the cold operating surface, or by placing the patient on a warm-water circulation blanket or heating pad. The use of a forced air heater, raising the environmental temperature, heating intravenous fluids and covering the patient with blankets will also help to reduce the risk of hypothermia (Evans *et al.*, 1973; Camus *et al.*, 1997; Machon *et al.*, 1999).

External heating is usually ineffective as a means of raising core temperature in hypothermic patients, because sluggish peripheral blood flow does not carry the warmed cutaneous blood centrally. Skin burns may result. Sluggish peripheral blood flow is the result of peripheral vasoconstriction and shock (Oncken et al., 2001).

Cutaneous warming may induce a peripheral vasodilation moving warm central blood peripherally and cold peripheral blood centrally that may result in acute cardiac failure. The most effective method of warming patients is the installation of warmed fluids into the peritoneal and pleural cavities. Maintenance of a warm environment during surgery is imperative (Kongsayreepong et al., 2003).

Induction of anaesthesia

Anaesthesia may be induced by means of an intravenous, intramuscular, oral or inhalation route. Usually the intravenous and/or inhalation route is used.

Regardless of the induction method chosen, monitoring of the patient is of paramount importance throughout the induction period. To ensure patient safety the heart rate, pulse strength, respiratory rate and depth, mucous membrane colour and capillary refill time should be checked frequently. Familiarity of the anaesthetist with the anaesthetic agents being used is important. It is seldom beneficial to anaesthetize a critically ill patient with a new drug that the anaesthetist may have heard or read about but has never tried before.

Intravenous anaesthetic agents are carried by the cardiovascular system to the central nervous system. Here they must cross the blood–brain barrier in order to induce anaesthesia. Substances with high lipid solubility will cross the blood–brain barrier rapidly, while those with a low solubility will not. It should be borne in mind that the brain receives a large proportion of blood for its size. Recovery from the anaesthesia is then dependent on the redistribution of the anaesthetic agent from the central nervous system to other compartments (muscles, fat) within the body. This redistribution is dependent on cardiovascular function and the chemical properties of the drug used. Ultimately the drug is metabolized and excreted.

Injectable agents

Thiopental
Thiopental is an alkaline solution that causes tissue necrosis if injected perivascularly. In order to avoid tissue necrosis it is suggested that a 2.5% solution of thiopental is used and that a catheter is inserted into the vein. Should perivascular injection occur, the area should be infiltrated with an equal volume of saline. Lidocaine should be added for its analgesic properties and to neutralize the alkalinity. Corticosteroids may be added to reduce the resulting inflammatory reaction.

Thiopental produces profound respiratory depression when administered rapidly intravenously. This is seen as a short period of apnoea (induction apnoea). Ventilator support should be provided if there is any concern for the patient's well-being. The cardiovascular effects of thiopental include direct myocardial depression, a reduction in cardiac output, vasodilation,

sensitization of the myocardium to adrenaline, and arrhythmias. It is not uncommon for arrhythmias to occur immediately following induction (i.e. ventricular premature contraction and ventricular bigeminy) (Muir, 1977a,b). Slow administration of the drug may reduce these side effects. Bolus dosing may cause a dramatic drop in blood pressure. Thiopental has no analgesic properties. Muscle relaxation does occur in a dose-dependent manner and is related to anaesthetic depth.

Propofol
Propofol is a potent respiratory depressant (similar to thiopental). The degree of respiratory depression is entirely dose-dependent. Induction apnoea may be avoided by administering the dose over a longer period of time (Muir and Gadawski, 1998). Propofol is a vasodilator but other cardiovascular effects are minimal. Propofol does not possess analgesic properties and produces muscle relaxation in a dose-dependent manner. The major disadvantage of propofol is the formulation: the oil emulsion is an ideal growth medium for bacteria (Crowther et al., 1996) and, if aseptic techniques are not observed, bacteria readily grow within this medium; this can result in the administration of bacterial endotoxins and bacteraemia.

Propofol is particularly useful when rapid recovery is required after a short anaesthetic. Brachycephalic dogs benefit from this during the recovery period and for this reason barbiturates are generally avoided in these breeds. Sight hounds have a reduced ability to metabolize and redistribute barbiturates and hence propofol is the drug of choice in these animals.

Ketamine
Ketamine is a dissociative anaesthetic and appears to disrupt the nervous pathways in the cerebellum and the reticular activating system. This results in a distinct type of anaesthesia known as dissociative anaesthesia or catalepsy. Reflex responses are exaggerated rather than depressed. For this reason it may be difficult to determine anaesthetic depth. Pharyngeal and laryngeal reflexes persist throughout anaesthesia, which may make endotracheal intubation difficult. Sensitivity to sound, light and other stimuli may result in what is perceived to be a light anaesthetic plane. Muscle tone increases and muscle rigidity is common. This can make surgery difficult if a muscle relaxant is not given. One advantage of ketamine is that it may be given by both intravenous and intramuscular routes.

Ketamine causes respiratory depression, which is seen as a reduction of both tidal volume and respiratory rate. The cardiovascular effects are mixed. Heart rate, blood pressure and cardiac output are usually increased as a result of an increase in sympathetic tone. However, ketamine is a direct myocardial depressant and these effects tend to predominate in patients with myocardial disease or in patients who cannot increase their sympathetic tone (Sprung et al., 1998). Ketamine generally causes an increase in salivation. The eyes become dry and fish like and it is important to protect the corneas with ocular lubricants. Ketamine is usually combined with a muscle relaxant (benzodiazipines, thiazines or phenothiazines). Ketamine has good analgesic properties.

Etomidate

Etomidate is structurally unrelated to any of the other anaesthetic agents. Induction with etomidate produces minimal changes in cardiovascular function (Nagel *et al.*, 1979; Brüssel *et al.*, 1989) and respiratory depression is dose-related. Muscle tone tends to increase with etomidate and it is advisable to premedicate with a muscle relaxant. Another major problem with the use of etomidate is suppression of the adrenal–cortical axis (Kruse-Elliott *et al.*, 1987).

Inhalational agents

Inhalational agents represent an occupational safety risk for people working in the dental room. Scavenging should be utilized to prevent exposure of staff to waste anaesthetic agents. These systems may be active or passive but their function should be checked regularly.

Halothane

Halothane is a commonly used inhalation agent. It causes myocardial depression, decreases cardiac output and also sensitizes the myocardium to catecholamines. Vasodilation occurs in a dose-dependent fashion. Halothane also causes dose-related respiratory depression with a drop in tidal volume and respiratory rate. It produces dose-dependent muscle relaxation but has no analgesic effect. Halothane is also a trigger for malignant hyperthermia. Forty percent of halothane may be metabolized.

Isoflurane

Isoflurane results in only small decreases in cardiac output and does not sensitize the myocardium to adrenaline. However, it is a potent dose-dependent vasodilator and causes respiratory depression. Isoflurane has muscle-relaxing properties but does not have analgesic properties. Very little (0.2%) isoflurane is metabolized.

Enflurane

Enflurane demonstrates dose-dependent cardiovascular and respiratory depressant effects. At equipotent doses, enflurane causes a greater drop in cardiac output and blood pressure compared with halothane and isoflurane. Enflurane is not a potent sensitizer of the myocardium to adrenaline and is hence less arrythmogenic than halothane. Two to eight percent of enflurane is metabolized.

Maintenance of anaesthesia

Following the induction of anaesthesia, the anaesthetist has two responsibilities:

1. To ensure that the patient remains in a pain-free state and anaesthetized to an appropriate depth.
2. To ensure that vital functions are maintained.

The monitoring of vital functions is more crucial than the maintenance of anaesthetic depth. In addition to monitoring the patient's vital signs and reflexes, the anaesthetist should ensure that rough handling or careless positioning while under anaesthesia does not compromise the patient. Care should be taken when the patient is moved. Checks must be made on the ET tube and the tubes of the anaesthetic machine to ensure that these do not become collapsed, kinked or disconnected. Interference with normal chest movement may occur in small patients when heavy instruments or hands are placed on the chest. Care should also be taken to ensure that all monitoring devices are connected properly and that these are not disconnected during the procedure.

Records

Complete and accurate medical records form an important part of a patient's file. They are legally required and should include a complete record of the anaesthetic period. This should involve details of the patient (identification, owner's details and procedure), information about the drugs administered (drug, dose, route and time of administration) and vital signs (signs monitored and their values). Relevant preoperative information should also be recorded.

The vital signs should be recorded every five minutes even though they are monitored continuously. Any abnormal events should be recorded (time and nature of event) and appropriate measures taken to correct the abnormality. Details as to non-standard procedures should be recorded (time and procedure). The times of induction, start of surgery, end of surgery and end of anaesthesia should be recorded. This monitoring form should be completed into the recovery period.

Incidents and accidents

Before an anaesthetic machine is used, it is essential that the machine is inspected to ensure patient and operator safety. An anaesthetic problem resulting from malfunction of the anaesthetic machine will be regarded as negligence. Monitoring is vital to supply the anaesthetist with enough information to give a warning before an anaesthetic accident happens. An anaesthetic incident is any event that occurs during an anaesthetic period that could be potentially harmful or have a negative outcome for the patient. An incident may happen acutely or result from a slow decompensation of a vital organ system. An anaesthetic accident, resulting in patient suffering, will result when an anaesthetic incident has occurred and has not been rectified in time. The time between an incident and an accident determines the safety factor and severity of a particular incident.

The patient's vital signs should indicate how well the patient is maintaining basic circulatory and respiratory function during anaesthesia. Neurological reflex responses give the anaesthetist valuable information on the depth of anaesthesia.

With modern medical science have come a host of machines to aid the monitoring of patients. These machines have not replaced the clinical judgement of a skilled anaesthetist but do enable closer monitoring of vital signs and give advanced warning of anaesthetic incidents and accidents. This in turn has made anaesthesia safer. Electronic surveillance (e.g. ECG machines, oscillometric blood pressure monitoring equipment and pulse oximeters), although convenient, should not be relied on to give a complete picture of patient status. Instruments are subject to power failures, interference from artefacts and loss of contact with the patient.

Monitoring of vital signs

Vital signs that should be monitored during anaesthesia include heart rate and rhythm, blood pressure, central venous pressure, capillary refill time mucous membrane colour, blood loss, respiratory rate and depth, blood gases and temperature.

Cardiovascular monitoring

Heart rate and rhythm can be monitored by palpation of the heart through the chest wall, palpation of an artery, auscultation of the chest and an electrocardiogram (ECG). The pulse may be detected at any one of several locations, including the femoral, lingual, carotid and dorsal pedal arteries. The pulse should be strong and synchronized with the ECG. The presence of a beating heart does not necessarily imply that circulation is adequate. The heart rate must be assessed in conjunction with pulse strength or blood pressure. Blood pressure reflects the perfusion pressure of circulation through the body. A rough estimate of blood pressure may be obtained manually by determining the strength of the peripheral pulse. Non-invasively measured blood pressure is not accurate but an average of five or more readings improves accuracy. It is important to monitor blood pressure in patients with renal and cardiac disease, and in other medically compromised patients.

The capillary refill time (CRT) is the rate of return of colour to a mucous membrane after the application of gentle digital pressure. It gives an indication of the adequacy of perfusion and 1–2 seconds is normal. The observation of purple or blue mucous membranes indicates cyanosis. Cyanosis during anaesthesia is usually the result of respiratory failure or upper airway obstruction and must be addressed immediately. Pale mucous membranes indicate blood loss, anaemia or poor perfusion. Bright pink mucous membranes with a rapid CRT are indicative of hyperdynamic shock. A slow CRT is indicative of hypoperfusion and shock. A normal CRT can occur in patients with shock.

Respiratory monitoring

Adequate ventilation is vital to maintain oxygenation and ensure an adequate uptake of the inhalational anaesthetic agent. The rate and depth of respiration (tidal volume) determine alveolar ventilation. The rate is easily determined by observation of the animal's chest or movement of the reservoir bag. To determine the depth of respiration, closer observation of the rebreathing bag is required to assess the degree of collapse of the bag during inspiration. Tidal volume decreases by at least 25% in most anaesthetized animals. The anaesthetized animal's breathing should be smooth and regular. Difficult or laboured breathing indicates the presence of an airway obstruction.

Ventilation is normally driven by the partial pressure of carbon dioxide in the blood. As alveolar ventilation decreases, arterial carbon dioxide rises. The arterial partial pressure of carbon dioxide in normal lungs correlates well with expired carbon dioxide. A capnograph measures the expired percentage of carbon dioxide and enables assessment of ventilatory function. As carbon dioxide is produced in peripheral tissues and transported by circulation to the lungs, capnography also gives an assessment of circulation.

Pulse oximetry allows for assessment of arterial oxygenation in the body. Arterial oxygen saturation decreases rapidly when patients with decreased alveolar ventilation are breathing room air. For spontaneously breathing patients on room air, pulse oximetry gives a good indication of alveolar ventilation. Normally under anaesthesia, 100% oxygen is administered and pulse oximetry is no longer a reliable indication of alveolar ventilation. Under these circumstances, pulse oximetry indicates more about the ability of the lungs to transfer oxygen to haemoglobin. For example, pulmonary oedema, shunts and atelectasis will decrease saturation and a decrease in the pulse oximetry reading indicates pulmonary damage.

Temperature

Throughout anaesthesia, the animal's temperature should be maintained as close as possible to normal. Temperature loss is greatest in the first 20 minutes of any anaesthetic period, and the anaesthetist should be concerned with preventing temperature loss. Hypothermia will result in a prolonged recovery, as it slows the rate at which liver enzymes metabolize anaesthetic drugs. Shivering increases the patient's oxygen demands during the recovery period and can lead to hypoxia in some animals. The patient's temperature should be routinely monitored every 30–60 minutes.

Urine production

A patient should produce 1–2 ml of urine/kg/hour. In critical cases it might be prudent to catheterize the animal and monitor urine production. Urine production is dependent on an adequate blood pressure and blood supply to the kidneys. A decrease in urine production usually occurs in shock, hypotension and cardiovascular collapse.

Eye protection

The eyes should be protected from drying out; this is a particular problem with ketamine anaesthesia. Artificial tears or another suitable ocular lubricant should be applied at the beginning of the anaesthesia and regularly throughout the anaesthesia to prevent drying of the cornea.

Recovery from anaesthesia

The recovery period is defined as being from the time the anaesthetic is discontinued until the patient regains its ability to maintain its own homeostasis. The length of recovery depends on:

- *The length of anaesthesia.* Generally the longer the anaesthesia, the longer the recovery

- *The patient status*. Longer recoveries are expected in compromised patients
- *The anaesthetic agent given*. Patients receiving barbiturate anaesthetic may exhibit prolonged recoveries
- *Hypothermia*. Hypothermic patients take longer to metabolize drugs and therefore experience longer recovery times.

Recovery should occur in an area where the patients can be continually monitored. Vital signs should be recorded every 5 minutes until the patient leaves the recovery area or until the patient is fully conscious. This area should have the facilities of an intensive care unit and appropriate therapy should be applied as required, according to correct principles. Analgesics should be administered to patients to prevent pain. Opioids are usually appropriate if pain is severe. Oxygen supplementation is particularly useful for compromised and geriatric patients. These patients are prone to hypoventilation during recovery. Brachycephalic dogs (especially Bulldogs) are prone to upper airway obstruction in the postoperative period; they should be placed in sternal recumbency during recovery and the ET tube only removed once a strong swallowing reflex is present. Intravenous fluids should be given as required. The animal's body temperature should be monitored and appropriate measures taken if it is hypothermic.

Extubation should be performed once the patient has regained its swallowing and gagging reflexes. Cats should be extubated at a deeper plane to avoid laryngospasm.

Patients that have undergone jaw fracture repair may not be able to eat in the postoperative period. For these patients the placement of a nasogastric or pharygostomy feeding tube is necessary. These tubes can be placed at the end of surgery or during recovery. The technique for a pharyngostomy or oesophagostomy feeding tube is identical to that of pharyngostomy intubation except that the tube is advanced down the oesophagus and not the trachea (for further information see *BSAVA Manual of Canine and Feline Head, Neck and Thoracic Surgery*).

Analgesia

Almost all procedures performed on a patient are painful. This pain could be mild and short lived (e.g. intravenous cannulation) or severe and protracted (e.g. a fractured jaw). As a general rule of thumb, if it is painful to you it is painful to your patient and they should receive an analgesic.

Pain causes suffering. Pain results in increased postoperative complications either directly or indirectly, with a resultant increase in morbidity, prolonged convalescence and increased hospitalization. Pain decreases food intake and increases catabolism with an inefficient use of available energy. It enhances the stress response, delays healing and impairs respiration, leading to hypoxia, hypercapnia and acidosis. Pain in the gastrointestinal tract results in hypomotility,

ileus, nausea and vomition. Some patients may mutilate themselves. These negative effects require pain to be actively managed.

Nociception is the first stage in the perception of pain. Peripheral free nerve endings are the simplest pain receptors in the body. Widely distributed throughout the body, superficial layers of the skin, periosteum, arterial walls, joints, flax and tentorium of the cranial vault, they are responsible for most of the pain perception. Other pain receptors include mechanosensitive pain receptors, thermosensitive pain receptors and chemosensitive pain receptors. The latter are responsive to bradykinin, serotonin, histamine, potassium ions, acids, prostaglandins, acetylcholine and proteolytic enzymes. Impulses are carried to the central nervous system by pain fibres. They are classified into fast and slow pain fibres. Acute sharp pain is transmitted by fast pain fibres classified as $A\delta$ fibres, which conduct at 6–30 m/second. Chronic pain is carried by slow pain fibres, or C fibres, which conduct at 0.5–2 m/second.

Continuous stimulation of sensory nerves results in hypersensitization of the nervous system to pain. Sensitization occurs both peripherally and centrally.

Severe pain requires immediate attention. NSAIDs may take up to an hour before an effect is seen, making them unsuitable for acute-onset severe pain. Ideally an intravenous formulation of an opioid should be used. Morphine, after an intravenous loading dose, takes 8–10 minutes to reach peak effect. If pain is not controlled, an additional bolus may be given every 8–10 minutes until the pain is controlled. In cats, excitement may be seen with doses of morphine above 0.5 mg/kg and a sedative or tranquillizer (benzodiazepines or phenothiazine) should be given. Fentanyl has a faster equilibration time of approximately 2 minutes and additional boluses may be repeated every 2 minutes.

The type of pain determines which analgesic drugs are more effective. Inflammatory type pain is best treated with NSAIDs. Surgical pain presents as a number of different types, including inflammation and somatic. Use of multiple drugs enables the exploitation of the synergistic activity of combination therapy. A synergistic activity has been found between NSAIDs and opioids. It therefore makes sense to use both types of drugs to control pain. This means that less of each individual agent is used, resulting in a reduction of side effects.

Uncontrolled pain leads to neuropathic pain or hypersensitivity. This type of pain is difficult to control with conventional analgesic drugs. Local anaesthetic blocks are a very useful technique for analgesia.

Opioids

Opioids form a fundamental part of any analgesic protocol. They dull the appreciation of pain without the loss of consciousness. High doses of strong opioids result in a loss of consciousness. The response to pain is altered such that pain is still perceived but the threshold for pain transmission to the brain is greatly increased. There is evidence that opioids act both pre- and post-synaptically. They exert their effect through inhibition of the release of excitatory neurotransmitters and hyperpolarization of neurons. A high concentration of opioid receptors is found in the dorsal horn of the spinal cord, explaining their analgesic action (Siddall and Cousins, 1995). Stimulation of mu receptors results in analgesia, sedation, hypothermia, miosis, bradycardia, euphoria and cardiovascular and respiratory depression, while stimulation of the sigma receptors causes indifference, delirium, ataxia, tachycardia and mydriasis. Respiratory depression is caused in the main by stimulation of the mu_2 receptors, whereas stumulation of the mu_1 receptors results in supraspinal analgesia and euphoria. Stimulation of the kappa receptors results in spinal analgesia, reversal of respiratory depression, physical dependence and sedation. Opioids demonstrate different affinities for opioid receptors. Opioids are used to control moderate to severe pain (Regan and Peng, 2000).

Mixed agonist–antagonists and partial agonists have different affinities for opioid receptors, leading to complex pharmacological effects. With true agonists, the dose of opioid can be titrated until the pain is controlled. This is unlike agonists–antagonists and partial agonist opioids, which have a ceiling effect after which they reverse the opioid effect.

Opioids reduce initial responses to pain but do not prevent 'winding up'. N-methyl D-aspartate (NMDA) antagonists do not prevent initial pain but do prevent wind-up. A combination of these substances has great potential, especially for intrathecal (cerebrospinal fluid) use. An antinociceptive synergism has been reported with local anaesthetics, NSAIDs and opioids.

Adverse reactions to opioids are either dose-dependent or unpredictable:

- Respiratory depression occurs due to depression of the bulbopontine respiratory centres. This is dose-related and the patient becomes dependent on a hypoxic driver for ventilatory control. Pain is an effective antagonist to respiratory depression. Excessive doses of mixed agonists–antagonists produce moderate to severe respiratory depression, unlike the apnoea caused by true agonists. The incidence of respiratory depression after axial opioid administration is low
- Vomition is frequently seen with the use of opioids but can sometimes be avoided by the concurrent use of ACP (Valverde et al., 2004)
- Bradycardia can occur following the administration of high doses and should be treated with atropine
- Histamine release has been described with morphine and pethidine usage. This histamine release is associated with pruritis, urticaria, hypotension and decreased systemic vascular resistance. The newer synthetic opioids, such as fentanyl and sufentanil, have had no such effect
- Opioids may affect vagal nerve tone and result in bradycardia
- Opioids reduce gastrointestinal motility, increase tone in the pyloric antrum and duodenum and reduce propulsive peristalsis

- Tolerance of, and dependence on, opioids is rare. In humans, only four out of 11,882 patients became addicted after analgesic use of opioids. Acute tolerance may develop when opioids are given in non-painful conditions
- Neurological signs have been reported after the use of pethidine. These effects are mainly due to norpethidine, an active metabolite
- All opioids induce nausea and vomition by direct stimulation of the chemoemetic trigger zone
- Opioids increase the tone of the urinary sphincter and inhibit the detrusor muscle, resulting in urine retention
- Opioids are only advisable in cranial trauma if ventilation is controlled, as the increased arterial carbon dioxide levels through respiratory depression raise intracranial pressure.

Neuroleptanalgesia usually consists of an opioid in combination with a tranquillizer. The effect seen is dependent on the drugs used. The opioids most commonly used are morphine and fentanyl derivatives. These are usually combined with ACP, $alpha_2$ agonists or benzodiazepines.

Non-steroidal anti-inflammatory drugs
The recent advancements in NSAIDs have brought with them agents capable of controlling moderate to severe acute pain. These newer generations of NSAIDs are sometimes superior to opioids. They can contribute significantly to pain management where the control of scheduled substances is problematic. However, the use of NSAIDs is associated with several risks and these must be borne in mind. The most important of these risk factors are gastrointestinal ulceration and renal compromise. Cats appear to be more prone to the adverse effects of NSAIDs than humans or dogs. This means that drugs safe for human use may not be safe in cats and dogs and those safe in dogs may not be safe in cats.

NSAIDs are seldom used on their own but are often combined with opioids or other drugs, due to their synergistic effects. Most NSAIDs take approximately 45–60 minutes to take effect and therefore additional analgesia needs to be given in this bridging zone. Opioids are a good choice for the bridging zone.

Their administration reduces the inflammatory reaction at the site of trauma, reducing the peripheral hypersensitivity response. In surgical cases, this effect can be used pre-emptively to aid in the management of pain. It is important to administer NSAIDs both before and after surgery to obtain the best benefit from pre-emptive analgesia.

- The ideal indication for NSAIDs is pain in well hydrated normotensive young to middle-aged animals with normal renal function and no evidence of gastric ulceration or haemostatic abnormalities.
- Older animals given NSAIDs should be monitored for adverse side effects.
- NSAIDs should be used with caution when creatinine levels are raised. Urine specific gravity

(normal >1.030 in dogs, >1.035 in cats) may be useful in decision making.

- NSAIDs should not be given to patients with known renal insufficiency, dehydration, hypotension, relative and absolute hypovolaemia, ascites, heart failure, thrombocytopenia, known coagulation deficiencies, gastric ulceration or any gastrointestinal disturbances, haemorrhage in non-compressible areas or with the concurrent use of corticosteroids.
- These drugs should not be given to shock or trauma patients on presentation.
- Patients with asthma or pulmonary disease may deteriorate due to inhibition of prostaglandin E_2 (PGE_2) production.
- Gastric ulceration can occur with all NSAIDs and prophylaxis should be instituted. Drugs that can be used are sucralfate 250–500 mg p.o. q8–12h in cats, 1–2 g p.o. q6–8h in dogs, misoprostol (2–5 μg/kg p.o. q8h) and ranitidine (3.5 mg/kg p.o. q12h, 2.5 mg/kg i.v. q12h).

The use of NSAIDs is covered in more detail in the *BSAVA Manual of Canine and Feline Anaesthesia and Analgesia*.

Alpha$_2$ agonists

Alpha$_2$ receptors are present in the spinal cord, which in part explains the effective analgesic properties of alpha$_2$ agonists (Siddall and Cousins, 1995). This class exerts marked analgesia that usually lasts as long as the sedative effects are present. They may be particularly useful for the control of severe pain that is not responding to conventional analgesic agents or during recovery from anaesthesia of patients with emergency delirium.

These drugs are associated with major changes in cardiovascular and respiratory function after their administration. Following the intravenous administration of an alpha$_2$ agonist, vasoconstriction rapidly ensues and results in hypertension. Baroreceptors sense the rise in blood pressure and slow the heart rate, with a reduction in blood pressure. The reduction in heart rate and vasoconstriction cause a significant reduction in cardiac output. A number of cardiac arrhythmias have been described following the administration of alpha$_2$ agonists (atrioventricular and sinoatrial blocks). The respiratory pattern is characterized by periods of apnoea followed by brief hyperventilation. These agents should be used with caution in compromised patients.

The cardiorespiratory side effects can be reduced by using lower doses (1–2 μg detomidine/kg) administered over a longer period of time.

NMDA receptor antagonists

NMDA receptors and the excitatory amino acids that bind to them are responsible for the development of wind-up (Siddall and Cousins, 1995). NMDA antagonists are capable of inhibiting the development of wind-up in the treatment of patients with central hypersensitivity (Siddall and Cousins, 1995; Ilkjaer *et al.*, 1996). NMDA receptors have been implicated in the development of opioid tolerance and the administra-

tion of an antagonist may prevent this (Siddall and Cousins, 1995). The most commonly used NMDA antagonist is ketamine (Siddall and Cousins, 1995). Ketamine is thought to have primary analgesic action (Ilkjaer *et al.*, 1996).

Local and regional anaesthesia

Indications

The use of local anaesthesia is indicated in exodontics (simple and open extraction techniques), periodontal surgery and oral surgery.

Local and regional anaesthesia has been found to inhibit systemic effects of pain by preventing propagation of the pain sensation. There are four regional anaesthesia sites commonly used in veterinary dentistry namely:

- The mental block
- The inferior alveolar (mandibular) block
- The infraorbital block
- The maxillary block.

The mental block

The needle (with its bevel facing the mandible) is placed either just caudal to the lip frenulum or passed medial to the lip frenulum and directed at the middle mental foramen (usually situated at the level of the apex of the mesial root of mandibular premolar 2. The needle may be introduced into the mental foramen (Figure 3.4) or the anaesthetic agent can be infused at the opening of the foramen and localized by digital pressure (Figure 3.5). If injecting into the canal care must be exercised to inject slowly so as not to cause neuropraxia as a result of pressure in the confines of the canal. It is essential to aspirate prior to administration of the anaesthetic agent to ensure the drug is not delivered intravenously.

Effect: Superficial injection will anaesthetize the buccal soft tissues and lower lip rostral to the foramen, while intracanal infusion will also anaesthetize the ipsilateral canine and incisors as well as the lip and oral mucosa rostral to this site.

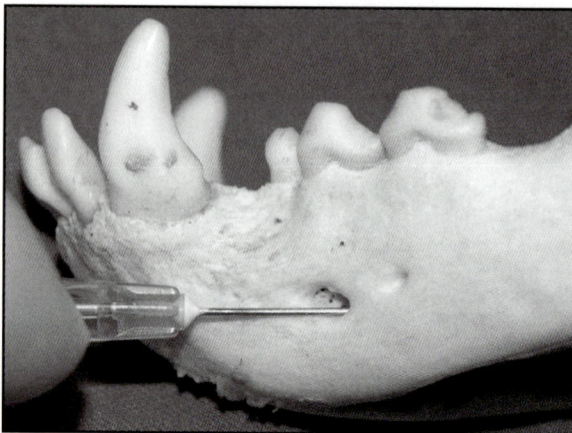

3.4 Mental block. The needle is advanced beneath or caudal to the lip frenulum into the middle mental foramen.

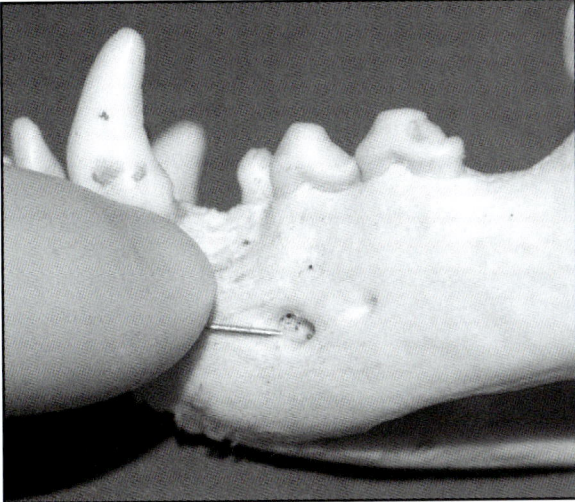

3.5 Superficial mental block. The needle is advanced to the middle mental foramen with the needle bevel facing the mandible.

The inferior alveolar (mandibular) block

This block can be performed percutaneously or intraorally. Either way the caudal opening of the mandibular canal, the mandibular foramen, is palpated intraorally; usually the neurovascular bundle can be palpated digitally with ease. When injecting intraorally, once the neurovascular bundle has been isolated, the needle is passed submucosally with the bevel of the needle facing the mandible until it is at the level of the mandibular foramen and the anaesthetic agent is deposited at that site (Figure 3.6). Using the percutaneous approach, the neurovascular bundle is isolated as in the intraoral approach and the needle is inserted percutaneously just medial to the mandible with the bevel facing the mandible, and the anaesthetic agent deposited at the mandibular foramen (Figure 3.7). Digital support helps localize the anaesthetic agent in this area.

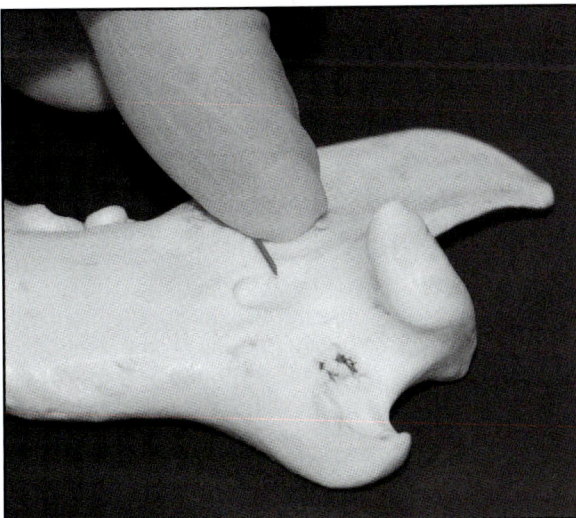

3.6 Mandibular block: intraoral approach. The mandibular foramen is identified digitally and the needle advanced submucosally with the bevel facing the mandible. Digital pressure over the tip of the needle restricts the anaesthetic to the injection site.

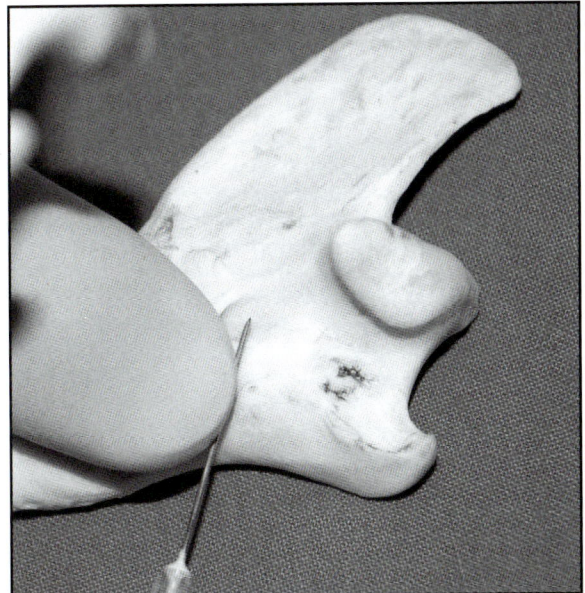

3.7 Mandibular block: percutaneous approach. The mandibular foramen is identified intraorally and the needle inserted percutaneously medial to the mandible and submucosally to the mandibular foramen.

Effect: Injection at the mandibular foramen will anaesthetize all teeth in the ipsilateral mandible, the oral mucosa, buccal soft tissues and lip on that side.

The infraorbital block

The needle (with its bevel facing medially) is directed medial to the infraorbital neurovascular bundle and into the canal (Figure 3.8). (An arterial pulsation is often visible intraorally just rostral to the infraorbital canal.) Aspiration must always be performed prior to injection of local anaesthetic agent to prevent intravascular injection that may cause cardiac dysrhythmias or ineffective anaesthesia due to systemic administration of the drug.

Effect: Superficial injection will anaesthetize the oral mucosa rostral to the infraorbital canal, the ipsilateral teeth rostral to the maxillary fourth premolar and the upper lip and oral mucosa.

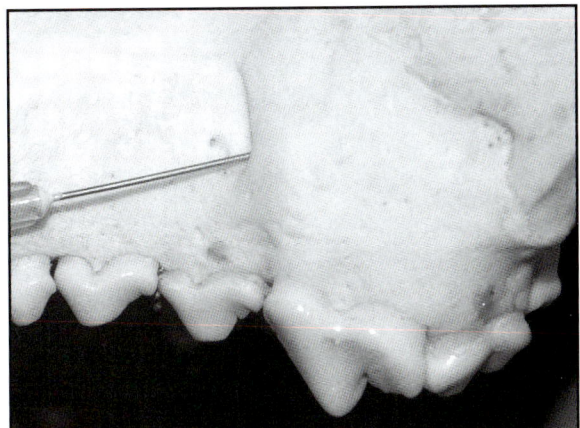

3.8 Infraorbital block. The needle is inserted into the infraorbital canal, medial to the infraorbital neurovascular bundle. Digital pressure keeps the anaesthetic agent localized.

The maxillary block

This block can be performed via the infraorbital canal (Figure 3.9) or percutaneously. Via the infraorbital canal a longer needle is used than that for the infraorbital block and the anaesthetic agent deposited deeper at the level of the bifurcation of the infraorbital nerve bundle. Via the percutaneous route the needle is placed caudal and ventral to the rostral zygomatic arch and inserted to a depth of about 25 mm (depending on the patient size) (Figure 3.10).

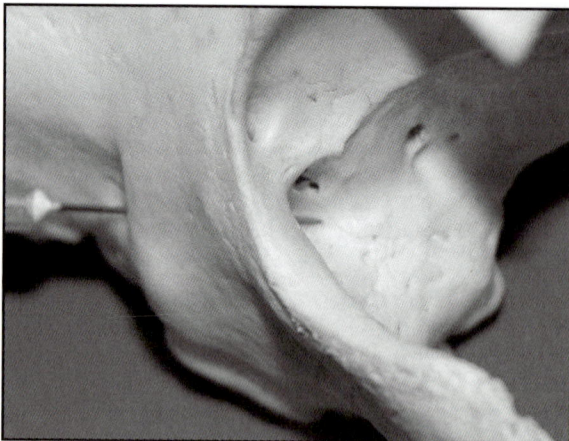

3.9 Maxillary block: intraoral approach. The needle is placed as in Figure 3.8 and advanced to the level of the distal root of the maxillary carnassial tooth (PM4).

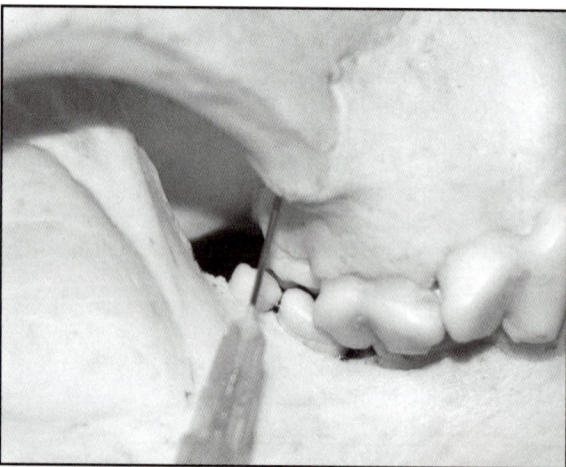

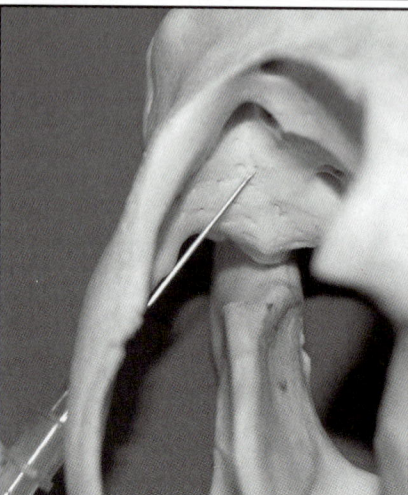

3.10 Maxillary block: percutaneous approach. The needle is inserted in the notch created by the rostral zygomatic arch and the maxilla and directed to the maxillary foramen.

Effect: Anaesthesia of all ipsilateral maxillary teeth, oral mucosa, buccal soft tissues and lip.

Local anaesthetic drugs

Local anaesthetic drugs block the initiation and propagation of nerve impulses; nerve action potentials are inhibited by the blocking of sodium ion channels in the neuronal cells. This leads to membrane stabilization and electrical activity inhibition in both sensory and motor nerves. Most local anaesthetic drugs potentiate the effect of injectable and inhalational anaesthetics, thereby providing an anaesthetic-sparing effect enabling use of lower doses of these drugs (Figure 3.11).

$$[BH^+] / [B] = 10^{(pKa-pH)}$$

Therefore: $[BH^+] = [B] \times 10^{(pKa-pH)}$

Dissociation formulae for local anaesthetic agent: where $[BH^+]$ is the concentration of the cationic form (active form); $[B]$ is the concentration of the uncharged base form (form in which the drug must be to pass into the nerve); pKa is the pKa value of the anaesthetic agent and pH is the pH of the tissue fluid.

The anaesthetic agent must be in the cationic form $[BH^+]$ to be effective. To be able to pass into the nerve sheath it must be in the base form $[B]$. When tissue is inflamed the pH of the tissue fluid decreases; for example if the tissue fluid pH decreases to 6 and the pKa of the anaesthetic agent is 8, $[BH^+] = [B] \times 100$. This means that there will be much less anaesthetic agent in the base form rendering it ineffective as there is insufficient to get to the site of action.

3.11 Mode of action of local anaesthetic drugs.

The most commonly used local anaesthetic drugs are:

* *Lidocaine.* Rapid onset effect with duration of 60–120 minutes
* *Bupivacaine.* Intermediate to slow onset of effect with duration of 3–10 hours. May cause cardiac side effects if injected intravascularly
* *Ropivacaine.* Similar onset and duration to bupivacaine but less cardiotoxic
* *Mepivacaine.* Onset similar to lidocaine but duration of 1.5–4 hours.

These agents belong to the amino-amide group. Increased lipid solubility results in increased effect and duration of the local anaesthetic. Local anaesthetics are weak bases with pKa values in the range of 8–9. The uncharged base form is the form that most easily penetrates and passes through biological membranes to arrive at the action site. At physiological pH the local anaesthetic takes on a cationic form that is the locally active form. The amide group of local anaesthetics binds to proteins, leading to increased duration of activity as well. Changes in tissue pH will affect the ionization of the anaesthetic drug and interfere with its effect.

Alpha$_2$ agonists (e.g. medetomidine) may be combined with local anaesthetic agents for local or regional anaesthesia and can be delivered locally or systemically, providing enhanced peripheral nerve blocking of increased duration.

Nerve function inhibition as a result of local anaesthetic effect occurs in the following order: pain, warmth, touch, deep pressure and motor function. It is therefore possible to block pain without blocking motor function. Proximal areas are innervated by more superficial nerve fibres and will therefore be blocked sooner than more distal structures that are innervated by deeper nerve fibres (the anaesthetic agent taking longer to reach these structures).

In vitro the addition of bicarbonate to the anaesthetic drug has led to faster onset of activity and a lower volume required for effect. This is probably due to there being more drug delivered in the base form but this is not yet commonly performed in practice.

The first signs of local anaesthetic toxicity are neurological. In humans, tinnitus is the first sign seen, followed by convulsions and seizures. The neurological signs are not usually fatal. Cardiovascular collapse through vasodilation and the negative inotropic effects (calcium channel-blocking effects) follow and can result in death. Resuscitation following an overdose with a local anaesthetic is usually unsuccessful. The maximum dose of local anaesthetic that can be administered should be calculated and this dose not exceeded. Maximum doses are:

- Lidocaine 10 mg/kg
- Bupivacaine 0.75 mg/kg
- Ropivacaine 1.5 mg/kg.

References and further reading

Abede W (2002) Herbal medication: potential for adverse interactions with analgesic drugs. *Journal of Clinical Pharmacy and Therapeutics* **27**, 391–401

Ang-Kee MK, Moss J and Yaun C-S (2001) Herbal medicines and perioperative care. *Journal of the American Medical Association* **286**(2), 208–216

Beal MW, Brown DC and Shofer FS (2000) The effects of perioperative hypothermia and the duration of anesthesia on postoperative wound infection rate in clean wounds: a retrospective study. *Veterinary Surgery* **29**, 123–127

Brüssel T, Theissen JL, Vigfusson G, Lunkenheimer PP, van Aken H and Lawin P (1989) Hemodynamic and cardiodynamic effects of propofol and etomidate: negative inotropic properties of propofol. *Anesthesia and Analgesia* **69**, 35–40

Camus Y, Delva E, Bossard AE, Chandon M and Lienhart A (1997) Prevention of hypothermia by cutaneous warming with new electric blankets during abdominal surgery. *British Journal of Anaesthesia* **79**, 796–797

Cashman JN (1996) The mechanisms of action of NSAIDs in analgesia. *Drugs* **52** (Suppl. 5) 13–23

Collard JA (1958) Unusual reaction to chlorpromazine hydrochloride in a bitch. *Australian Veterinary Journal* **34**, 90

Crowther J, Hrazdil J, Jolly DT, Galbraith JC, Greacen M and Grace M (1996) Growth of microorganisms in propofol, thiopental, and a 1:1 mixture of propofol and thiopental. *Anesthesia and Analgesia* **82**, 475–478

Dahl JB (1994) Neuronal plasticity and pre-emptive analgesia: implications for the management of postoperative pain. *Danish Medical Bulletin* **41**(4), 434–442

Evans AT, Sawyer DC and Krahwinkel DJ (1973) Effect of a warmwater blanket on development of hypothermia during small animal surgery. *Journal of the American Veterinary Medical Association* **163**(2), 147–148

Hodges PJ and Kam PCA (2002) The peri-operative implications of herbal medicines. *Anaesthesia* **57**, 889–899

Ilkjaer S, Petersen KL, Brennum J, Wernberg M and Dahl JB (1996) Effects of systemic N-methyl-D-aspartate receptor antagonist (ketamine) on primary and secondary hyperalgesia in humans. *British Journal of Anaesthesia* **76**, 829–834

Kongsayreepong S, Chaibundit C, Chadpaibool J, Komoltri C, Suraseranivongse S, Suwannanonda P, Raksamanee E, Noocharoen P, Silapadech A, Parakkamodom S, Pum-In C and Sojeoyya L (2003) Predictor of core hypothermia and the surgical intensive care unit. *Anesthesia and Analgesia* **96**, 826–833

Kruse-Elliott KT, Swanson CR and Aucoin DP (1987) Effects of etomidate on adrenocortical function in canine surgical patients. *American Journal of Veterinary Research* **48**(7), 1098–1100

Lundeberg T (1995) Pain physiology and principles of treatment. *Scandinavian Journal of Rehabilitation Medicine* **32**, 13–42

Machon RG, Raffe MR and Robinson EP (1999) Warming with a forced air warming blanket minimizes anesthetic-induced hypothermia in cats. *Veterinary Surgery* **28**, 301–310

McCormack K (1994) The spinal actions of nonsteroidal antiinflammatory drugs and the dissociation between their antiinflammatory and analgesic effects. *Drugs* **47** (Suppl. 5), 28–45

Meyer EK (1997) Rare idiosyncratic reaction to acepromazine in dogs. *Journal of the American Veterinary Medical Association* **210**(8), 1114–1115

Muir WW (1977a) Electrocardiographic interpretation of thiobarbiturate-induced dysrhythmias in dogs. *American Journal of Veterinary Research* **170**(12), 1419–1424

Muir WW (1977b) Thiobarbiturate-induced dysrhythmias: the role of heart rate autonomic imbalance. *American Journal of Veterinary Research* **38**(9), 1377–1380

Muir WW and Gadawski JE (1998) Respiratory depression and apnea induced by propofol in dogs. *American Journal of Veterinary Research* **59**(2), 157–161

Nagel ML, Muir WW and Nguyen K (1979) Comparison of the cardiopulmonary effects of etomidate and thiamylal in dogs. *American Journal of Veterinary Research* **40**(2), 193–196

Oncken AK, Kirby R and Rudloff E (2001) Hypothermia in critically ill dogs and cats. *Compendium on Continuing Education for the Practicing Veterinarian* **23**(6), 506–520

Regan JM and Peng P (2000) Neurophysiology of cancer pain. *Journal of Molecular Cellular Cardiology* **7**(2), 111–119

Siddall PJ and Cousins MJ (1995) Pain mechanisms and management: an update. *Clinical and Experimental Pharmacology and Physiology* **22**, 679–688

Skinner CM and Rangasami J (2002) Preoperative use of herbal medicines: a patient survey. *British Journal of Anaesthesia* **89**(5), 792–795

Sprung J, Schuetz SM, Stewart RW and Moravec CS (1998) Effects of ketamine on the contractility of failing and nonfailing human heart muscle *in vitro*. *Anesthesiology* **88**(5), 1202–1210

Tessier DJ and Bash DS (2003) A surgeon's guide to herbal supplements. *Journal of Surgical Research* **114**, 30–36

Tyburski JG, Wilson RF, Dente C, Steffes C and Carlin AM (2001) Factors affecting mortality rates in patients with abdominal vascular injuries. *Journal of Trauma* **50**, 1020–1026

Urquhart E (1993) Central analgesic activity of nonsteroidal antiinflammatory drugs in animal and human pain models. *Seminars in Arthritis and Rheumatism* **23**(3), 198–205

Valverde A, Cantwell SL, Hernandez J and Brotherson C (2004) Effects of acepromazine on the incidence of vomiting associated with opioid administration in dogs. *Veterinary Anaesthesia and Analgesia* **31**, 40–45

4

Operator safety and health considerations

Judith Deeprose

Injuries at work are an unpleasant prospect. The reality is that within the veterinary dental workplace hazards are present and some pose a significant risk of harm to the veterinary dental team. Veterinary practitioners are ethically, morally and legally bound to provide themselves and their co-workers with a safe workplace. This especially applies to women of childbearing age. Some basic preparation can maintain a safe working environment and prevent injury to veterinary dental surgeons, their co-workers and their patients. The main factors to consider when reviewing operator and veterinary dental team safety and health are:

- Legal requirements, including Health and Safety legislation and the Control of Substances Hazardous to Health (COSHH)
- Working conditions, including ventilation, lighting, personal protective equipment and ergonomic surgery design considerations
- Oral microbial exposure and cross-infection control
- Equipment safety
- Operator safety in relation to the use of dental equipment and materials (see Chapter 5 for additional details)
- Radiographic safety.

Legal requirements

A veterinary surgeon's responsibility for health and safety in the workplace is governed by the Health and Safety at Work etc. Act 1974 (HSW Act). The act seeks to protect all those at work – employers, employees and the self-employed – as well as members of the public who may be affected by the work activities of these people. In particular a veterinary practitioner should:

- Provide a working environment for employees that is safe, without risks to health and with adequate facilities and arrangements for their welfare at work
- Maintain the place of work in a safe condition
- Provide and maintain safe equipment, appliances and systems of work
- Ensure that dangerous or potentially harmful substances or articles are handled and stored safely
- Provide the necessary instruction, training and supervision to ensure health and safety.

Health and Safety legislation is increasingly risk driven. Recent legislation places a specific obligation on employers to assess the risks to their employees and others who might be affected by their work activities. The requirement to assess risks can be general, as in the Management of Health and Safety at Work Regulations 1999, or specific, as in the Control of Substances Hazardous to Health Regulations 2002.

The Health and Safety Executive (HSE) is the statutory body responsible for enforcing the HSW Act and providing an advisory service. Any workplace is liable to a HSE inspection, which will include examination of the premises and equipment with particular attention to anything posing obvious potential danger, e.g. radiographic equipment, autoclaves, electrical appliances and gas cylinders. Inspectors will not undertake technical testing of equipment but will request to see evidence of the safety checks that have been carried out.

It is good practice to have a written health and safety policy that is brought to the attention of all employees, ideally with each employee having their own policy document.

A risk assessment is no more than a careful examination of the contents of the workplace and the potential to cause oneself and others harm. It helps the practitioner to identify what precautions are required to prevent or minimize the risk of injury and/or ill health. Risk assessment is a practical exercise to identify hazards, or anything that can do harm, and assess the risk, or the chance of harm actually being done, associated with that hazard. The following approach will help in carrying out a risk assessment in the practice setting.

1. Look for the hazards. Manufacturer's instructions (for equipment and products) and material safety data sheets (for chemical products and hazardous substances) are important in helping to identify hazards and risks. Suppliers of equipment and chemicals have a legal obligation to supply Health and Safety information.
2. Decide who might be harmed and how.
3. Evaluate the risks arising from the hazard and decide whether existing precautions are adequate or if more should be instituted. For each significant hazard, it needs to be decided whether the risk is high, medium or low. Even after all precautions have been taken some risk

Significant hazards	Those at risk	Existing controls or action required
Examination		
Risk of: Contamination with blood and saliva Bite injuries	Veterinary dentist Veterinary dental team co-worker Clients	Protective clothing, including protective eyewear, mask or face shield, gloves and head covering Appropriate patient restraint Sedation or anaesthesia of patient Provide muzzles for handling of fractious animals
Restorative procedures		
Risk of: Eye injury from debris Aerosol production and splatter Contamination with blood and saliva	Veterinary dentist Veterinary dental team co-worker Other patients and staff	Protective clothing, including protective eyewear, mask or face shield, gloves and head covering Use of rubber dam where practical Good ventilation High-volume aspiration (suction)
Eye injury		
Risk of: Flying debris and splatter from rotary instruments Splashing during the cleaning of instruments instruments	Veterinary dentist Veterinary dental team co-worker Patient	Use of protective eyewear during clinical procedures for operator, co-workers and patient Use of protective eyewear when cleaning instruments and equipment prior to sterilization Use of high-volume aspiration for procedures using rotary and those creating an aerosol Use of rubber dam where practical, to restrict the operative field

4.1 Example risk assessments carried out in respect of examinations, restorative procedures and eye injuries.

may remain. Can the risk be eliminated altogether? If not, what should be done to control the risk so that harm is unlikely? Whatever is reasonably practical should be implemented to keep the workplace safe by minimizing all the risks.

4. Record the findings.
5. Review the assessment periodically (for example, when new equipment or materials are introduced) or at least every five years to ensure that the precautions are still effective.

Examples of risk assessments carried out in respect of examinations and restorative procedures together with a general risk assessment with respect to eye injuries are detailed in Figure 4.1.

Control of Substances Hazardous to Health

The COSHH Regulations were introduced to protect workers against ill health and injury caused by exposure to hazardous substances. The Regulations require elimination or reduction of exposure to known hazardous substances in a practical way.

Manufacturers of hazardous substances are required to display an orange and black warning symbol on the label and packaging of any substance that is classified as hazardous and provide material safety data sheets containing more detailed information (Figure 4.2). The labels will also state how the substance is toxic, harmful, corrosive or irritant.

Substances that are classified as hazardous include:

- Substances with an occupational exposure limit (OEL) (e.g. mercury)

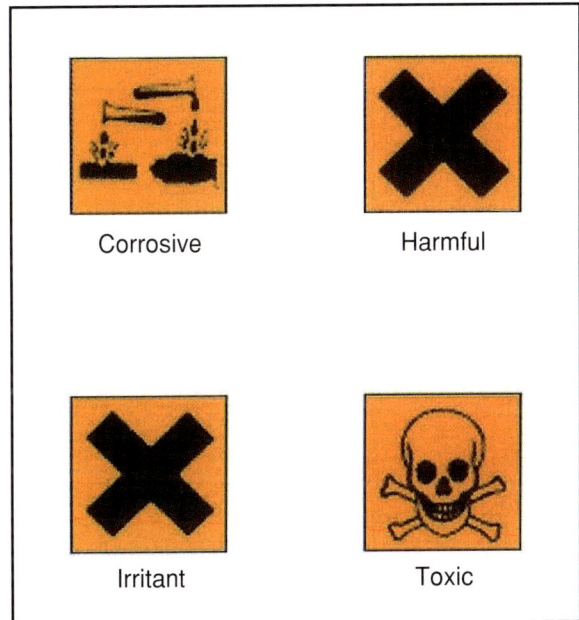

Corrosive   Harmful

Irritant   Toxic

4.2 Warning symbols for hazardous substances.

- Biological (infectious) agents directly connected with the work
- Any type of dust in significant quantities
- Any other substance classed as hazardous (e.g. latex).

A COSHH assessment should include identification of hazardous substances and a consideration of the risks. Particular attention should be paid to:

- Acids (e.g. phosphoric acid used in the conditioning of enamel and dentine)

- Adhesives (may contain xylene or toluene, which are classified as harmful)
- Blood and saliva (infectious agents)
- Disinfectants, strong detergents and other cleaning agents (may be harmful or irritant)
- Latex gloves (risk of allergy)
- Mercury (toxic by inhalation and contact)
- Solvents (various ill-health effects)
- Radiographic chemicals (irritating to eyes and skin and possibly the respiratory system).

Most modern restorative and impression materials pose negligible risk and so will not normally need to be included in a COSHH assessment.

Factors to be taken into account when the risks are assessed include how often the substance is used, how much is used, how people may be exposed to it and who could be affected. The assessment should be recorded and reviewed, and decisions made about what precautions are required. It is important to ensure that precautions are followed and controls maintained.

Examples of COSHH assessment forms for a ready-to-use radiographic developer and phosphoric acid are detailed in Figure 4.3.

Exposure limits

There are two types of exposure limits for hazardous substances:

- Occupational exposure standards (OESs)
- Maximum exposure limits (MELs).

MELs are set for substances for which safe levels are difficult to achieve in practice. Exposure to these

Ready-to-use developer	
Composition	Hydroquinone
Handling/storage	Avoid inhalation of vapour. Ensure adequate ventilation. Avoid eye and skin contact. Wear suitable protective clothing. Store in a cool, dry, well ventilated area in tightly closed labelled containers
Disposal	Do not allow product to enter drains, sewers or water courses
Hazard identification	Irritant to eyes and skin
Health effects	Eyes: may cause irritation Skin: may cause irritation and redness, repeated contact may cause sensitization Ingestion: may be harmful if swallowed, seek medical advise immediately
First aid measures	Eyes: irrigate with water for at least 15 minutes, seek prompt medical attention Skin: remove contaminated clothing, wash with soap/cleanser, seek medical attention if irritation persists Ingestion: DO NOT induce vomiting. Drink plenty of water, seek immediate medical attention Inhalation: move to fresh air and rest. If recovery is not rapid seek immediate medical attention
Protective measures	Safety glasses or chemical goggles are recommended if eye contact is probable. Rubber gloves are recommended. Avoid inhalation of vapour. Use in well ventilated areas
Control measures	Ensure adequate ventilation
Emergency action	Spillage: ventilate area, wear gloves and safety glasses, isolate spillage, absorb with inert material, scoop up and place in container for disposal Fire: toxic fumes are produced when these substance are involved in a fire
Etching gel	
Composition	Phosphoric acid
Use	Conditioning of enamel and dentine
Storage	General storage – above 0°C and below 40°C
Disposal	Drain to sewer with large volumes of water
Health effects	Eyes: severe eye irritation, damages eyes Skin: destructive to skin, may cause irritation Ingestion: possible irritation, destroys tissue
First aid measures	Eyes: flush immediately with water, seek medical attention Skin: flush immediately with water for at least 15 minutes Ingestion: DO NOT induce vomiting. Drink large amounts of water or milk, seek medical attention
Protective measures	Protective eyewear and gloves
Control measures	Keep away from strong bases, chemical reaction when mixed together
Emergency action	Spillage: clean up with damp cloth Fire: not flammable

4.3 Example COSHH assessment forms for a ready-to-use radiographic developer and phosphoric acid.

substances has, or is liable to have, serious health implications for workers. Few substances used in dentistry are assigned a MEL but one example is glutaraldehyde, which has a MEL of 0.05 parts per million (ppm) for both short- and long-term exposures.

Where the manufacturer's material safety data sheet refers to an OES or MEL, practitioners are obliged to meet the requirements of those exposure limit standards to ensure a safe working environment.

Working conditions

Dental procedures produce a microbial aerosol. For this reason they should be performed in a separate room with good light and good ventilation. Walls and surfaces must be impervious and easily cleaned.

Ergonomics is the study of the efficiency of people in their working environment. It involves all the factors that affect how the human body moves, operates and responds to the forces associated with specific tasks. The veterinary dental surgery can be a difficult physical working environment. Surgeons often adopt awkward and uncomfortable working positions, performing fine and exacting work.

Surgery layout
Ergonomic considerations should be made when planning the surgery layout, which should also be simple and uncluttered to aid infection control.

- There should be sufficient free space to allow people to move around with ease and workstations should be arranged so that surgery can be carried out comfortably.
- The operator's area should have access to the turbines, three-in-one syringe and slow handpiece, and the operating light be within arm's reach. Ideally, an assistant's area would contain the suction lines, perhaps a second three-in-one syringe, curing light, dental materials and a designated area for clinical waste disposal and the decontamination of instruments.
- The surgery layout should be arranged to reduce manual handling. Manual handling of the patients, especially the lifting and carrying of the unconscious or sedated animal, can be hazardous. Many manual handling injuries are cumulative and build up over time rather than being caused by a single handling event.
- The surgery layout must also consider the requirement to scavenge anaesthetic gases.

Lighting and ventilation
Lighting should be sufficient to enable the operator to work safely and without eyestrain. The use of an overhead dental operating light is highly recommended. It should be equal to or brighter than the background light, but not by more than three times. If the operating light is too bright, eye fatigue may occur.

Air turbines, ultrasonic scalers and air/water syringes can produce splatter reaching a distances of over 2 m and an aerosol containing tooth particles,

bacteria, fungi and possibly viruses and oil. Aerosol can be an irritant to the lungs when inhaled and harmful to the eyes. Risks are considerably reduced by good ventilation and the use of high-volume suction, facemasks and protective spectacles. Ventilation must also be adequate where hazardous substances are in use, such as in the X-ray film developing area.

Surgeries and other enclosed workplaces must be ventilated by fresh or purified air. Usually an open window will suffice (open windows must be protected by an anti-escape device to ensure that conscious patients do not escape) but in some cases it may be necessary to install an extraction fan. Ventilation systems should exhaust to the outside of the building without risk to the public and without recirculation into the veterinary facility or any public building. Ventilation systems should supply fresh air at a rate not below 5–8 litres/second per occupant but the creation of draughts should be avoided. Recycling air conditioning systems are not recommended. High-volume aspiration systems will also reduce the risk of infection by eliminating aerosols. Darkrooms should be suitably ventilated.

Working position
There is a high incidence of musculoskeletal pain related to poor posture in health care professionals. This is especially true in the field of dentistry. Space constraints, unsuitable seating, poor lighting and sustained or awkward working positions will result in poor posture and consequently in back, neck and shoulder pains and strains together with stress and fatigue. Upper limb disorders, including repetitive strain injury (RSI), can also occur as a result of poorly designed work areas.

Pain tends to occur when the spine cannot maintain its natural curvature. Pain in the lower back, shoulders and neck increases as a direct function of time seated in a poor position. Correct posture, aided by good surgery design incorporating the latest advances in ergonomic furniture, is essential for the veterinary dental practitioner to reduce immediate discomfort and also to reduce the risk of long-term musculoskeletal disorders.

Veterinary dentistry should be carried out in the seated position to provide support for the lower back. The optimum postural position will maintain the neutral 'S' shape of the spine by angling the hips at 45 degrees to the spine. This places the anterior and posterior thigh muscles in balance, with the lumbar spine in a backwards concave curve (lordosis) and with no undue stress on the musculoskeletal system (Figure 4.4).

A conventional flat chair requires the hips to bend at 90 degrees to the spine. The hips can easily accommodate bending up to about 60 degrees to the spine with comfort, but to 'give' the extra 30 degrees the hamstring muscles at the back of the thigh have to pull the pelvis backwards. This forces the lumbar spine to adopt an unnatural and uncomfortable 'C' shape with convex curvature (kyphosis). The extra force generated compresses the vertebrae together, creating excessive pressure on the discs, in particular the fourth and fifth lumbar discs in the lower spine (Figure 4.5).

Clinical veterinary dental practice is performed in front of the body, resulting in the clinician reaching the

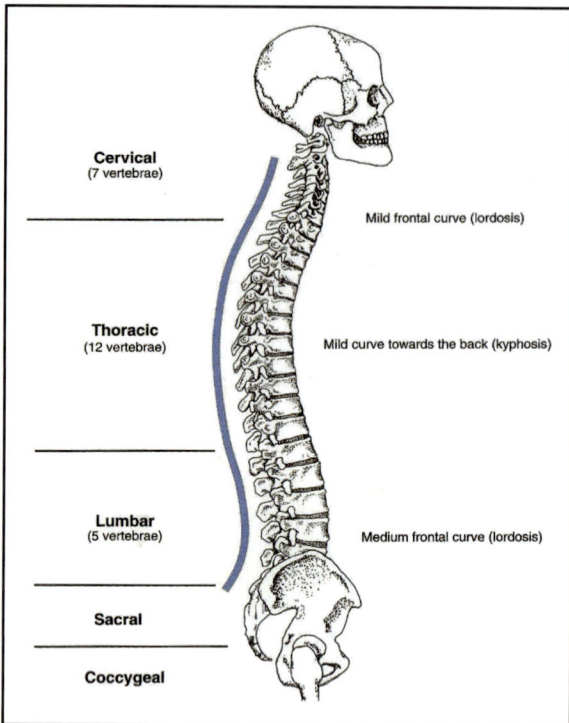

4.4   Human spinal column in normal standing position. (Reproduced with permission from Bambach Saddle Seat (Europe) Ltd.)

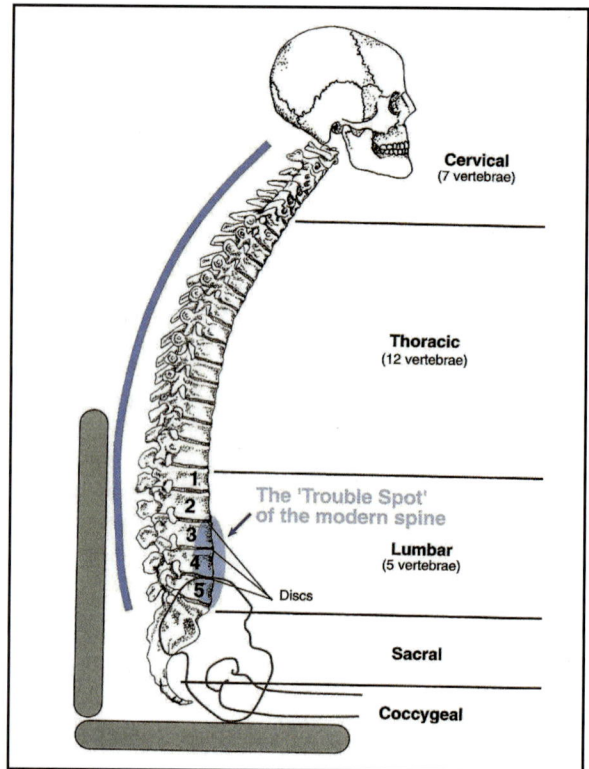

4.5   Human spinal column in a flat-seated position during a reach-forward activity, showing lumbar kyphosis. (Reproduced with permission from Bambach Saddle Seat (Europe) Ltd.)

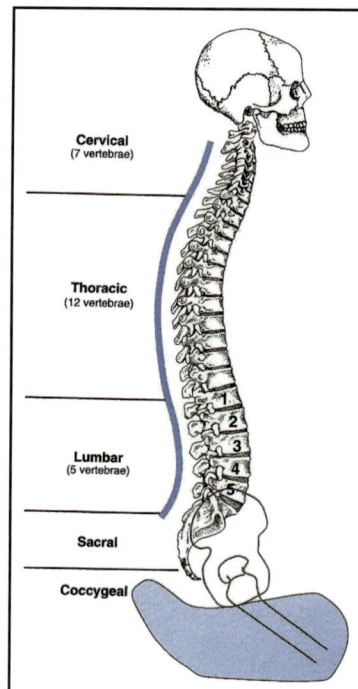

4.6   Human spinal column in a saddle-sitting position, showing maintenance of normal spinal curvature even in a reach-forward activity. (Reproduced with permission from Bambach Saddle Seat (Europe) Ltd.)

torso forward. Because the body's centre of gravity is supported behind the ischial tuberosities ('sit bones') on a conventional flat seat, the lack of support in front of the body causes the practitioner to achieve body support through the arms by leaning on the operating table. This inhibits free arm movement, hinders the accuracy of hand movements and can result in pain in the arms and neck. Discomfort may also occur as a result of the hard front edge of the seat impeding circulation to the legs and feet.

RSI appears to be caused by insufficient oxygenated blood getting to muscles and tendons that are undergoing continuous, sustained and repetitive work – a situation worsened if they are held in an awkward strained position (such as on a conventional flat chair.) The poor blood flow can gradually lead to the muscles losing their elasticity and reducing in length. This causes the tendons to stretch and do work that they were not designed to perform. The result can be pain, inflammation and injury.

The ideal working position is one that would reproduce a position, whilst the operator is seated, that would promote a stable, upright pelvic orientation, maintaining neutral spinal curvatures even when leaning forward to work. One way to achieve this is by the sit-stand or saddle-sitting position (Figure 4.6). In this position the spine is maintained in an unstrained posture, with abnormal intradiscal pressures minimized, so that the back, head, neck and shoulder girdle are all free to work in a balanced neutral position. The feet are beneath the body's centre of gravity, providing support without the need for arm rests. This provides a mechanical advantage for the forearms and hands during delicate movements. An open hip posture when seated helps to maintain good blood circulation.

Other ergonomic factors to consider are adjustability of the operating table height and patient positioning.

Magnification systems
The incidence of musculoskeletal and neurological disorders will also be reduced with the use of ergonomically designed magnification systems. Together

with proper illumination, they will encourage good posture and reduce the need for prolonged periods of over-flexion of the neck. This in turn will avoid neck and shoulder pain, eyestrain, muscle strain and headaches.

There are many variables to consider when choosing a magnification system:

- Working distance (distance between the eyes and the working area)
- Depth-of-field (difference between nearest and farthest distances within which the object stays in focus). The range of focus needs to be large enough to allow the clinician to move the head freely within the required working range
- Inter-pupillary distance
- Convergence angle (the pivotal angle aligning the two oculars to allow them to point at an identical distance and angle, normally preset by the manufacturer).

The most important ergonomic factors are weight, frame design and declination angle. Clinically the latter is the most important. The declination angle is defined as the angle of the line of sight made with neutral eye position and the actual line of sight made by the declined eye chosen by the clinician (Figure 4.7). The operator must be able to select and adjust the correct declination angle to reduce neck fatigue. With too small an angle the chin tips into the chest; with too big an angle the operator declines the eyes or tips the neck backwards.

- First-generation magnification systems are single lens magnifiers. These can be clipped on to spectacles or worn on a headband. They are inexpensive but do have limitations. They simply magnify, and simple enlargement does not always deliver a pin-sharp image, especially at higher magifications. They can also promote poor posture as a result of excessive head tilt, which over time can cause chronic neck pain.
- Second-generation magnification systems have preset declination angles (Figure 4.8). They can be through-the-lens (TTL) or front-lens-mounted (FLM).
- Third-generation FLM magnification systems allow adjustment of the declination angle to enable the operator to obtain the most comfortable working position.

Illumination sources that clip on to the magnification systems are also available. This concentric lighting (from between the eyes) provides illumination in line with the telescopes and therefore with the line of sight. The exact area where the operator is looking is perfectly illuminated.

Cross-infection control should not be ignored and sealed oculars on the loupes and a hygienic flat wipe-clean front control panel on the light source are important requirements.

Specialist practitioners are also moving towards the use of surgical (operating) microscopes. These

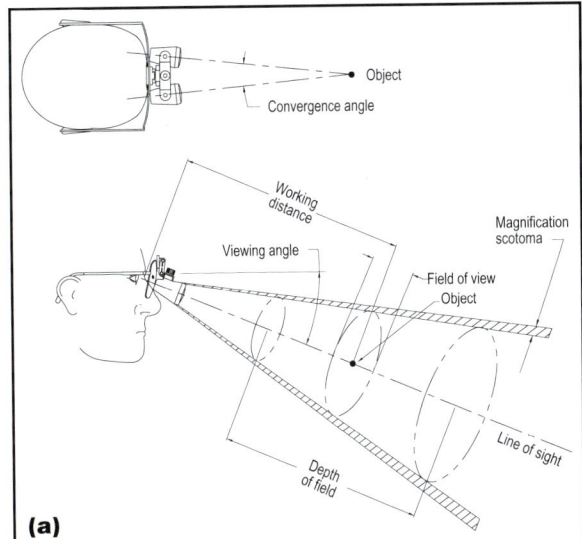

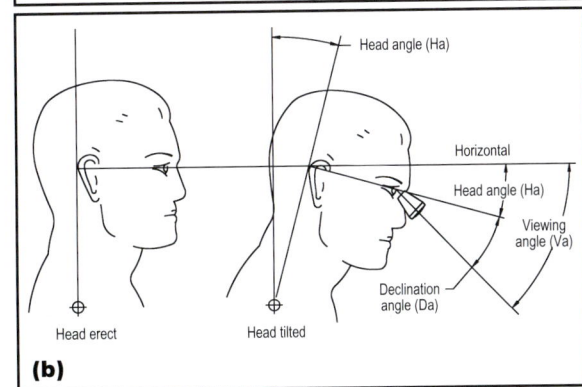

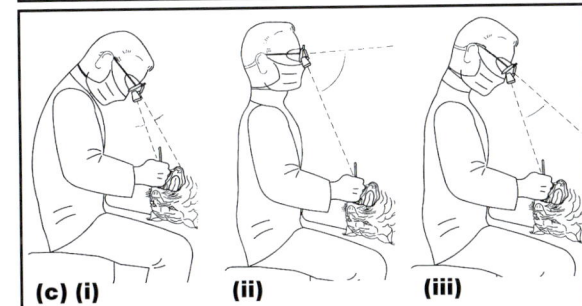

4.7 **(a)** Magnification terminology. **(b)** Declination angle. **(c)** Declination angle and postural changes associated with a declination angle that is (i) too small, (ii) too large and (iii) optimal. (Reproduced with permission from DP Medical Systems Ltd.)

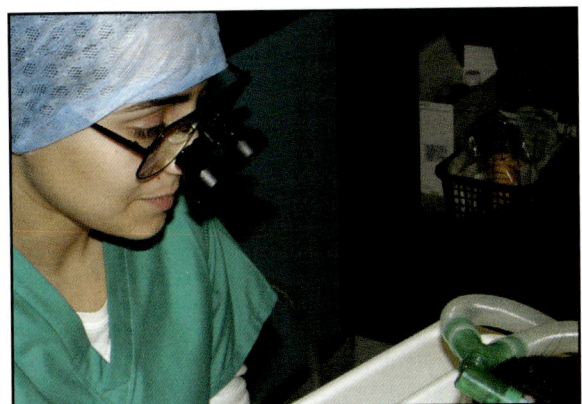

4.8 Example of a second-generation magnification system.

provide greater magnification for some of the more intricate endodontic procedures.

Scavenging of anaesthetic gases

At high concentrations, i.e. several ppm, all anaesthetic agents reduce activity of the nervous system, leading to anaesthesia. Veterinary personnel will be exposed to much lower concentrations daily but chronic exposure to trace levels of waste anaesthetic gases has been associated with spontaneous abortion, birth defects, neoplasia, hepatic disease, renal disease, neurological disturbances, haemopoietic changes, infertility and pruritus (Smith, 1993). OESs at which there are no significant risks to health have been set for four anaesthetic agents (nitrous oxide, enflurane, isoflurane and halothane) (Figure 4.9).

Anaesthetic agent	OES over an 8-hour time-weighted average
Nitrous oxide	100 ppm
Enflurane	50 ppm
Isoflurane	50 ppm
Halothane	10 ppm

4.9 OESs for nitrous oxide, enflurane, isoflurane and halothane.

Veterinary practitioners are responsible for ensuring that their own and their staff's exposure to gaseous anaesthetic agents by inhalation is reduced to the OES. To estimate exposure, consideration needs to be given to the amount of time personnel are exposed to the anaesthetic agent and how well the room is ventilated. Personal sampling can be undertaken by taking weighted air samples from the breathing zone of those personnel most at risk of exposure.

The main sources of pollution are leaks from the breathing circuit. An appropriately inflated, cuffed endotracheal (ET) tube not only keeps anaesthetic gases contained but also eliminates inhalation of aerosolized microorganisms by the anaesthetized patient. Personnel must be instructed in safe anaesthetic practices (see Chapter 3). Visual checks should be performed at least weekly to ensure that scavenging and ventilation equipment is working properly. Servicing in accordance with the manufacturer's recommendations should be undertaken. Operation of scavenging equipment should be reviewed to ensure that it is being used correctly. Staff should be made aware of the possible health risks, understand why scavenging and ventilation are important and be instructed in proper equipment use.

Gas cylinders should be stored, if possible, in external well ventilated stores, preferably with piped supplies to the point of use. If internal storage is the only option, the cylinders should be stored within a fire-resistant enclosure with ventilation through an external wall to a safe place outside the building. Stocks should be kept as low as possible and any flammable gases should be kept away from sources of ignition and not stored with oxygen.

Oral microbial exposure and cross-infection control

Veterinary practitioners have a duty to take appropriate precautions to protect patients and members of the veterinary team from the risks of cross-infection. There is an obvious need for surgery staff to be thoroughly instructed in handling, decontamination and disposal of instruments to avoid cross-infection and injury from the instruments or from the sterilizing equipment. Basic training in surgery procedures should identify the risks and how they are to be avoided.

Employers must provide protective equipment and clothing for use during operative procedures, to minimize the risk of exposure to oral pathogens and debris. Employers must also ensure that the protective clothing and equipment are being used in the correct manner. Personal protective equipment (PPE) made or sold in the UK must carry the European Conformity 'CE' mark to indicate it has been satisfactorily type-examined by an approved body.

Good ventilation, the use of high-volume suction and the wearing of facemasks and protective spectacles will considerably reduce the risks associated with aerosol inhalation and ocular contamination. Rinsing the patient's mouth with an antiseptic oral rinse prior to treatment will reduce microorganism contamination of the aerosol.

Masks

Masks (Figure 4.10) do not confer complete microbiological protection from aerosol inhalation; they provide 95% filtration efficiency for particles 3–5 microns in diameter but do stop splatter from contaminating the face.

Masks are recommended for all operative procedures and should be changed after every patient. Some literature suggests that they should be used for only a maximum of 20 minutes in areas of high humidity and a maximum of 60 minutes in dry climates before being changed.

Masks should not contact the mouth whilst they are being worn, as the moisture generated will reduce the filtration efficiency of the mask. Some plastic face shields provide good protection from debris and enable the operator to wear a magnification system underneath (Figure 4.10b). A mask is still required when a simple face shield is worn. One-piece mask and splatter guards are available.

Eye protection

Eye protection (Figure 4.10) should be worn by those working in close proximity to the patient during treatment, to protect against foreign bodies (e.g. tooth and restoration particles), splatter and aerosols that may arise during operative procedures, especially scaling (manual and ultrasonic) and when using rotary instruments. The wearing of protective spectacles is also important to prevent ocular injury from fractured high-speed burs. Eyewear should have full lenses and side protection; half lenses do not provide sufficient protection.

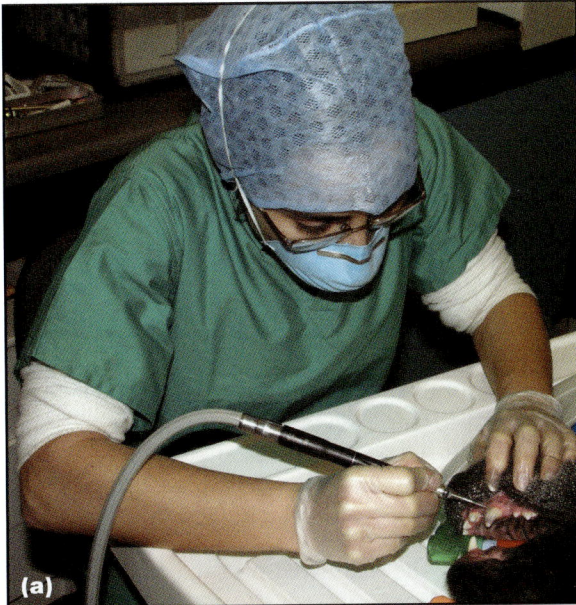

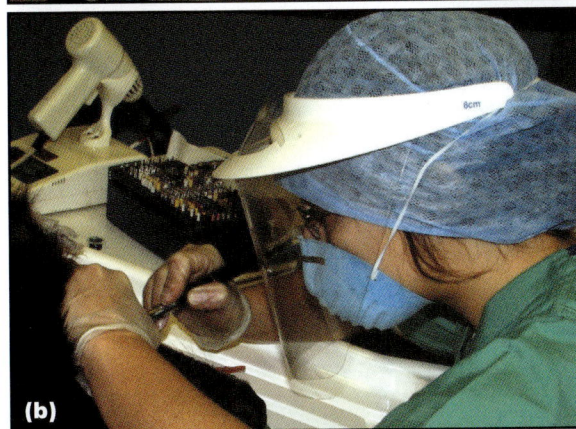

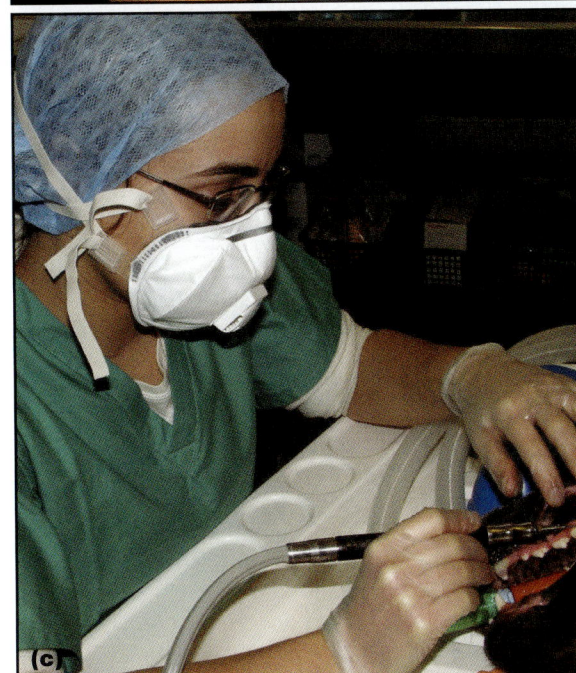

Hand protection

The care of hands is vital to infection control: lacerated, abraded and cracked skin can offer a portal of entry for microorganisms.

Gloves must be worn for all clinical procedures and treated as single-use items. They should be donned immediately before contact with the patient and removed as soon as clinical treatment is completed. Used gloves must be disposed of as clinical waste.

The following are recommendations for hand care during clinical sessions:

- Operators should have short nails
- Rings, jewellery and watches should be removed
- All cuts and abrasions should be covered with waterproof adhesive dressings
- Hands should be washed methodically, using good quality liquid soap preferably containing an antiseptic. A full hand wash and drying is recommended before donning gloves
- Gloves should be removed and hands washed after each patient
- An emollient hand cream should be used regularly to prevent the skin from drying.

Skin damage resulting from repeated washing can lead to irritant contact dermatitis. Damaged skin is associated with changes in the composition of microbial flora of the hands, such as colonization with more species and an increase in the prevalence of certain microorganisms.

Alcohol-based hand-rubs

Alcohol-based hand-rubs and gels can be used as an alternative to hand washing. Alcohol itself is not a cleansing agent and visible contaminants must be removed with soap and water or a detergent-based solution. Most alcohol-based hand-rubs contain emollients to reduce the drying effect on the skin. Alcohol combined with other antimicrobials (such as an alcohol and chlorhexidine combination) has been found to be very effective against microorganisms.

Gloves

There are a variety of gloves available. Good quality single-use gloves (to European standard BS EN 455 parts 1 & 2) should be worn for all clinical procedures, as they protect against contact with blood, saliva and other tissue fluids. They must be changed after every patient.

The gloves should be well fitting and powder free. Powder can contaminate radiographs, disperse allergenic proteins into the surgery atmosphere and interfere with wound healing. The powder in some gloves can also retard or even prevent the polymerization of some restorative and impression materials. The gloves should also be 'hypoallergenic' and 'low protein' to reduce the likelihood of allergy.

Allergic contact dermatitis is rare but, if it develops, it can be serious enough to cause the person to cease working. Irritant contact dermatitis is more common and can be avoided by careful choice of glove and hand disinfectant and meticulous hand care.

Heavy-duty gloves must be worn when handling disinfecting agents, cleaning solvents and radiographic processing chemicals to protect against burns or skin irritation.

Protective clothing

Protective clothing should be worn only in the surgery and not taken into eating areas. Uniforms should avoid any features that could collect mercury or be caught on equipment. Contaminated clothing should be washed in a washing machine using a biological detergent and a hot wash cycle (at least 65°C). Suitable shoes should be worn that protect against spillage, irritants and other substances.

Rubber dams

Rubber dam isolation of teeth also offers substantial advantages and should be used wherever practical. It enhances the quality of the operative environment, virtually abolishes saliva and blood splatter and reduces the bacterial load of the aerosols. When working without a rubber dam, the use of high-volume suction is advisable.

Disposables

The use of disposable covers and barriers for objects, equipment and surfaces will help in the prevention of cross-infection (Figure 4.11). They are particularly useful in cases such as feline immunodeficiency virus (FIV)-positive cats. Covers are to be considered as single-use items and changed after each patient. Suitable barriers include plastic film (sheets or bags) and aluminium foil and can be used on the following:

- Patient support sand bags
- Operating table
- Dental X-ray tube head
- X-ray control panel
- Overhead dental light handles
- Operator chair handles
- Dental handpieces and connecting tubing

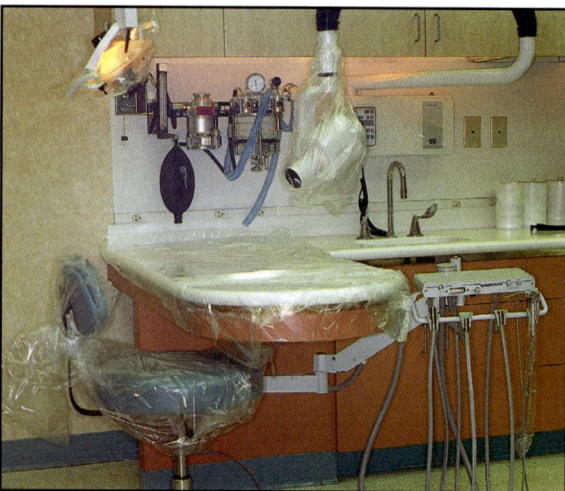

4.11 Inexpensive, disposable barriers prevent patient cross-infection and minimize clean-up time between patients. Sites of placement are dictated by operator gloved hand contact, e.g. X-ray control panel, X-ray tube head, chair and light handles.

- Instrument table and tray
- Three-in-one air syringe and tubing. A single use disposable tip for attachment to the three-in-one syringe is also available.

Equipment safety

Electrical equipment must be in good working order at all times. User checks, formal visual inspection and combined inspection and testing should be carried out at appropriate intervals.

User checks are simple visual checks of the equipment and its cable and plug for damage before use. A more detailed formal visual inspection, including where possible the removal of the plug cover to check for signs of internal damage, should be carried out on an annual basis. This can be performed by practitioners provided that they have sufficient knowledge and training and know how to avoid damage to themselves. Earthed equipment should also have an occasional combined inspection and test by an appropriately trained person to identify faults that cannot be found by visual checks alone (three years is suggested as an appropriate time interval).

All personnel who use autoclaves within the practice should be thoroughly trained in their use. The Pressure Systems Safety Regulations 2000 were introduced to reduce the risk of serious injury from the release of stored energy as a result of a pressure system failure. Periodic safety examination of the vessel must be carried out in addition to regular maintenance checks following the manufacturer's instruction.

The design of some dental equipment requiring a water supply means that it is possible for contaminated water to be drawn back through the water lines to the mains water supply (back siphonage). Mains supplied water services must be protected from contamination by back siphonage (The Water Supply (Water Fittings) Regulations 1999). The level of protection required depends upon the risk posed. The presence of blood and saliva from the dental environment requires the highest level of protection.

Interrupting the water supply to the relevant surgery equipment by a physical break (air gap) will prevent the possibility of backflow. The delivery system (dental handpiece, three-in-one syringe and ultrasonic scaler), wet line suction apparatus and automatic radiographic processors all require an air gap for protection against back siphonage. Manufacturers can provide equipment with an integral air gap but this must be checked.

All dental unit water lines and air lines should be fitted with anti-retraction valves to help to prevent contamination of the lines, but these valves cannot be relied upon to prevent infected material being aspirated back into the tubing.

Most dental water lines will harbour biofilm, which acts as a reservoir of microbial contamination and may be a source of known pathogens. Aerosolization of contaminated water can result in potentially hazardous situations, especially if the water lines have become contaminated with, for example, *Legionella* (Challacombe and Fernandes, 1995; Walker *et al.*, 2000).

To reduce or eliminate the problem of contaminated dental unit water lines, the following precautions should be adopted:

- The ultrasonic scaler, triple syringe and handpiece should be supplied with bottled water (a 'clean water' system)
- Disinfectants can be introduced into the water supply to reduce the bacterial load. The manufacturer's advice on the type and strength of disinfectant should be followed
- Sterile polyionic fluid should be used where surgical flaps or other surgical access into body cavities is anticipated.

Noise in the dental operatory is generated by compressors, handpieces, suction units and both sonic and ultrasonic scalers. A noise level of 75 decibels is considered 'safe', but even these 'safe' levels can be irritating and contribute to increased stress levels. Every effort should be made to limit noise pollution.

All handpieces commonly used produce high frequency noises, the frequency of which should not approach or exceed the 'safe' level of 75 decibels. Newer handpieces are manufactured with improved noise reduction.

Quiet oil-cooled compressors, such as on the base of a cart, can be sited near the operator but noisier oil-free compressors should be isolated away from work areas. These units may be sited in the building loft or an outdoor shed. Compressor reservoir tanks must be emptied on a regular basis to prevent rust being formed by the condensate.

Operator safety in relation to the use of dental materials

Mercury

Mercury is one of the most hazardous substances that dentists use on a regular basis. The use of mercury amalgam as a restorative material is declining and it is rarely used in veterinary dentistry. However, in certain circumstances it can be a very useful material. Careful dispensing, handling and disposal will help to avoid the potential hazards of mercury.

All those involved in the handling of mercury in any form should understand its potential hazards. Mercury may gain access to the body through the skin on contact, through ingestion and via inhalation as a vapour. Personnel must receive specific training in safe handling procedures in respect of the preparation of mercury for use and how to deal with mercury spills, including the safe disposal of contaminated materials. Routine personal hygiene is essential to minimize the possibility of absorbing mercury via skin contact and a mask should be worn to decrease exposure to particulate amalgam. The use of high-volume suction during placement and removal of amalgam restorations will reduce the exposure to mercury vapour. The overall risk of mercury contamination is minimized greatly by using pre-dispensed capsules; these limit

the handling of liquid mercury and reduce the possibility of a liquid mercury spill.

Commercial agents are available to absorb spilled mercury and amalgam waste should be stored in a sealed, labelled container under a mercury-suppressing solution or paste. The disposal of waste amalgam, waste mercury and used amalgam capsules is controlled: the materials must be collected by a person licensed to carry such waste.

The UK Mercury Screening Service can provide further advice. There is a HSE Guidance Note MS12 ('Mercury: medical guidance notes') that provides general information on working with mercury, including OELs, clinical effects of chronic and acute poisoning, prevention and health surveillance.

Other materials

Restorative materials, such as glass ionomers or composites, have the capacity to be light-cured. Operator control of polymerization is achieved with the use of curing lights that operate in the wavelength range of 400–450 nm. Lights with a high-energy output have good penetration and a good depth of cure but, to avoid retinal damage and prevent a distracting after-image in the operator's visual field, the operator must be careful to limit retinal exposure. This can be achieved with the use of small orange, red or yellow tinted translucent shield tips fitted to the filter; these are convenient but some light can still shine out. Larger handheld shields may be used to eliminate exposure of the eye to unshielded light (Figure 4.12).

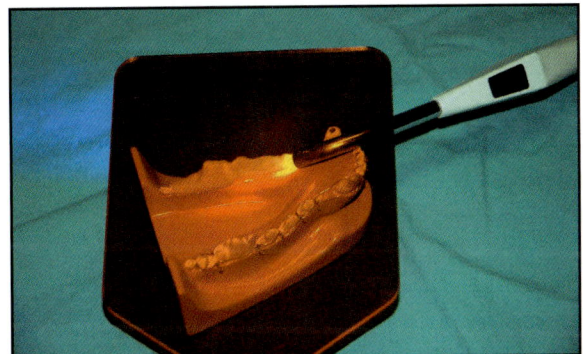

4.12 To avoid retinal damage, exposure of the eye to the high intensity blue light must be avoided.

Radiographic safety

Whilst the ionizing radiation dose delivered to individual patients is low, the collective dose delivered in a dental operatory over a period of time is significant because of the large numbers of radiographs taken. Veterinary surgeons have obligations under current legislation and also as part of good working practice to ensure the safety of all staff involved in the taking and processing of radiographs and of the patients. The Ionising Radiations Regulations 1999 (IRR99) are concerned with the protection of workers and patients. The Ionising Radiation (Medical Exposure) Regulations 2000 (IRMER) impose requirements for patient protection. Compliance with IRR99 and IRMER will minimize the risks from ionizing radiation for both patients and workers.

A radiation protection adviser (RPA) is appointed to provide advice on complying with legal obligations, including the periodic examination and testing of all radiographic equipment, risk assessment, contingency plans, staff training and the quality assurance programme.

A risk assessment, carried out with the help of the RPA, will identify the precautions necessary to restrict the exposure of patients and those involved in taking radiographs. It should be reviewed every five years, or more frequently if changes to working methods or new types of equipment are introduced.

A radiation protection file should hold as much information as possible about the procedures in place to ensure radiation protection within the practice.

Before a radiograph is taken, an assessment must be made as to whether an individual exposure is justified. Steps must be taken to eliminate exposures that have no merit and to optimize all those exposures that are justified. The benefits must outweigh the detriment of the exposure: new information to assist future management is mandatory. For every radiograph, the dose from the exposure should be kept as low as reasonably practicable (ALARP) for the intended diagnostic procedure. Written guideline exposure settings must be in place for every type of exposure and kept close to the X-ray equipment. Each radiograph must then be subjected to clinical evaluation, with quality assurance programmes in place to ensure consistently accurate diagnostic information.

A controlled area should be defined around the dental X-ray equipment and no one, with the exception of the patient, should enter this area whilst radiographs are being taken. The RPA will help to define the area, which is normally within 1.5 m of the X-ray tube and the patient and within the primary X-ray beam until it has been sufficiently attenuated by distance or shielding. It should not normally extend beyond the X-ray room or surgery.

Operators and staff must stand well outside this controlled area – preferably 2 m or more from the X-ray tube and the patient and well out of the direction of the primary beam. The control panel of the equipment should have a light to indicate that the main power is on. A warning light should be fitted to give a clear indication that an exposure is taking place and remain illuminated for the duration of the exposure. Audible warnings should work in the same way as the visual warning light. It is advisable that all staff vacate the room whilst radiographs are being taken but the operator must be able to see the X-ray tube warning light and the patient throughout the exposure. Other personnel must be prevented from entering the controlled area whilst the exposure is occurring.

Personal dose meters should be provided for veterinary practice staff. The dose meter wear period may be up to three months. The results should be recorded and discussed periodically with the RPA. The results of personal monitoring must be kept for at least two years.

Film processing should consistently produce good quality radiographs, to avoid the need for repeat exposures.

Radiographic developer and fixer are potentially irritating to the eyes and skin and possibly the respiratory system. They should be handled with care and heavy-duty gloves should be worn when working with these chemicals. Radiographic processing chemicals are classified as special waste and must be collected by a waste collection agency licensed to collect and dispose of this chemical waste.

Maintenance and testing

Suppliers and installers of dental X-ray equipment are required to provide adequate information about its proper use, testing and maintenance. The equipment must be subjected to the following tests:

- Critical examination and report by the installer
- Acceptance test to provide baseline values for subsequent routine tests
- Routine tests to confirm that there are no significant changes to equipment or its location and to include representative patient dose tests.

Summary

- The veterinary dental practitioner has an ethical, moral and legal duty to be aware of job-related hazards and to eliminate or minimize the associated health risks.
- Practical precautions must be in place to protect the veterinary team and the patient from potentially harmful materials, equipment and infectious medical waste.
- Most dental materials routinely used in veterinary dentistry present a low risk to the veterinary health care team and patients.
- Oral microbial exposure via splatter and aerosolization is a significant hazard. Personal protective equipment for the entire veterinary dental team using barrier protection is mandatory.
- An ergonomically designed workstation will enable veterinary dentistry to be performed more safely, efficiently and effectively and protect against chronic musculoskeletal and neurological disorders in the veterinary dentist.

References and further reading

British Dental Association (BDA) website: www.bda.org
BDA (2003) *Radiation in dentistry* – Advice sheet
BDA (2003) *Risk assessment in dentistry* – Advice sheet
BDA (2004) *Health and safety law for dental practice* – Advice sheet
Challacombe SJ and Fernandes LL (1995) Detecting *Legionella pneumophilia* in water systems: a comparison of various dental units. *Journal of the American Dental Association* **126**, 603–608
DeForge DH (2002) Physical ergonomics in veterinary dentistry. *Journal of Veterinary Dentistry* **19**(4), 196–200
Gorrel C (2004) *Veterinary Dentistry for the General Practitioner.* WB Saunders, Edinburgh
Smith J (1993) Anaesthetic pollution and waste anaesthetic gas scavenging. *Seminar of Veterinary Medicine and Surgery (South Africa)* **8**(2), 90
Walker JT, Bradshaw DJ, Bennet AM, Fulford MR, Martin MV and Marsh PD (2000) Microbial biofilm formation and contamination of dental unit water systems in general dental practice. *Applied Environmental Microbiology* **66**, 3363–3367
Wiggs RB and Lobprise HB (1997) *Veterinary Dentistry Principles and Practice.* Lippincott-Raven, Philadelphia

5

Dental instrumentation and equipment

John Robinson

The correct tools are required to be able to perform a job properly. This is especially so in the more challenging tasks such as tooth extraction in cats and dogs. This chapter describes the basic equipment that every small animal practice should have to be able to perform routine dentistry.

Each type of instrument is available in an array of patterns for use in human dentistry. A relatively small number of instruments are needed for dentistry in cats and dogs, as the range of tasks is less and the access to teeth is less restricted, so requiring less variation in pattern.

The supposedly same instrument from different manufacturers or suppliers commonly varies in some aspects. Even a small difference in design can make a huge impact on its suitability and functional effectiveness.

Grips

Dental hand instruments, scalers and drills are all held and used with the modified pen grip. Exceptions are extraction elevators, luxators and forceps, which are held in a palm grip.

Modified pen grip

The thumb and first finger grip the bottom of the handle and the middle finger is extended and placed on the instrument shank (Figure 5.1). This provides a firm grip with good tactile feedback and allows for easy rotation of the instrument. The handle passes between thumb and first finger and over the back of the hand. The ring finger and little finger are used to make a finger rest by making contact with a stable surface close to the tooth. A firm base allows fine control of the instrument.

Palm grip

The handle of the instrument sits in the palm of the hand, ideally with the end of the handle in the middle of the palm. The shank is held between the thumb and forefinger. With dental elevators and luxators, the forefinger should be extended and placed near the tip of the instrument.

Hand instruments

Dental examination

Dental explorer probe

This sharp-pointed instrument (Figure 5.2) is used to feel for irregularities in the tooth surface, such as enamel defects, pulp chamber exposures in fractured teeth, caries or feline odontoclastic resorptive lesions (FORLs). There are numerous patterns with different shaped shanks. The Shepherd's Hook pattern is frequently specified in veterinary texts. A pattern No. 6 with its simple, almost 90 degree bend is ideal for use in all small animal dentistry.

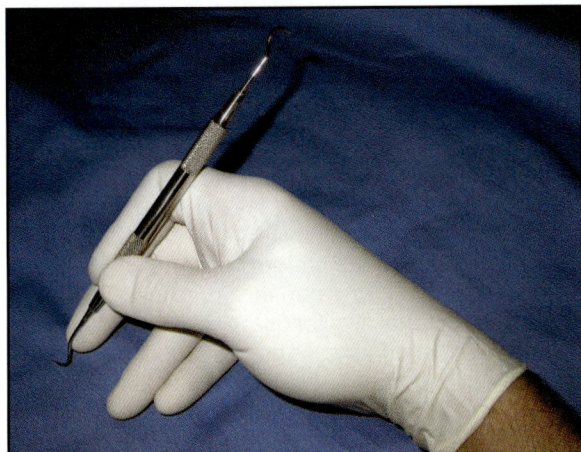

5.1 Modified pen grip.

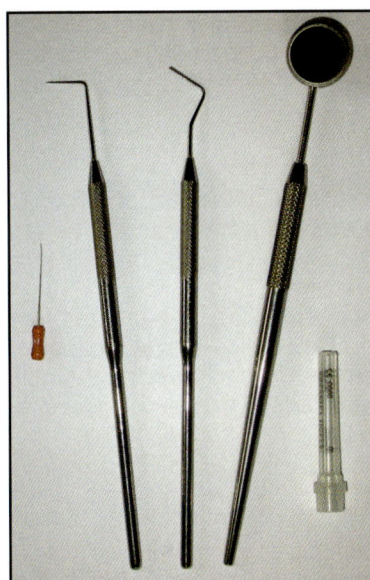

5.2 (Left to right): Pathfinder; dental explorer probe (No. 6); periodontal probe (Williams 14WB); mirror (size 3); needle cap as a mouth gag. (Courtesy of Big-O Veterinary Dental Supplies Company.)

Periodontal probe

A periodontal pocket-measuring probe is required for measuring the distance between the gingival margin and the gingival attachment to the tooth at all sites around the circumference of each tooth. It is also used to measure gingival recession and gingival hyperplasia and to assess furcation lesions. These measurements enable the maximum clinical periodontal pocket depth to be assessed and also the amount of attachment loss, the true and false pocket depths to be calculated. The instrument is a blunt-ended probe with markings along its length; it is simply a specialized ruler. The end is rounded and blunt so that soft tissues are not traumatized or penetrated. The shank needs to be of small diameter to allow easy insertion between the gingiva and tooth.

The markings are either engraved rings or surface colouring in black. The colouring can fade with repeated use. A probe with engraved rings that are coloured black provides clear markings for optimal reading. The Williams periodontal probe (Probe 14WB) (see Figure 5.2) is the most suitable. Screening probes that only have block markings (3 mm or 4 mm bands) are not recommended. In the cat, measurements need to be made in half millimetres, requiring a probe to have markings at least for each millimetre.

Before using any probe, the operator should ensure that they know what the markings represent by placing it alongside a ruler.

Pathfinders

The Pathfinder™ (Kerr) is a fine seeker probe (see Figure 5.2). It is useful in identifying small holes in teeth (e.g. in fractured teeth). The fine, flexible shaft can worm its way into the pulp canal, so verifying a pulp exposure.

Mouth mirrors

Changing the positioning of the animal usually allows direct visualization of most tooth surfaces, making the conventional use of dental mouth mirrors redundant. However, there are still some areas, such as the upper second molar in the dog, where a mirror will facilitate vision. Using a mirror can be easier than moving the animal. Mouth mirrors make good oral tissue retractors and can enable inspection of other sites, especially the nasopharynx.

> **PRACTICAL TIP**
> **Wiping the mirror surface on the buccal mucosa helps prevent its surface from frosting due to condensation.**

Mouth mirrors are available in a range of sizes. The most commonly available are size 4 (overall diameter approximately 23 mm) or the smaller size 3 (20 mm diameter). A size 3 would best suit cat and dog requirements (see Figure 5.2).

Other requirements

Mouth gags: A mouth gag enables improved access to the lingual surfaces of the teeth and caudal mouth.

Many designs are available and each usually comes in a range of sizes. The Grays mouth gag is commonly found in practice: there are two arms that slide along a bar with a spring around it. This type is quite bulky and heavy and is difficult to clean. Other types are the Smith Baxter and Swales. A sturdy needle cap, with the closed end cut off to make a tube of the desired length, makes a good gag that is cheap and disposable (see Figure 5.2).

When using a gag the mouth should not be opened too wide (just to the point of resistance) or kept open for long periods, as myositis or neuropraxia may result. The gag should be removed periodically.

Dental charts: All the findings of the dental examination should be recorded on a dental chart. There are a growing number of chart designs available. There are two basic layout types: one based on the 'open-mouth' representation of the teeth; and the other on the flattened projection layout (e.g. DentaLabels) (Figure 5.3). Some combine the open-mouth with additional lateral view projections.

A chart is used by drawing on abnormalities or placing notation against the pictorial representation of the teeth. A good chart should allow for multiple details to be clearly recorded at each tooth without using location arrows or the chart becoming cluttered. Some charts allow for several uses (recording the findings of several examinations of the mouth at different times) with the aim of direct comparison of some parameters. The problem with some multi-use charts is that there is only one drawing of the teeth and anything drawn on there is not dated. Single-use charts are therefore recommended.

The best chart design will depend on personal preference and type of use (general practice or specialist). Some computer software packages for veterinary practice include dental charts; they require a terminal at the place of dental treatment and are currently not user friendly.

Periodontal treatment

Calculus forceps

Extraction forceps or rongeurs can be used to crack off large chunks of calculus. Specific calculus forceps are available with one beak flattened and modified to reduce the risk of nipping the gum or tooth and so reducing the risk of iatrogenic trauma.

Hand scalers

Hand scalers are instruments for the removal of calculus from the tooth *above* the gumline, i.e. supragingivally.

Many inappropriate patterns of hand scalers have found their way into veterinary practice. There are many patterns available for use in human dentistry, but the range for veterinary use can be reduced as access to the teeth is better. The sickle-type scaler is recommended, especially the Hygienist pattern, H6/H7. It is a double-ended instrument, with each end being the mirror image with opposite curvature.

The shank is the rod that connects the working part

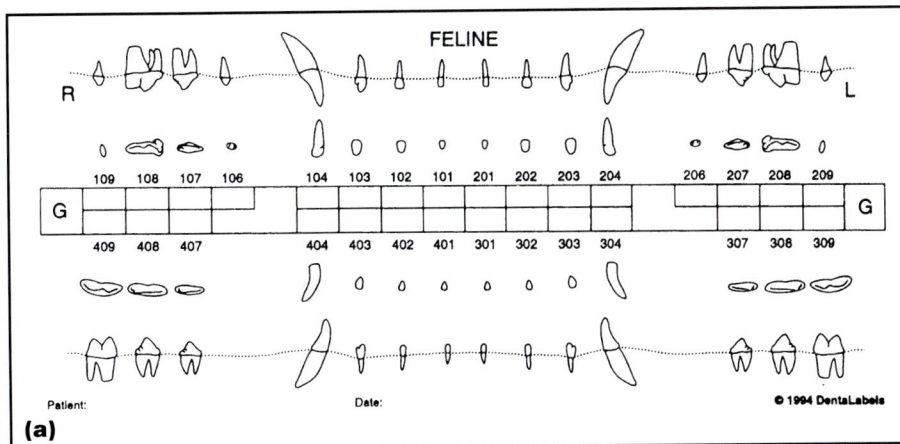

5.3
(a) Feline dental chart.
(b) Canine dental chart.
© DentaLabels, John Robinson.

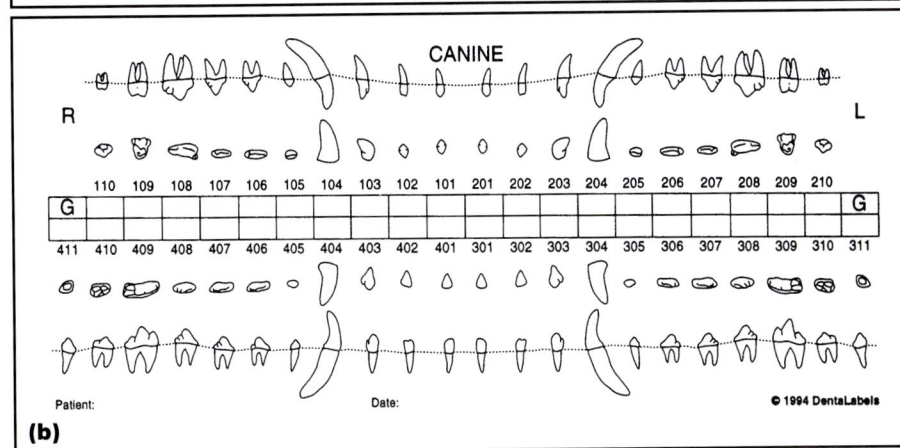

of the scaler to the handle and often has bends (off-sets). Different patterns of sickle scalers have different offsets to present the scaler blade to the tooth at different angles relative to the handle. The terminal part of the instrument is the blade – the working part – which is basically triangular in cross-section, with the upper surface being flat and having sharp edges on either side. In sickle scalers, the blade is a curved scythe shape. Scalers terminate, at the toe, in a sharp point (Figure 5.4).

To work efficiently, the instrument's sharp edges must be maintained. This is achieved by sharpening after every couple of uses.

The handle should have a large diameter to allow a comfortable finger grip; this is referred to as a 'balanced grip' handle. Cushioned handles made of silicone are available for greater operator comfort.

Curettes

A dental curette (see Figure 5.4) is a modified hand scaler for use *below* the gum line, i.e. subgingivally. The blade is smaller and semicircular in cross-section. The tip (or toe) is rounded rather than a sharp point. These modifications allow better access into the periodontal pocket and the rounded edges reduce unwanted tissue trauma.

Curettes are used to scale subgingivally (remove subgingival calculus in periodontal pockets) and to perform root surface debridement. They may also be used supragingivally. The instrument needs to be maintained in a sharp condition.

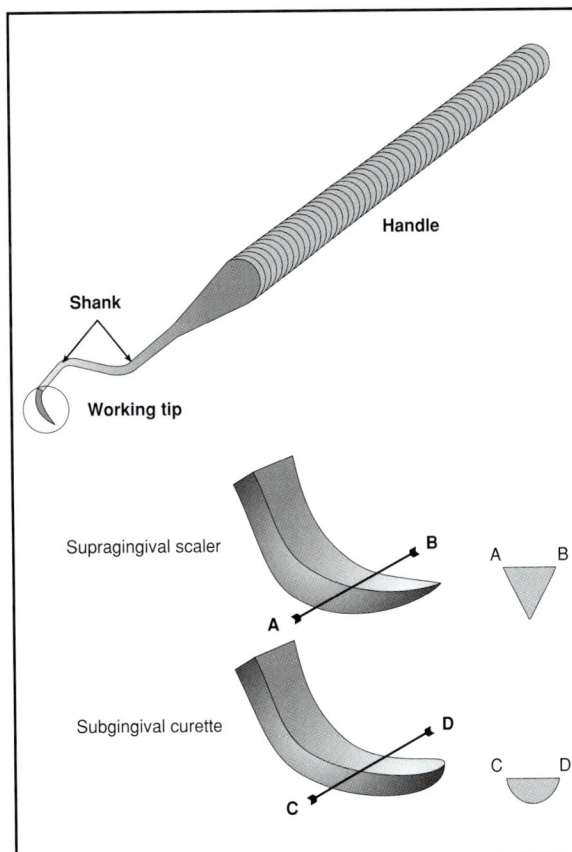

5.4 Hand scaler and curette.

The range of curette patterns available is even greater than that for hand scalers. Curette types are divided into universal and Gracey. In universal curettes, the flat top of the blade is at 90 degrees to the terminal portion of the shank; this changes to 70 degrees in Gracey curettes. The Columbia 4L/4R (universal) pattern or other patterns recommended for human incisor tooth use are good starting instruments. Patterns of a smaller number generally equate to curettes to be used on teeth towards the front of the mouth.

'After 5s' are curettes with extended shanks and even smaller toes, designed for use in deeper (>5 mm) periodontal pockets. In the animal situation, pockets of such depth normally indicate extraction of the tooth. After 5s may be useful in 3–5 mm pockets in smaller animal teeth or in furcation areas.

Arkansas sharpening stone
The sharpening of scalers and curettes requires a fine-grade sharpening stone, often made from Arkansas stone (a natural stone). The stones are either blocks with flat surfaces or rods with a rounded surface. A wedge-shaped stone with rounded ends, giving two different diameters of curvature, is also available for use on instruments of different sizes. The stone is used in conjunction with a light-grade engineering oil.

The scaler or curette is presented to the stone as it would be to a tooth surface and is repeatedly dragged over the surface to re-hone the working edge. Gracey curettes have a convex working surface that must be sharpened accordingly. Only very slight modifications should be made to the instruments using the fine stone. If a synthetic (ceramic) sharpening stone is used, water should be used as the lubricant to prevent clogging of the sharpening surface.

The sharpness of a scaler or curette can be checked by using it on a plastic stick (included in sharpening kits) or on a thumbnail to see if it 'bites' into the surface.

Polishing cups and brushes
Teeth should only be polished using a rubber polishing cup or polishing brush, in conjunction with a fine polishing paste, driven by a dental handpiece at approximately 3000 rpm.

The cup type should be 'soft', so that only a light force is required to flatten the edge. The edge of the prophylaxis cup needs to be flattened in use to allow polishing 1–2 mm subgingivally. This allows best use without excessive friction and so reduces the risk of heat trauma to the tooth. The rubber cups and brushes are available as 'pop-ons' to fit button attachments or with latch grip shanks (RA) or screw-on types (see later for different attachment types).

Polishing paste
Flour of Pumice powder made into a slurry with water should not be used to polish teeth. This compound is too rough and will scour the tooth surface, leaving microscopic scratches that will subsequently attract more staining and plaque build-up.

A fine polishing paste should be used. The paste will not feel gritty when rolled between finger and thumb tips.

Coarse-grade paste will clean the teeth but will also scour the surface. Coarse polishing paste should be used sparingly and followed by the use of a fine paste.

The paste should be decanted, in a single-use amount, to a suitable receptacle prior to treatment. This will avoid contamination of the remaining paste and the risk of cross-infection.

Paste holder
A Dappens dish acts as a small bowl to hold a single dose of polishing paste. Fixy daps® (Svenska) are plastic dishes with a glued base that stick to the back of the gloved hand or other convenient surface.

Polishing pastes are also available in single-use plastic pots, which fit into a finger ring to hold them on the hand.

Tooth extraction

Elevators
The Coupland's elevator is the origin of most dental elevators used nowadays. It was originally a bone chisel (or gouge) which was then adapted for tooth extraction. The working part is a shank, in line with the handle, that has a trough along one side which increases in depth towards the tip.

The end or tip should form a sharp edge (as in a kitchen knife rather than a scalpel), which can be square or rounded. With proper use the tip should not need sharpening, but if blunted or distorted it can be reshaped with a carpenter's chisel sharpening stone. The tip is sharpened on its convex surface.

Elevators are available with tips of different width, corresponding to the size of the tooth root (Figure 5.5).

The instrument is applied with a downward force to wedge the tip between the marginal bone and root. The curvature of the concave surface should be slightly less than that of the surface of the tooth root. The working action is a rotation around its long axis. The large diameter of the handle creates the mechanical advantage. A Coupland's elevator should not be struck and used like a chisel, nor used with a lever action.

Many variations to the basic Coupland's elevator design are available. Offsets have been put in the shank to give a different approach to the teeth. The tips have been notched with a 'V' or the edges serrated (e.g. Lindo-Levien patterns) to try to improve the grip on the tooth surface. The 'winged' elevators (Wiggs Winged elevators) have extended sides to wrap around the tooth more and these are proving very popular.

The elevator size should be appropriate for the

Size	Width of tip	Uses
Superslim	1.7 mm	All cat teeth (except canines), dog root remnants and very small teeth
No. 1	3.0 mm	Small dog teeth and cat canine teeth
No. 2	3.5 mm	Medium dog teeth
No. 3	4.0 mm	Larger dog teeth

5.5 Coupland's elevators.

tooth size but the actual pattern is a matter of personal preference. It is recommended to start with the basic pattern and try others, especially when a good purchase on the tooth is not obtained.

Luxators

Luxators, at first glance, look like Coupland's elevators. The tip is thinner and should have a sharper edge and the trough is shallower. However, the main difference is in the action of use. A luxator is designed to slip through the gingival sulcus and into the periodontal ligament space, working as a cutting device. The metal at the tip is too thin and weak to be used as a wedge with rotational forces. Luxators are used to begin the extraction technique prior to use of elevators and forceps. They are supplied in 1mm to 5mm tip widths, with straight or curved shanks. Luxators are sharpened on their concave surface.

Extraction forceps

The patterns of tooth extraction forceps required are 76N and 76 (Figure 5.6). These are almost straight forceps but with a slight offset of the beaks. The 76N has the same profile as the 76 but has narrower beaks to grip smaller teeth.

Used correctly, forceps are useful to complete loosening of the tooth and then remove it from the socket. The forceps should grip the tooth firmly and not swivel around the tooth, as this can result in tooth breakage. Forceps can easily apply excessive or improper forces and so break teeth. The forces should be rotational around the tooth's long axis and not lateral leverage. Small cat teeth can easily be crushed if gripped too hard.

Root tip picks

Root tip picks have a thin shank with a pointed tip. The shank can be straight or have a left or right curvature. The concept is that the fine tip can get purchase on the tooth root fragment by insertion between socket and tooth. Alternative instruments, such as the Superslim elevator (see Figure 5.6), may be more effective.

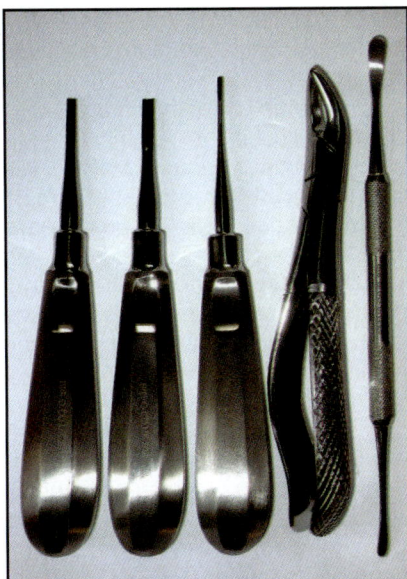

5.6

(Left to right): Coupland's elevator (No. 1); Coupland's elevator (No. 3); Superslim elevator; extraction forceps (pattern 76N); Goldman Fox periosteal elevator. (Courtesy of Big-O Veterinary Dental Supplies Company.)

Periosteal elevator

Specialized periosteal elevators are used in dentistry and oral surgery to raise mucoperiosteal and other soft tissue flaps (e.g. in surgical tooth extraction). Goldman Fox (see Figure 5.6), Molt or Howarth patterns are commonly used. All have a spoon-like blade, in line with the handle. The working side is flat with a concave curvature and the back side is rounded. The edge should be 'kitchen knife' sharp.

Cumine scaler

This double-ended instrument has a spoon-shaped end and a scaler end. The spoon-shaped end can be used as a curette on bone (removing granulation tissue from tooth sockets) or as a periosteal elevator. The scaler end is a heavy-duty version of a Jaquette scaler. Both ends can be used to crack off large calculus deposits.

Power equipment

Power scalers

Ultrasonic scalers

Ultrasonic scalers are so called because the tip vibrates at a frequency above human hearing range. Machines work at 25 kHz, 30 kHz or sometimes higher. The tips are made to vibrate, at small amplitude, by a mechanism contained in the handle.

In magnetostrictive-type scalers, the mechanism is an electric coil around a stack of laminated ferromagnetic strips or a ferrite rod. The tip vibrates in an elliptical path, with 80% being in line with the long axis of the handle and 20% across that axis. The Cavitron® and the Bobcat™ are examples of this type of scaler, with many other manufacturers using the same technology.

Odontoson scalers are also of the magnetostrictive type. They work at a higher frequency of 42 kHz but at a smaller amplitude of vibration. They have a ferrite rod rather than the metal stack of the Cavitron type. The tip moves in a circular motion, meaning that all sides of the tip are equally effective at scaling.

Piezoelectric-type scalers (Figure 5.7) use a piezo-

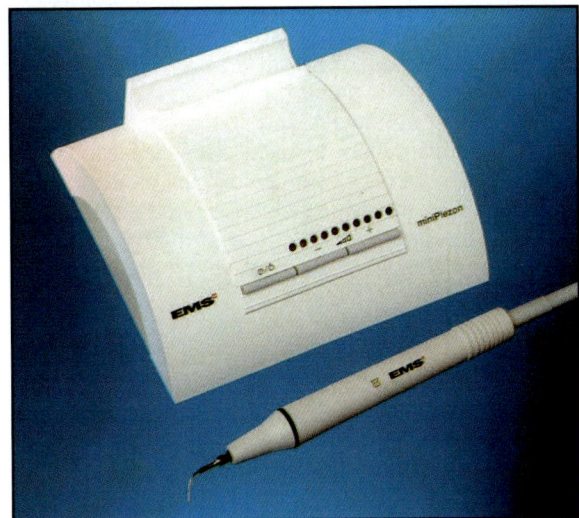

5.7 Mini Piezon (piezoelectric) scaler with universal tip. (Courtesy of Burtons of Maidstone.)

electric crystal system with piezoceramic discs that vibrate on a titanium shaft when a high frequency electric current is applied. The tip vibrates only in a linear direction, in line with the long axis of the handle. EMS Piezon and Cocoon (Satelec) are examples of this type of scaler.

To achieve an efficient and atraumatic scaling action, only the two areas on each side of the tip should be applied to the tooth, with light contact. The scaler tip should always be kept moving.

Coolant water: Metal vibrating at high frequency develops a lot of heat and the tip must be cooled with a copious stream of water to prevent thermal damage to the teeth and soft tissues. Sufficient water flow over the tip should keep it from becoming dangerously hot. If the tip is becoming too hot to touch, then either the water flow must be increased or the power setting (amplitude of vibration) reduced. Magnetostrictive scalers generate more heat than piezoelectric scalers, as the stack also heats up during function.

The high frequency vibration of the ultrasonic scaler tip results in cavitation within the coolant water. Cavitation is the production of microscopic bubbles which then implode, releasing energy. This aids the cleaning action and also has an antibacterial action, especially on anaerobic bacteria.

Health and safety: The water aerosol created when ultrasonic scalers are used is highly contaminated with bacteria and other microorganisms from the mouth. This creates a serious health hazard and necessitates protection for the operator and assistant (face shield, spectacles, mask and gloves). A zone of 2 m in radius should be regarded as contaminated from commencement of scaling until 2 hours after the last tooth is scaled. Ideally, an air-extraction system should be fitted in the dental treatment area (see Chapter 4).

Maintenance and hygiene: All types of tip for power scalers eventually become worn. A small loss of length at the tip will dramatically reduce the operating efficiency. Some manufacturers have cards with printed tip outlines which are then compared with the actual tip and show when replacement is required. If a tip is damaged or becomes bent it will not work effectively and so needs replacing. A bent tip cannot be straightened.

The scaler handpiece and tip need to be cleaned between each patient to avoid cross-infection. The optimum is to sterilize by autoclave but as a minimum they should be thoroughly cleaned and treated with a hard surface disinfectant (check with manufacturer's instructions for suitability).

Sonic scalers

These power scalers are driven by compressed air that rotates an eccentric rotor around the central shaft. The scaler handpiece fits on to an outlet on a standard air-driven dental unit, which also supplies the integral water spray. The frequency of vibration is much lower than in ultrasonic scalers, which means less heat generation at the tip and so greater safety in use. Even the best and most expensive models are much slower in scaling than ultrasonic scalers. They are probably best used for light scaling duties.

Tip types

Each power scaler has a variety of tip types. The fine, sickle-shaped type, sometimes called the universal or perio tip (see Figure 5.7), is a very useful pattern and can scale all supragingival surfaces and up to 2 mm below the gum line. The thicker and wider tips (beavertail or spade-shaped) are more robust but cannot access all areas of the teeth or scale subgingivally.

There are tips that are specifically sold for subgingival use. They have design features to enable the water coolant to get to the entire tip even when inserted into a periodontal pocket where the tip is surrounded by soft tissue and tooth. The user needs to be sceptical of the ability to achieve complete cooling of the tip. The heat generated at the tip during use can be assessed by pinching the tip, whilst the scaler is running, between finger and thumb to varying depths to mimic the periodontal pocket. The tip should remain cool to prevent thermal damage to the tooth and gingiva.

Rotosonic scaling burs

There are several shapes of flat-sided 'non-cutting' Rotosonic burs, which fit into high-speed dental (air rotor) handpieces. It has been proposed that these burs might be used for scaling teeth. Rotosonic burs do scale teeth very rapidly but it is impossible to use them without serious and irreparable damage to the tooth surface. They should never be used for scaling in veterinary dentistry.

Dental drill units

Air-driven dental unit

A basic air-driven dental unit should be considered a minimum requirement for small animal practice. Capital investment in an air-driven unit is highly recommended and is returned by a machine that will be used daily to make many procedures (including oral surgery) quicker and easier, thus saving time and effort. There are a number of optional additional features available with certain units.

The basic unit is made up of an air compressor, a control unit and the handpieces.

The control unit is commonly mounted on a frame with wheels, which is then referred to as the 'cart' (Figure 5.8). The compressor usually sits on the base of the cart but can be sited elsewhere and connected to the cart by an air hose (6 mm polypropylene high-pressure pipe). The control unit may otherwise be fixed to a wall or other secure surface either directly or using a wall bracket and pivot arms.

Control unit

The inputs to the unit are compressed air and water. The water usually comes from a bottle pressurized by the air compressor but can come directly from the mains. The latter requires a non-return valve and an in-line filter (see Chapter 4).

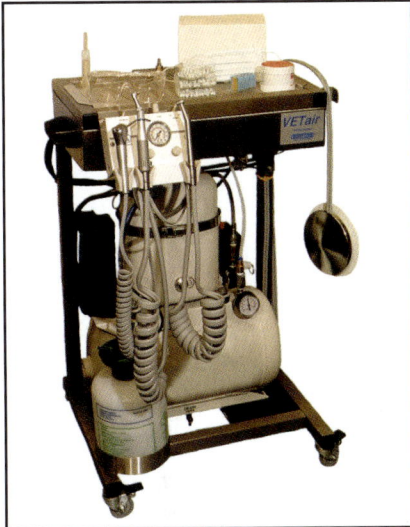

'Vetair' air-driven dental cart. (Courtesy of Burtons of Maidstone.)

The unit regulates the air and water to the outlets. Units may have two or three outlets. On two-outlet units there is a toggle switch to direct the air to the required outlet. On three-outlet units there are microswitches that open a valve when the handpiece is lifted from its cradle. The water flow to the outlets is adjusted by turning a knob on the unit.

There are separate valves to adjust the air pressure to each outlet. These are either inside the unit or small screws flush with the surface. They are intended to set up the system and not for regular adjustment. There is usually a pressure gauge on the unit to display the outlet air pressure. The correct pressure varies for different handpieces and air motors. Reference should be made to the manufacturer's instructions for the recommended operating pressure and the machine should be set accordingly. Operating pressure is usually about 30 psi (never exceed 35 psi: higher pressure will damage the mechanism of the handpiece and shorten its life). To check and adjust the operating pressure, the handpiece should be attached to the outlet and the foot pedal fully depressed and the gauge monitored.

The three-in-one syringe has two push-button valves: one for a jet of water and one for a jet of air. These are both unregulated from the supply. If both are pressed simultaneously a water spray is produced. The three-in-one syringe is indispensable for rinsing, to remove debris, and for drying to improve vision during examination and operative procedures. A dry tooth surface will show any irregularities and residual calculus more clearly than a wet surface.

Compressor

Oil-cooled compressors are quiet in operation and so can be sited near people, such as on the base of the cart. The alternative is an oil-free compressor (as used by garage mechanics), which is noisy and should be sited away from work areas and connected to the cart by long air hoses. The oil-free type is cheaper and virtually maintenance free. The oil-cooled type requires servicing and maintenance.

There should be an oil filter (trap) on the air outlet; this will show an early sign of seal deterioration.

Weekly compressor maintenance

- Drain water from air reservoir: turn compressor off and open screw valve on underside of air reservoir (tank) with a dish beneath to catch fluid.
- Check outlet air pressure on gauge on compressor: 60–80 psi (4–5 bar). To adjust: turn large knob on the regulator valve near to gauge. If adjustment is made, the outlet pressures on the control unit will need to be checked.
- Check oil level to line on bubble window (oil-cooled type only).

Handpieces

High-speed handpiece
The high-speed handpiece, also called the air-rotor or air-turbine handpiece, is recognizable by the high-pitched sound that people associate with 'the dentist's drill'. The cartridge in the head of the handpiece is driven by a jet of compressed air. The cartridge is a turbine, mounted on minute bearings, around a clutch mechanism that holds the shank of the bur. The turbine spins at between 350,000 and 400,000 rpm, depending on design and the actual air pressure. It is designed for high-speed, low-torque use and so should be used with the foot pedal fully depressed.

Features and options:

- Intergral water cooling jet, which exits at the drill head from one or more holes. A greater number of holes gives better water distribution and cooling action.
- Screw type or push-button. The push-button chuck negates the need for an additional tool to insert or remove burs. Push-button chucks can only work with bur shanks made to within a high tolerance of the correct shank diameter. If the bur does not insert easily or is not gripped, a different bur should be used.
- Three-hole Borden or four-hole Midwest coupling to hose (Figure 5.9).
- Additional swivel or quick-release coupling between the hose connection and the handpiece shank, allowing the handpiece to rotate independently of the delivery hose. This removes torsional forces on the operator's grip for easier operation.
- Fibreoptic lighting. A bulb is built into the handpiece coupling and the light is taken by fibreoptics to the drill head and illuminates the operative area.

Proper use:

- Check that the bur is fully home when inserted and gripped firmly.
- With screw-type clutch, do not over tighten.
- Use a light touch (brush action) and keep the drill at full speed (listen to the pitch).
- Do not extend the bur (only partly inserted into head) – greater lateral forces will damage the bearings.

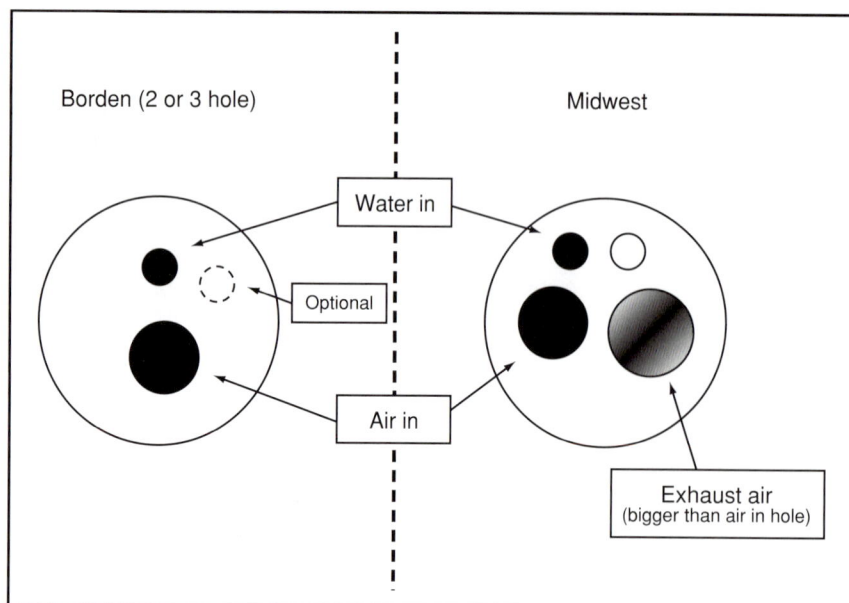

- Do not run the drill without a bur – this can damage the cartridge (even when oiling).
- Do not use bent or damaged burs.
- Store the handpiece with a blank (or bur) in place.

Maintenance:

- Clean the handpiece after every patient. Remove any blood or debris with a damp cloth or tissue, then either spray with a quality hard surface disinfectant or autoclave. Most handpieces can withstand autoclaving but it reduces the life of the bearings. It is important to follow the manufacturer's instructions regarding oiling and sterilizing procedures. Usually the instructions are to oil the handpiece before each autoclave cycle.
- Oil the handpiece regularly, after approximately ten patients or at least weekly. For basic handpieces: disconnect from tubing, insert two or three drops of handpiece oil into the air inlet hole (see Figure 5.9), reconnect and run for a while to push the oil through the turbine. For quick-release connections: detach at quick-release point and put oil into air inlet or use a can of spray oil with the same fitting as the male part of the coupling.
- Always check that there is copious water flow. The exit hole(s) may need cleaning with a fine wire or blast of air if debris becomes lodged (hard water may result in limescale accumulation if mains water is used).
- Check that the cover plate, which holds the cartridge in, at the back of the drill head is tight. This plate is either where the chuck inserts to change a bur or is the push-button for changing a bur.
- Check for worn or damaged bearings. Feel for play or wobble in the bur and check that the bur spins freely when turned with fingers.

Air motor

The air motor is a motor driven by compressed air. It usually has a Midwest connection (see Figure 5.9) to the supply hose. There is a collar on the motor near the hose connection which can be rotated. Moving this collar adjusts the direction (forward or reverse) and speed of the air motor. At the other end of the motor is a standard 'e-fitting' which connects to all slow-speed dental handpieces. The e-fitting is a tube around a central spinning drive shaft. The air motor speed has a maximum of 25,000–30,000 rpm.

Air motors should be lubricated, as for air turbine handpieces, by disconnecting and putting oil into the air inlet hole (the smaller inlet of the two large holes).

Slow handpiece

Slow handpieces are driven by an air motor and all attach by a standard e-fitting. There is a range of types of slow dental handpieces.

Contra-angle handpieces

Contra-angle handpieces are similar in shape to air-turbine handpieces, having a slight offset (bend) between the drill head and the handle. The burs are held perpendicular to the end portion of the drill shank. When the handpiece is held in a pen grip, the bur is presented at right angles to the resting surface. The burs are most commonly 'latch grip', so called because they have a key and slot in their end which is slotted into the handpiece and held by a latch that slides into the slot. Friction grip heads, as used with air turbines, are also available for contra-angle slow handpieces.

The head of the handpiece can be replaced with a prophylaxis (polishing) head. This has a 'button' on to which polishing cups or brushes connect. It also has a shroud under the button to prevent polishing paste getting into, and damaging, the gearing. Latch-key prophylaxis cups and brushes are also available, as are disposable (single-use) polishing heads.

Contra-angle handpieces are usually of a 1:1 gearing, meaning that the output speed is the same as the air motor speed. Speed-increasing handpieces, with gearing up to a ratio of 4:1 or 5:1, are available. The higher speed is better for sectioning multi-rooted teeth prior to extraction. Speed-reducing handpieces are only required for restorative dentistry but could be used for polishing purposes.

Straight or nose-cone handpieces

These take HP burs (Figure 5.10) that fit down the centre of the handpiece in line with its long axis. The burs are inserted and are then gripped when the top portion of the handpiece is twisted. A modification is the Doriot handpiece – a straight handpiece that takes various heads as attachments (e.g. prophylaxis heads, contra-angle heads). These lock on and are driven by a central shank that fits like an HP bur. Disposable plastic heads are available for polishing, including those that oscillate rather than rotate.

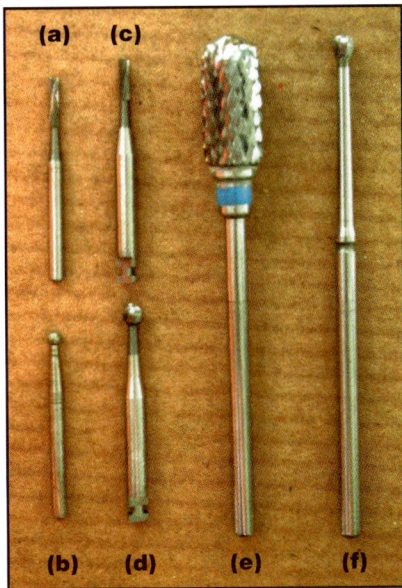

5.10 Different types of bur. **(a)** FG fissure bur (TC). **(b)** FG round bur (diamond). **(c)** RA fissure bur (TC). **(d)** RA round bur (TC). **(e)** HP acrylic trimmer bur (TC). **(f)** HP round bur (TC).

Maintenance

All slow handpieces should be oiled regularly by removing them from the air motor and applying oil to the e-fitting. This is best done by aerosol cans of oil with an e-fitting nozzle.

Micromotors

Micromotors are small electric motors that connect to an e-fitting handpiece. The motor is connected to a control box by a wire cord. The control box has a forward/reverse switch, an on/off foot pedal and a speed control knob. The following are features of micromotors, compared with air-driven units:

- No integral water for coolant (some models now have this feature)
- No three-in-one syringe
- Slower cutting compared with air turbine (even with speed-increasing handpieces)
- Shorter life expectancy – motors burn out, especially if stalled (or slowed due to excessive pressure in use) or with water ingress or if over-oiled
- Expensive repairs

- Lower purchase price (capital outlay) but more expensive in the long run
- Speed can be accurately controlled and constant (using dial).

Burs and handpiece accessories

Burs are manufactured in a huge range of sizes and shapes. For general veterinary use only a few patterns and sizes are needed.

- Fissure burs have a cylindrical or tapered shape with cutting surfaces on the side and often also on the end. A 'flat fissure' bur has parallel sides, whereas a 'tapered fissure' bur decreases in diameter towards the tip.
- Round burs have a ball-shaped cutting area attached at the end of the shank.

The cutting surface of a bur is made of stainless steel, tungsten carbide (TC) or diamond.

The TC and stainless steel types have cutting blades. A sharp TC bur will cut fastest of all dental burs. TC and stainless steel burs become worn and blunted with use and so should be regularly replaced with new ones. In use, the bur needs to be kept cool by copious water spray, because it will become blunt almost instantly if the surface metal becomes hot.

Cross-cut burs have grooves at right angles to the cutting blades, like rings around the bur. The cross-cuts are designed to reduce clogging with tooth debris and so maintain cutting efficiency.

Diamond burs have a coating of tiny sharp diamond fragments embedded in a resin on the bur shank. As the surface is worn down and diamond particles are lost, others are exposed to maintain cutting efficiency until there is no more coating. A copious water flow is required when using diamond burs, to prevent thermal damage to the teeth and to prevent clogging of the diamond grit with debris.

Bur shanks

The different shapes and patterns of bur are available with different shanks. The shank type is specific for the handpiece. There are three types: friction grip (FG); right-angle or latch grip (RA); and HP.

- FG is for air turbines and contra-angle handpieces with a FG head.
- RA is for most contra-angle handpieces (with a latch mechanism).
- HP is for straight handpieces.

Codes for burs

When ordering burs from a catalogue, there are multiple codes to identify the bur's features.

- There is a one to four digit number that gives the pattern and diameter size (e.g. 701 is a 1.2 mm diameter tapered fissure cross-cut bur). It is best to match this number to previous purchases.
- There is a three-digit ISO number that simply relates to the diameter in tenths of millimetres (e.g. 012 is 1.2 mm).

- The individual retail company will assign their own order code (up to six digits).

Bur care

All burs should be cleaned after use to remove any debris (e.g. tooth powder). They may need cleaning during use if the blades are clogged up, as this will dramatically reduce the cutting rate. Bur brushes are usually made of fine brass wires bundled in either a flat or round shape. All burs can be autoclaved.

Bur blocks are available to hold the burs and store them ready for use; bur blocks that can be autoclaved are also available. Stainless steel and TC burs should be kept dry or stored in special non-rusting disinfectant solutions (e.g. Rusnon solution).

Air polishing units

These units are stand-alone or attachments for air-driven units. They polish teeth and remove stains by firing a stream of non-hygroscopic sodium bicarbonate powder from a nozzle in the handpiece (in a similar action to sand-blasting). Ideally they should be used with a high-volume suction unit to remove the powder and prevent air contamination. The jet will traumatize surface epithelium if aimed at soft tissue. Care should be taken to avoid this and the soft tissue should be protected using a guard or by applying a gel (e.g. Vaseline).

Electrocautery units

An electrocautery unit is useful in dentistry for removing excess soft tissue, especially gingival hyperplasia. In addition to cutting soft tissue, it will cauterize and coagulate. The loop-shaped tip is recommended. Dental electrocautery units are less powerful than medical units and are a cheaper option. They should be used on oral tissues with due care, as thermal necrosis of soft tissues, teeth and alveolar bone are possible consequences of improper use.

Radiography

X-ray machine

A standard veterinary (medical) unit can be used for dental radiography, including intraoral techniques. However, a dental X-ray machine is recommended as it has the following advantages:

- It can be sited at the dental treatment area, avoiding the need to move the animal to another location
- The machine head is more manoeuvrable. The machine is moved around the animal's head. (With a veterinary unit the animal's body and head have to be positioned to allow for a vertical beam)
- A shorter focal–film distance (FFD) means markedly reduced exposure settings
- Most dental X-ray machines have fixed kilovoltage (kV) and milliamperage (mA), and so only have adjustment of exposure time.

Digital dental X-ray machines are becoming cheaper and may be economically viable for general veterinary practice. A dental X-ray machine is used in conjunction with different sized tablets (transducers), which replace the intraoral film. The tablet connects directly to a computer that uses specific software. The tablets are bulkier than dental film and so can be more difficult to position, especially in smaller mouths.

Digital radiography requires lower exposure settings than conventional radiography and so is safer. It also allows almost instant viewing of the image (no processing requirements) and the image can be manipulated on the computer to aid interpretation.

X-ray film

Dental X-ray film is non-screen, high-definition film. It requires higher exposure settings (relative to typical settings when using cassettes with intensifying screens) but gives a higher image quality. The film is contained in a moisture-resistant package that also contains a lead-foil backing and a paper or cardboard sheet.

The three most commonly available and used sizes are:

- Standard or adult periapical = 30 x 40 mm (size 2)
- Occlusal = 57 x 76 mm (size 4)
- Paediatric = 22 x 35 mm (size 0).

Dental film is commonly available in two speeds: D (ultra) and E (ekta). Film designated E is twice as fast as film designated D; it requires less exposure time (radiation dose) but at the expense of a small loss of quality. E-speed film cannot be developed in 'red' safe light conditions (some chair-side developers use red plastic windows and others orange) as the film will become fogged. E-speed film must be developed under an orange safe light.

Processing

Some veterinary automatic X-ray film processors cannot handle the small dental films unless they have mesh film carriers, as are used in dental automatic processors. Standard dental film can easily be processed manually using a four-bath system in a darkroom or in a chair-side light-safe box. Standard developer and fixer solutions may be used. The process can be speeded up by using faster solutions, such as 'Rapid Access' by Kodak.

Mono-processing films (self-developing): These are only available in adult periapical size. They are processed using a single developer and fixer solution. In some (e.g. ECO-30) the solution is contained in a separate compartment within the film package. The film is processed in the package, by breaking the seal between the two compartments and squeezing the solution into the film compartment. It is then massaged around the film for an approximate specified time (1 minute for ECO-30). No darkroom facility is required. The film must be thoroughly rinsed immediately after the package is opened to remove residual developer/fixer fluid and prevent artefact development. ECO-30 gives images of comparable quality to other dental film.

Developmental oral and dental conditions

Leen Verhaert

Occlusal patterns and malocclusion

Variations relating to the jaws and occlusion

There are a variety of dog and cat breeds, and what is considered normal occlusion for a Boxer would be highly abnormal for a Greyhound. A Boxer, having shortened maxillae but mandibules of normal length, has a normal occlusion for the breed, even if this occlusion is strictly speaking a severe malocclusion that may lead to mucosal damage. Humans have contributed greatly to the incidence and severity of malocclusions, due to selective breeding of dogs and cats for show purposes. Unfortunately for the animals, there is a tendency to select for extreme and exaggerated types: small breeds are getting smaller; Persian cats and Bulldogs have faces shortened to the extent that they can hardly breathe. One can see a change in skull type over time in several breeds, because some skull types are found 'more desirable' or 'more typical for the breed'; for example, many present-day Rottweilers have a severely shortened, broad maxilla and mandible, leading to rotation and crowding of teeth.

Three basic skull types exist:

- *Mesocephalic*: medium jaw length and medium muzzle width. Most dog and cat breeds fall into this category
- *Dolichocephalic*: long jaws evidenced by abnormally large interdental spaces and a narrow muzzle. Examples are Greyhound, Rough Collie, Siamese and Oriental Shorthair cat
- *Brachycephalic*: short, broad skull. Examples are English and French Bulldog, Shih Tzu, Cavalier King Charles Spaniel, Persian and Exotic Shorthair cat.

Terminology

Relating to the jaws:

- *Prognathia*: one jaw is in a forward (rostral) relationship relative to the other jaw
- *Retrognathia*: one jaw is in a caudal relationship relative to the other jaw
- *Brachygnathia*: shortened jaw.

The adjective 'mandibular' or 'maxillary' should be added to describe the condition more precisely (e.g. mandibular prognathia, maxillary retrognathia; in both cases the mandible is relatively longer than the maxilla, or the maxilla is relatively shorter than the mandible).

Relating to the teeth: The most commonly used prefixes are:

- *mesio-* (towards the dental arch midline)
- *disto-* (away from the dental arch midline)
- *labio-* (towards the lips)
- *bucco-* (towards the cheek)
- *linguo-* (towards the tongue)
- *palato-* (towards the palate).

These prefixes are used with the terms:

- *-version* (tipping)
- *-cclusion* (occlusal relationship with the counterpart of the tooth).

For instance: linguoversion means that a tooth is tipped towards the tongue; labioversion means that the tooth is tipped towards the lip.

Normal occlusion

Normal mesocephalic occlusion in the dog (Figure 6.1) is characterized by the following:

- *Incisors*: scissor bite; upper incisors are rostral to lower incisors, with the incisal tips of the lower incisors touching the cingula of the upper incisors
- *Canines*: mandibular canine evenly spaced between the upper third incisor and upper canine
- *Premolars*: interdigitation; the cusp tips of the premolars oppose the interdental spaces of the opposite arcade, with the mandibular first premolar being the most rostral ('pinking shear' effect)
- *Carnassial teeth*: the mesiobuccal surface of the mandibular first molar occludes with the palatal surface of the maxillary fourth premolar; the distal occlusal surface of the mandibular first molar occludes with the palatal occlusal surface of the maxillary first molar. The second and third mandibular molars occlude with the distal part of the occlusal surface of the maxillary first molar and with the occlusal surface of the maxillary second molar.

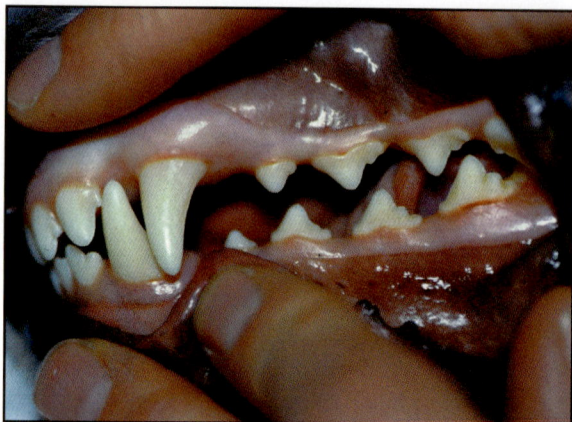

6.1   Normal mesocephalic occlusion in the dog: incisor scissor bite; mandibular canine evenly spaced between the upper third incisor and upper canine teeth; normal premolar interdigitation. © Leen Verhaert.

Dolichocephalic breeds show a similar occlusion, though the premolar teeth will have abnormal spacing with wider interdental spaces due to the relatively longer jaw. These breeds, however, have a functional occlusion that follows the general outline of the mesocephalic occlusion.

Most brachycephalic breeds have, according to breed standards, a malocclusion due to a shortened maxilla, and a normal mandible. The upper incisors occlude lingually to the lower incisors with premolars and molars exhibiting rotation and/or reduced interdental spaces and overlapping. Some brachycephalic breeds (e.g. Cavalier King Charles Spaniel) have a normal incisor scissor bite occlusion because the mandible is bowed ventrally as a result of dental interlock, thus decreasing the jaw length discrepancy between upper and lower jaws.

The incisor and canine occlusion in the mesocephalic cat is the same as in the dog. The premolar and molar occlusion in the cat is as follows:

- The most rostral premolar is the maxillary second premolar
- The buccal surface of the mandibular first molar occludes with the palatal surface of the maxillary fourth premolar
- The maxillary first molar does not occlude with another tooth.

Causes of malocclusion

Malocclusion is by definition an abnormality in the position of the teeth. Malocclusion may cause discomfort or pain and may be the direct cause of severe oral pathology, such as oronasal fistulation.

The development of the occlusion is determined by genetic and environmental factors. Jaw length, tooth bud position and tooth size are inherited and wide variations exist. For instance, small dog breeds often have large teeth in comparison with jaw size (Gioso, 2001), which could easily lead to crowding and malocclusion. The development of the maxilla, the mandible and the teeth are genetically independently regulated. Non-harmonious development of the upper jaw, lower jaw and teeth will result in malocclusion.

Environmental factors may influence the genetically determined occlusion: jaw growth may be altered by hormonal (endocrine) disorders, trauma or functional modification. Normal function (occlusion and mastication) plays an important role in normal jaw growth in the dog. Trauma to the bone or the soft tissues may result in growth disturbance. Facial trauma needs to have significant consequences to cause malocclusion (e.g. scarring, abnormal bone healing).

Various events during development and growth, such as trauma, may alter tooth bud position, leading to a dental malocclusion. A single tooth or a few neighbouring teeth are likely to be affected, and will often show developmental disorders other than malposition. Persistent deciduous teeth are associated with malpositioned permanent teeth. Persistence of deciduous teeth is likely to be an inherited condition and, subsequently, malposition of teeth secondary to this condition is indirectly inherited.

Specific genetic mechanisms regulating malocclusion are unknown. A polygenic mechanism is most likely and explains why not all siblings in successive generations are affected by a malocclusion to the same degree, if affected at all. It has been claimed that around 50% of malocclusions are acquired (Shipp and Fahrenkrug, 1992) but there are no data to substantiate such a claim in dogs. Establishing the aetiology of a malocclusion (developmental *versus* inherited) may be difficult or even impossible. The most reasonable approach to evaluate whether a malocclusion is hereditary or acquired has been suggested as follows:

- Skeletal malocclusions in dogs are considered inherited unless a developmental cause can be reliably identified
- Pure dental malocclusion in dogs should be given the benefit of the doubt and not be considered inherited, unless a breed or family predisposition exists (e.g. rostrally displaced upper canine teeth in Shetland Sheepdogs).

Diagnostic approach to malocclusions

Malocclusion may result from the malposition of teeth (dental malocclusion), jaw size discrepancy (skeletal malocclusion), or a combination of both.

Skeletal malocclusion

Most orthodontic problems where veterinary attention is sought are encountered in dogs that are supposed to have a normal incisor scissor bite. The first diagnostic step is to determine whether the malocclusion has a skeletal component. Most skeletal malocclusions are considered inherited and ethical considerations play a major role in treatment decision making.

Rotation and crowding of premolars is an indication of jaw shortening (Figure 6.2a); excessive space between premolars is an indication of jaw lengthening (Figure 6.2b). Skeletal malocclusion may exist even though jaw length discrepancy is not obvious on clinical examination. A thorough examination is necessary and should include a critical assessment of jaw length, premolar–molar occlusion and occlusion of the canine teeth.

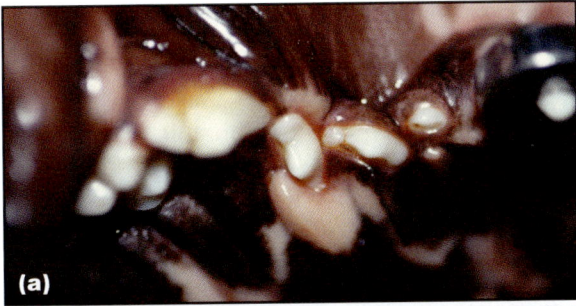

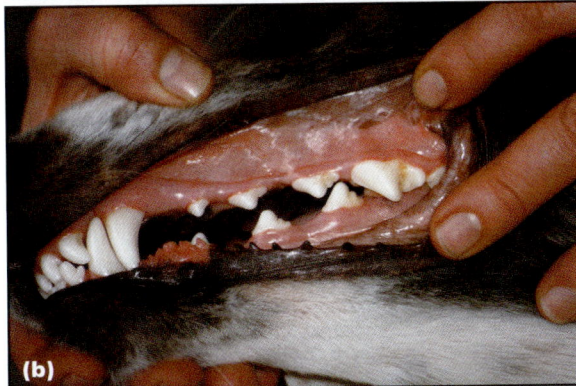

6.2 Jaw length assessment. **(a)** Shortening of a jaw is evidenced by rotation of premolars. **(b)** Lengthening is evidenced by abnormal spacing between premolars. © Leen Verhaert.

Jaw length: It is important to note the existence of major jaw length discrepancy. This is indicated by either bowing of the mandible, or excessive shortening (evidenced by rotation of teeth) or lengthening (evidenced by abnormally wide spacing between premolars) of either jaw. It should be remembered that both jaws may be shortened or lengthened to the same extent, leading to a normal occlusion.

Premolar–molar occlusion: Loss of normal interdigitation, premolar distocclusion (premolars caudally displaced relative to their counterparts) or mesiocclusion (premolars rostrally displaced relative to their counterparts) and open bite (abnormal spacing between upper and lower jaw due to bowing of the mandible) are all signs of a skeletal malocclusion (Figure 6.3).

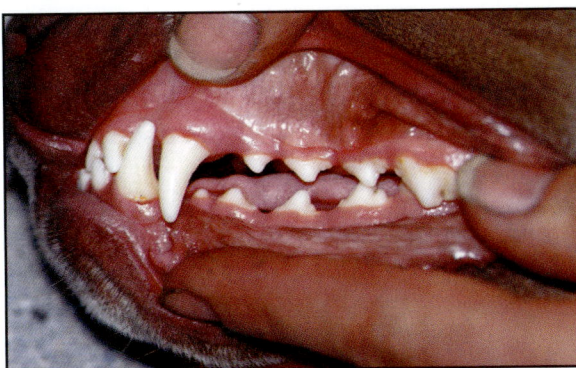

6.3 Skeletal malocclusion in a Weimaraner. The mandible is relatively longer than the maxilla. Normal interdigitation is lost; the mandibular premolars are rostrally displaced relative to their maxillary counterparts. Lower canine is tight against upper third incisor © Leen Verhaert.

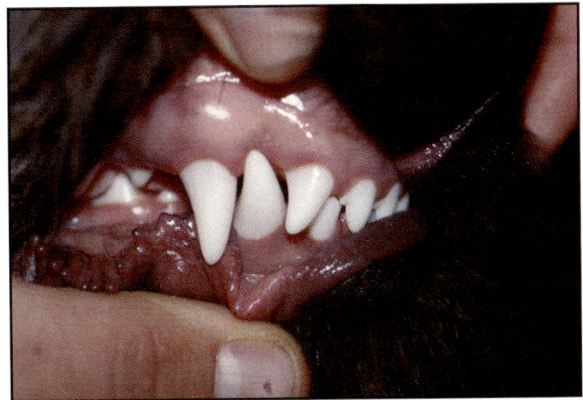

6.4 Normal canine occlusion. The lower canine tooth crown is evenly spaced between the upper third incisor and upper canine teeth. © Leen Verhaert.

Occlusion of the canine teeth: The lower canine tooth should be evenly spaced between the upper third incisor and upper canine teeth, without touching either of them (Figure 6.4). When occlusion of the canines is incorrect, a skeletal malocclusion is usually present.

Common malocclusions in dogs

Rostral (anterior) cross bite and edge-to-edge incisor relationship

Rostral cross bite is the term commonly used where one, several or all upper incisors occlude lingually to the mandibular incisors (Figure 6.5). Rostral cross bite is a common condition in dogs of all sizes and head shapes. It is also commonly seen in brachycephalic cat breeds (e.g. Persian, Exotic Shorthair and British Shorthair).

This condition may be a dental malocclusion if only the incisor teeth are affected, and may be caused by persistence of deciduous incisors. Therefore, if the deciduous teeth are still present while the permanent teeth are erupting, the deciduous teeth should be extracted as soon as possible to avoid this type of malocclusion (see also 'Disorders of eruption and shedding' later).

However, in most cases rostral cross bite has a skeletal origin, evidenced by abnormal premolar and canine occlusion. Full assessment of jaw length, pre-

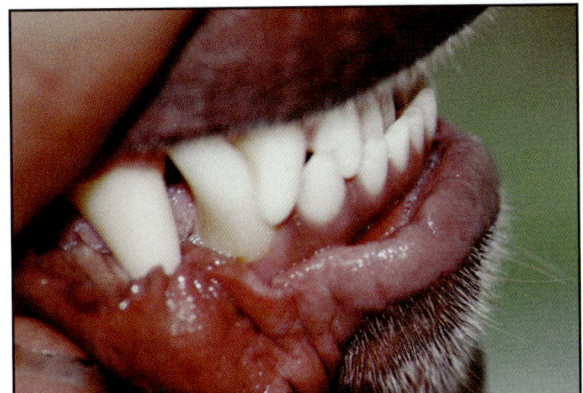

6.5 Rostral cross bite. The maxillary incisors occlude lingually to the mandibular incisors. This is the same dog as shown in Figure 6.3, indicating a skeletal malocclusion in this dog. © Leen Verhaert.

molar–molar occlusion and occlusion of the canine teeth is mandatory before orthodontic treatment is considered. Most animals with a rostral cross bite will have a prognathic mandible. Orthodontic treatment in these cases is mainly for cosmetic reasons and should not be performed.

Caudal (posterior) cross bite
This condition is most commonly seen in breeds with dolichocephalic skulls. The normal buccolingual relationship of the carnassial teeth is reversed: the upper fourth premolar occludes lingually to the lower first molar (Figure 6.6). In these cases, the lower first molar will accumulate more plaque and calculus than the upper fourth premolar.

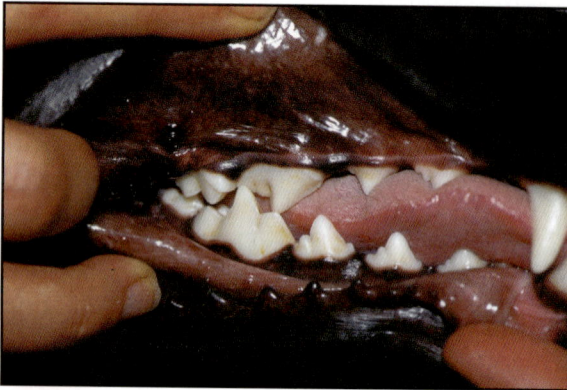

6.6 Caudal cross bite. The upper fourth premolar occludes lingually to the lower first molar.
© Leen Verhaert.

Prognathic mandible and retrognathic maxilla
The mandible is relatively longer than the maxilla and some or all of the mandibular teeth are rostral to their normal position (Figure 6.7). The normal interdigitation in the premolar region is lost, due to a rostral position of the mandibular premolars. Depending on the degree of malocclusion, the incisor occlusion may be normal, or there may be a level bite or a rostral cross bite. The lower canines may be touching the upper third incisors, or they may be rostral to the upper third incisors.

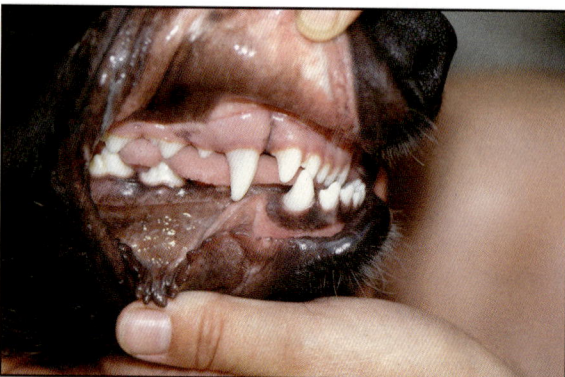

6.7 Prognathic mandible. The mandible is relatively longer than the maxilla. Mandibular premolars are rostrally displaced, a rostral cross bite is present and the mandibular canines are rostral to the upper third incisors. Although there is a severe malocclusion, this dog had a comfortable bite and treatment was unnecessary.
© Leen Verhaert.

Treatment is indicated in those cases where the lower canines force the upper third incisors into an abnormal, uncomfortable position.

Prognathic maxilla and retrognathic mandible
When the mandible is short compared with the maxilla, the mandibular canine teeth may not be able to occlude rostrally to the maxillary canine teeth (Figure 6.8a). A very painful condition may result, depending on the length difference between upper and lower jaw, and the width of the lower jaw and inclination of the lower canines. Most of the time the lower canines will occlude with the palate (which can result in an oronasal fistula) (Figure 6.8b) or with the palatal or palatodistal side of the upper canine, leading to pathological attrition of the occluding teeth. This is one of the worst and most painful malocclusions seen in dogs and it should not be left untreated. Sometimes the mandibular canines occlude caudally to the maxillary canines, and in these animals the bite is functional and comfortable and treatment is not necessary.

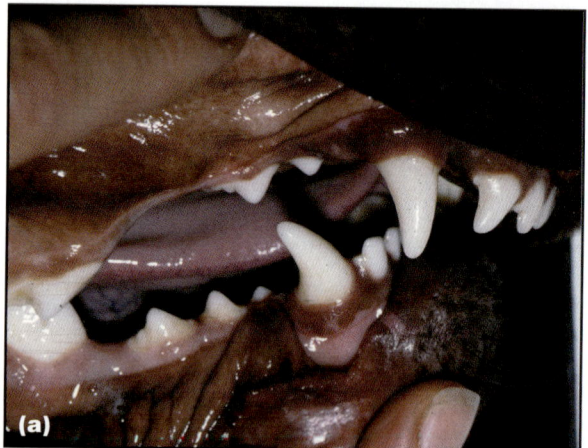

(a)

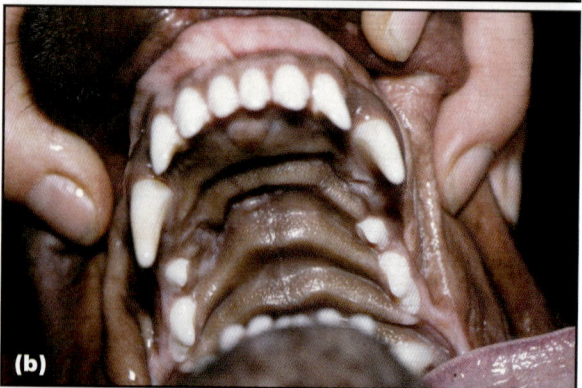

(b)

6.8 Labrador with a retrognathic mandible. The mandible is short compared with the maxilla, leading to a painful malocclusion. **(a)** There is major jaw discrepancy. In this Labrador both jaws are abnormal: there is excessive space between second and fourth premolars, indicating elongation of the maxilla; and there is insufficient space between mandibular third premolar and mandibular first molar to accommodate a (missing) fourth premolar, indicating jaw shortening. **(b)** A deep pit can be seen on the palate distal to the left upper canine tooth, caused by the crown tip of the maloccluding left mandibular canine. The right mandibular canine in this dog occluded distally to the maxillary canine, not causing any soft tissue injury. © Leen Verhaert.

Wry bite

Wry bite is the result of unequal arch development. In a mild form, a one-sided prognathic or retrognathic bite develops. In severe cases, the whole head may be asymmetrical, and the midline may be clearly deviated (Figure 6.9). Wry bite may be associated with an open bite (inability to bring the incisors into occlusal contact). Wry bite is a skeletal malocclusion of genetic or traumatic (usually early in life) origin.

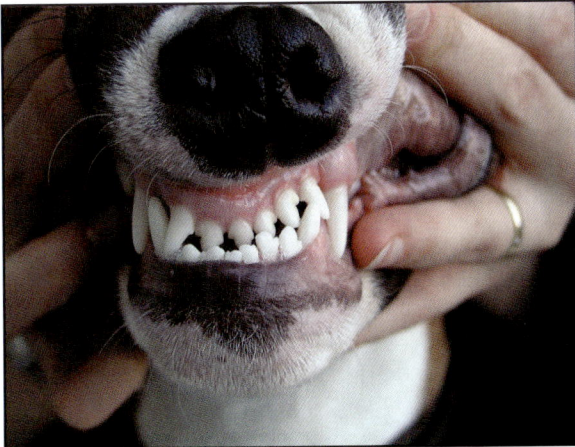

6.9 Wry bite, with clearly deviated midline. © Leen Verhaert.

Rostroversion/mesioversion of the upper canine tooth

Also known as lance or spear canine, this condition is seen mainly in toy and small breeds and is often associated with persistence of the deciduous canine teeth. A breed predisposition in Shetland Sheepdogs has been reported. Affected dogs should not be used for breeding.

The upper canine tooth is severely displaced rostrally, often hitting the upper third incisor tooth (Figure 6.10a). If left untreated, severe periodontal disease (due to plaque retention) and lip ulceration from pressure of the crown tip may result. Furthermore, the crown of the rostroverted upper canine occupies the diastema that is normally present between the upper canine and third incisor to accommodate the crown of the lower canine tooth. Therefore, the lower canine tooth will be pushed labially due to the occlusal force of the upper canine tooth (Figure 6.10b). This can lead to ulceration of the upper lip.

Linguoversion or lingual displacement of the lower canine tooth

This is a common malocclusion seen in a variety of breeds, often incorrectly named 'base narrow canines'. It may be due to a skeletal abnormality (micrognathia, narrow mandible) or to a dental abnormality (linguoversion of the lower canine). Persistent deciduous canines may cause linguoversion of the permanent canines.

When there is no jaw length discrepancy, the lower canine teeth may hit the palate or the diastema between the upper canine and third incisor teeth (Figure 6.11). In cases of a retrognathic mandible or micrognathic mandible, the canine teeth most often are also

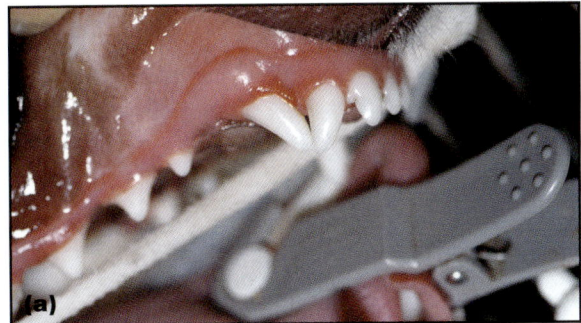

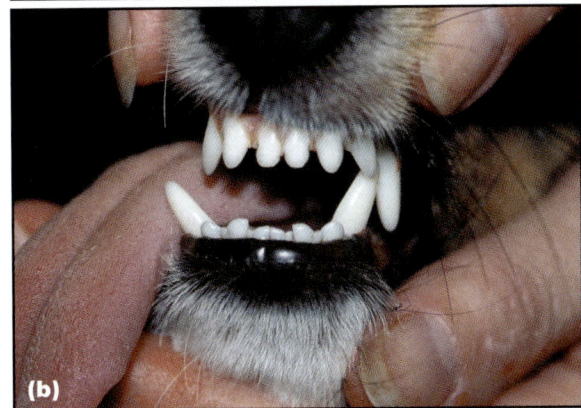

6.10 Rostroversion/mesioversion of upper canine tooth in a Shetland Sheepdog. **(a)** The upper canine tooth is rostrally deviated, hitting the upper third incisor. **(b)** The crown of the mesioverted tooth occupies the diastema that is normally present to accommodate the crown of the lower canine tooth, forcing the lower canine tooth labially. © Leen Verhaert.

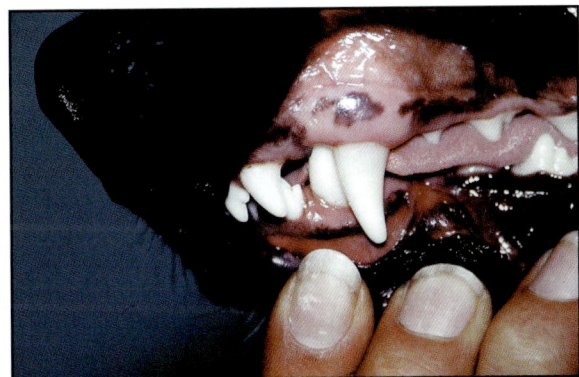

6.11 Linguoversion of mandibular canine tooth in a German Shepherd Dog. The left mandibular canine tooth occludes mesiopalatally to the maxillary canine, causing soft tissue trauma to the palatal mucosa. This condition should not be left untreated. In this particular dog it was corrected using the 'rubber ball' technique. © Leen Verhaert.

lingually displaced and may hit either the palate, which may lead to an oronasal fistula, or the palatal or palatodistal side of the upper canine teeth, leading to pathological attrition of the occluding teeth. This is a painful condition that should not be left untreated.

Tooth rotation and crowding

Individual teeth may be rotated. Rotation and crowding of premolars is an indication of jaw shortening. Supernumerary teeth may be rotated and cause crowding and may need to be extracted.

Treatment of malocclusions affecting the deciduous dentition

Deciduous teeth involved in a functional malocclusion should be extracted as early as possible, i.e. at 6–8 weeks of age. This is particularly true in cases of a retrognathic mandible or an excessively narrow mandible, where the deciduous lower canine teeth impinge on the palate, or the lower deciduous canines occlude caudal to the upper canines (Figure 6.12). Extracting maloccluding deciduous teeth before eruption of their permanent counterparts is termed interceptive orthodontics. By extracting the maloccluding lower deciduous canines, discomfort and possible pain are eliminated. Furthermore, extraction of the lower canines that may interfere with forward growth of the short mandible allows expression of the full genetic growth potential of the jaw (the development of dental interlock-induced malocclusion will thus be prevented). However, one should not expect a skeletal malocclusion in the deciduous dentition to be corrected by extraction of interfering teeth. In most cases the permanent teeth will show a similar malocclusion.

Extraction of deciduous canine teeth is not an easy procedure and should be done with great care. Deciduous teeth have long and narrow roots that fracture easily (the roots usually comprise two-thirds to three-quarters of the length of the tooth). Preoperative radiographs should be taken to assess the morphology of the deciduous teeth roots and to determine the position and stage of development of the permanent counterpart. An open (surgical) extraction technique is strongly recommended. The reader is referred to Chapter 11 for more information on open extraction techniques.

A common practice, unfortunately still used by breeders, is to cut the crowns of deciduous teeth with nail clippers, so that they will not interfere with jaw growth. This is malpractice and should never be done. It leads to pulp exposure, pulpitis and eventual pulp necrosis, which may affect the permanent tooth bud that develops in the region of the apex of the deciduous tooth. Possible consequences are enamel defects and even necrosis of the developing tooth (see 'Structural defects' later).

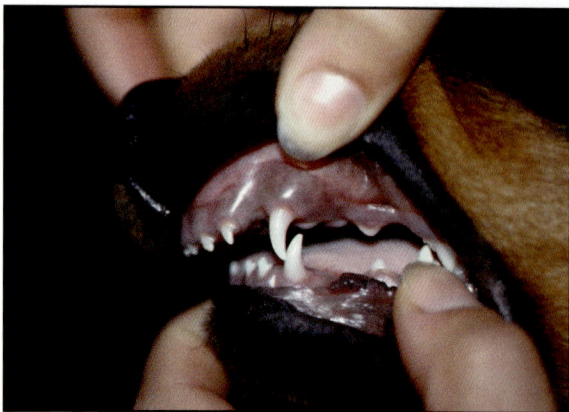

6.12 Retrognathic mandible in a 7-week-old puppy. The lower deciduous canines impinge on the palate distal to the upper deciduous canines. The maloccluding deciduous teeth should be extracted to eliminate pain and discomfort (interceptive orthodontics), and to prevent dental interlock-induced malocclusion. © Leen Verhaert.

Furthermore, a necrotic deciduous canine may be the portal of entry for tetanus spores. Many dogs affected by tetanus have a fractured, necrotic deciduous tooth as the portal of entry of the disease.

Treatment of malocclusions affecting the permanent dentition

Ethical considerations

Only those malocclusions causing discomfort, pain or any associated oral pathology should be treated. Treatment options include extraction, crown shortening or orthodontics. In many instances extraction or crown shortening is preferable to orthodontics.

When a skeletal malocclusion is diagnosed, and a developmental cause for the malocclusion cannot be reliably identified, the condition is considered to be at least in part hereditary. In human orthodontics, whether a malocclusion is genetic or acquired will not influence treatment planning. This is in contrast with veterinary orthodontics, where aesthetics and ethics are directly linked. The aim of any treatment is to make the animal comfortable, and the bite functional. Cosmetic considerations should not play a role. Inherited malocclusions in dogs and cats should not be orthodontically corrected to a perfectly normal occlusion, unless the animal is neutered. This will avoid propagation of the malocclusion in the breed. If treatment is necessary for the welfare of the animal, either a non-conservative treatment method should be chosen (such as extraction or crown reduction), or one may opt for imperfect correction so that the animal cannot be shown. In any case, genetic counselling is of major importance.

Principles of orthodontic movement

Orthodontic movement of teeth can be described as movement as a result of prolonged application of pressure to a tooth. This will result in remodelling of the bone surrounding the tooth. Bone is resorbed at the compression side and new bone is formed at the tension side. Bone lysis will occur more rapidly than bone formation, therefore a retention time to keep the tooth in the new position is usually necessary.

The optimal force is the force that will move the tooth most rapidly into the desired position with the least tissue damage and the least discomfort. Magnitude of force, distribution of force and duration of force are important factors that need to be considered. The ideal force is one that is light and continuous. Heavy continuous force is the most damaging to the tooth and its supporting tissues and should not be used. It may lead to pulpal disruption, tooth root resorption, ankylosis of the tooth and possibly even avulsion of the tooth (i.e. the tooth may be pulled out of the alveolus).

Certain teeth can be used as anchorage to move other teeth. It is important to realise that the total root surface area of the anchoring teeth should be larger than the root surface area of the tooth that needs to be moved. It may be necessary to include more than one tooth in the anchorage unit to avoid movement of the anchor.

Patients that need orthodontic treatment should be referred to someone with expertise in orthodontics; therefore, most orthodontic treatment options will only be outlined here. Only one relatively new technique, the 'rubber ball' technique for correction of lingually displaced mandibular canine teeth, will be described in detail (Verhaert, 1999).

Rostral cross bite

Rostral cross bite does not usually cause functional problems in dogs and cats. The abnormal occlusal contact may cause trauma to the teeth or the mucosa lingual to the lower incisors, and in these cases crown reduction or extraction of some teeth may be indicated. Orthodontic treatment of rostral cross bite is rarely indicated except for correction of a cosmetic defect. This is to be considered unethical.

Prognathic mandible and retrognathic maxilla

Treatment is indicated in those cases where the lower canines force the upper third incisors into an abnormal, uncomfortable position. The most sensible approach is to extract the smallest of the maloccluding teeth, i.e. the third incisor(s).

In brachycephalic cats, the lower canines may traumatize the upper lip. The best option in these cases is surgical crown reduction of the mandibular canine(s).

In cases of major jaw length difference, treatment is usually unnecessary. Techniques have been described to shorten the mandible by cutting away part of the jaw, but these are inhumane and should not be used.

Rostroversion/mesioversion of the upper canine tooth

Treatment options include:

- Extraction of the affected tooth
- Orthodontic correction with power chain.

Rostrally displaced maxillary canines are usually moved using orthodontic brackets or buttons and an elastic chain. Use of multiple anchor points is recommended to reduce the risk of movement of the anchor tooth. Affected animals should not be used for breeding, and neutering of those animals is highly recommended.

Linguoversion or lingual displacement of the lower canine tooth

Surgical/non-surgical crown shortening: Non-surgical crown reduction consists of crown shortening without exposing the pulp. When the trauma to the palate is only minor, this is a valid treatment option. After crown reduction, the dentinal tubules should be sealed to avoid inflammation of the pulp.

Surgical crown reduction consists of crown shortening, partial pulpectomy, pulp capping and surface restoration of the mandibular canines. These teeth will usually require standard root canal treatment at a later date, and should be radiographically monitored in the long term. This treatment should be left to someone skilled in veterinary dentistry, with expertise in endodontics. Crown shortening of the mandibular canines is the most valid treatment option if major jaw discrepancy exists, though extraction of these teeth is another option.

Orthodontic correction: Several orthodontic treatment modalities are available for correction of lingually deviated or displaced mandibular canines. The most widely used technique is the use of inclined planes placed in the maxilla. These appliances are available in different forms: direct acrylic inclined plane, indirect acrylic or a metal inclined plane. In young, growing dogs the use of a telescoping inclined plane is preferable, to overcome the problem of jaw growth inhibition by fixed appliances. All these appliances are functional devices that rely on the dog actively closing its mouth. Active devices that are placed in the mandible are also used. Examples are the expansion screw, W-wire and the modified quad-helix appliances.

Removable orthodontic device ('rubber ball' technique): In properly selected cases (young dogs with no major jaw discrepancies) the 'rubber ball' technique (Verhaert, 1999) has a high success rate, with correction of the malocclusion within 4 weeks in most cases. This often eliminates the need for more complex orthodontic techniques involving multiple anaesthetics. A beneficial side effect of the technique is the strong bond that is usually formed between owner and animal during the course of treatment.

This technique for correcting uncomplicated cases of lingually displaced/deviated mandibular canines involves stimulating the dog to play, as often as possible, with specific rubber toys of correct size and shape (Figure 6.13). Accurate diagnosis is critical for successful treatment. No major jaw discrepancy should be present. The diastema between the maxillary third incisor and canine should be wide enough to accommodate the mandibular canine tooth. The idea behind the technique is that the act of playing and chewing on a suitable object might force the teeth into a more appropriate position (mimicking a fixed orthodontic device).

The most appropriate objects for this technique are toys with a round or conical shape (e.g. a ball or a rubber toy). Ropes or handles should not be present when the toy is used for the specific purpose of moving the canines; dogs tend to pick up toys the easiest way, e.g. by the rope if it is present.

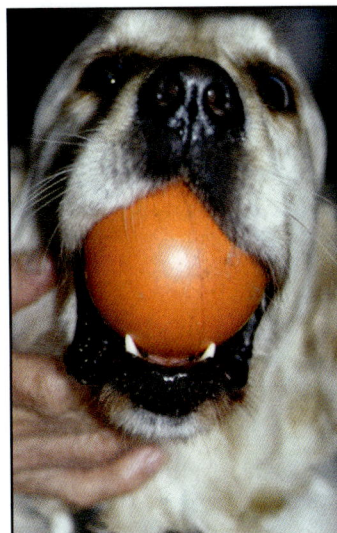

6.13 'Rubber ball' technique for correction of lingually displaced mandibular canine teeth. The correct size of toy is larger than the distance between the mandibular canine teeth, so that is applies lateral pressure while the dog plays. This is illustrated in this photograph of the true inventor of the technique – the author's Golden Retriever. © Leen Verhaert.

The toy size is important. Too small a toy will not make contact with both mandibular canines at the same time and also might be held too caudal in the mouth, not touching the canine teeth at all. Too large a toy might cause intrusive rather than lateral tipping pressure and might be uncomfortable for the dog. A toy of the correct size sits between and just behind the canine teeth and is larger than the distance between the mandibular canine teeth, principally applying laterally directed pressure to the teeth while the dog plays (see Figure 6.13). As a guideline: for small dogs the ball should have a diameter of 4 cm, for larger dog breeds 6–8 cm and for giant breeds more than 8 cm.

The composition and consistency of the object are important. The toy should be made of hard rubber, with just a little give. Too soft a toy is unlikely to apply enough pressure and would be rapidly destroyed by chewing. Toys that are too hard or abrasive could damage the teeth. The toy should have a smooth surface to avoid excessive tooth wear (abrasion).

Active play for 15 minutes three times a day is the recommended minimum, but longer and more frequent episodes are preferable. The owner is advised to play with the dog as often as possible, and to take away all other toys. Assuming a one-week learning phase before the treatment becomes effective, two further weeks are needed before any benefit from the treatment is likely to be seen. Occlusion is checked after 3 weeks, and then monthly as necessary. If no movement is seen after 3 weeks, other treatment methods should be considered.

This technique works best in dogs younger than 7 months of age, and the most rapid correction of malocclusion is seen when the teeth are not yet fully erupted. The major advantages of the technique are that it is best used at an age when a fixed appliance is not indicated, it is inexpensive and it has not shown any side effects in a large series of patients.

It is advisable to obtain full pre- and post-treatment impressions and radiographs, as with any orthodontic technique, but most owners do not want their dogs to be anaesthetized just for that. As a compromise, hard wax bite registration wafers can be used to record crown tip positions in most conscious dogs. Photographs should be taken to record the degree of malocclusion, taking a rostral, left and right view of each case. Although this technique is not invasive, genetic counselling in cases needing this kind of treatment should not be overlooked.

Complications of orthodontic treatment

Orthodontic treatment can have a variety of deleterious effects.

- Soft tissue trauma may result from pressure of the device, especially if it is poorly designed. Good oral hygiene is essential. The procedure should not be initiated if the owner is not willing to perform meticulous daily plaque control while the device is in the animal's mouth.
- Use of a high continuous force may lead to pulpal disruption, resulting in pulp necrosis, and should therefore be avoided.
- Use of too high forces may also lead to root resorption and tooth ankylosis. Even with slight forces, root resorption and tooth ankylosis cannot always be avoided. In one study in humans, 28.8% of orthodontically treated incisors showed root resorption after treatment (Trope and Chivian, 1994).
- Orthodontic treatment may result in abnormal displacement of teeth (e.g. movement of anchorage teeth, over-correction of target teeth). High continuous forces may even lead to avulsion of anchorage or target teeth. Tissue necrosis may be such that the tooth is no longer attached in the alveolus and can be simply pulled out of the socket.
- Discomfort and pain have been reported in humans. Therefore, it is likely that dogs and cats treated with a fixed appliance may experience discomfort and pain as well.

Developmental disorders of teeth

Developmental dental disorders may be due to abnormalities in the differentiation of the dental lamina and the tooth germs leading to anomalies in number, size or shape, or due to abnormalities in the formation of the dental hard tissues leading to anomalies in structure.

Developmental dental disturbances may be inherited, but they may also be acquired or idiopathic. They may be congenital (i.e. present at birth) but may also occur later on, during the formative stage of the teeth (up to 4 months of age).

Variation in number

Decrease: anodontia, oligodontia and hypodontia

Anodontia (congenital absence of teeth) and *oligodontia* (only a few teeth present) are rare conditions, often associated with generalized disorders. *Hypodontia* (one or a few teeth missing) is a common condition. An example of a systemic disorder associated with hypodontia/oligodontia in the permanent dentition is ectodermal dysplasia in the hairless breeds, such as the Chinese Crested Dog (Figure 6.14).

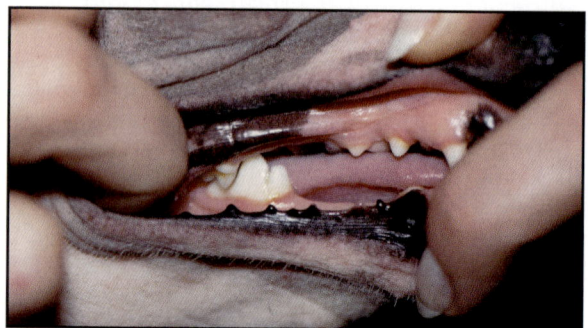

6.14 Chinese Crested Dog with a 'normal' dentition for this breed. Due to the ectodermal dysplasia that causes the specific skin characteristics, most of the premolar teeth are missing. Note that the second upper premolar is a deciduous tooth that is still present due to absence of the permanent counterpart. © Leen Verhaert.

Hereditary factors are often involved in the congenital absence of teeth, but teeth can also be missing as a result of disturbances during the initial development phase as a result of trauma or infection.

Hypodontia in the permanent dentition is more frequent than in the deciduous dentition. When a deciduous tooth is congenitally missing, its permanent successor is usually missing too, though not necessarily (Nik Noriah Nik-Hussein and Zubaidah Abdul Majid, 1996). Premolars and incisors are the most frequently affected teeth.

Clinical significance and treatment: Radiography is essential to differentiate missing teeth from impacted and embedded teeth. Hypodontia is mainly a cosmetic issue. Differentiation between possible hereditary and proven traumatic causes is important for breeding dogs.

Increase: supernumerary teeth and hyperdontia
Extra teeth can occur in the deciduous and/or the permanent dentition. Supernumerary teeth may be inherited, but this condition can also be caused by disturbances during tooth development. They are more prevalent in the incisor and premolar region. Additional incisor teeth are common in brachycephalic breeds. Supernumerary teeth can, but do not necessarily, have a normal shape and size.

Clinical significance and treatment: Supernumerary teeth may cause disturbances in eruption, crowding and deviation of adjacent teeth (Figure 6.15). In addition, crowded teeth may accumulate more plaque, predisposing them to periodontal disease. In these cases extraction needs to be considered. The tooth that is most abnormal in size, shape or position is usually the one to be extracted. Radiographs are mandatory before extraction of any of these teeth. When the condition does not cause clinical problems, treatment is unnecessary. The owner needs to be advised of the possible heritability of the disorder.

Alteration in size
Alterations in the size of teeth are of limited clinical importance in dogs and cats.

- *Macrodont* teeth are those that are larger than normal.
- *Microdont* teeth are those that are smaller than normal.
- *Peg* teeth are small, conical-shaped teeth.

Teeth present in dogs with ectodermal dysplasia are often small and of simple conical shape. Sometimes supernumerary teeth are smaller than normal. Alterations in tooth size are usually only cosmetic problems, although a macrodont tooth may need to be extracted because of interference with a comfortable occlusion.

Alteration in shape

Gemination, fusion and concrescence
Gemination is defined as an attempt to make two teeth from one enamel organ. In single-rooted teeth, the result is a structure with two completely or incompletely separated crowns with a single root and root canal. In two-rooted teeth, the resulting structure will have two crowns (completely or incompletely separated) and

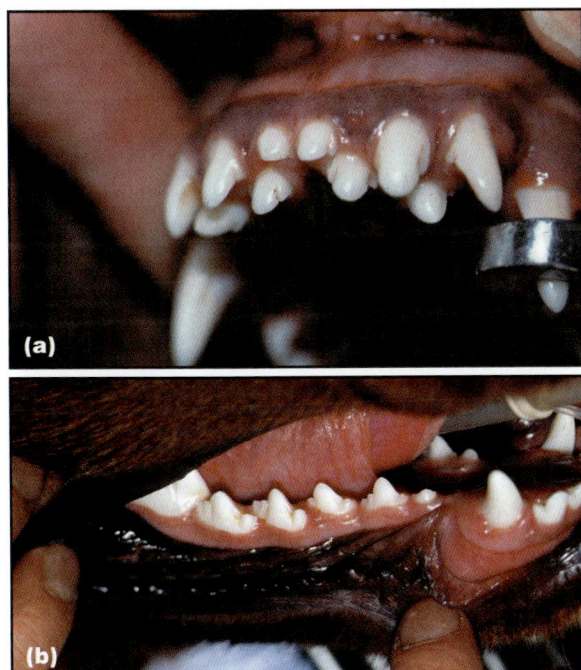

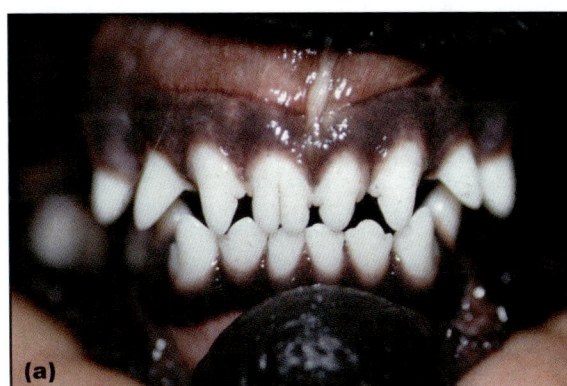

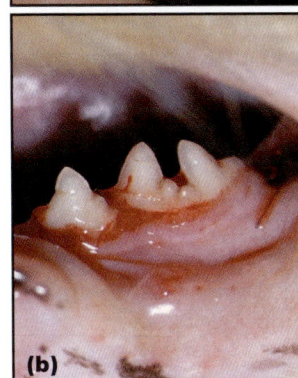

6.15 Supernumerary teeth commonly cause crowding and malocclusion. **(a)** Crowded supernumerary incisors in a Rottweiler. This particular dog had ten upper and eight lower incisors and a supernumerary upper first premolar. **(b)** Supernumerary premolars in an Irish Setter. The premolars are rotated due to lack of space. Several related Irish Setters have been presented with this condition, suggesting a hereditary aetiology in this case. © Leen Verhaert.

6.16 Gemination and fusion. **(a)** Gemination of an upper incisor in a dog, resulting in a longitudinal groove in the crown. **(b)** Gemination of a lower fourth premolar, or fusion between a lower fourth premolar and a supernumerary fourth premolar, in a cat. The resulting structure had three roots. © Leen Verhaert.

three roots (Figure 6.16). Occasionally complete cleavage or twinning is seen (two teeth from one enamel organ). Gemination is seen most often in the incisor region. The aetiology is unknown, but trauma has been suggested as a possible cause, as has a familial tendency. Gemination is seen in the deciduous as well as permanent dentition.

Fusion is the joining of two tooth germs, resulting in a single large tooth. Fusion may involve the entire length of the teeth, or only the roots, depending on the stage of development of the teeth at the time of the union. The root canal can be shared or separate. The aetiology is unknown, but trauma and a familial tendency have both been suggested as possible causes. Fusion is seen in the deciduous as well as permanent dentition. It may be difficult or even impossible to differentiate fusion of supernumerary teeth from gemination.

Concrescence is the fusion of adjacent already formed teeth by cementum. It may take place before or after eruption. It is thought to arise from trauma or crowding of teeth.

Clinical significance and treatment: Gemination, fusion and concrescence usually do not require treatment. When they do need treatment (e.g. for periodontal or endodontic disease), preoperative radiography for planning of treatment is essential. Geminated or fused teeth may have a different number of roots and root canals than expected.

Dilaceration

Dilaceration refers to a sharp bend, curve or angulation in the root or crown of a tooth. The cause is usually acute mechanical trauma during the development of the tooth. The trauma may change the position of the already mineralized portion of the tooth, and the remainder is then formed at an angle. The curve or bend may occur anywhere along the length of the tooth. Hereditary factors are thought to be involved in only a small number of cases.

Clinical significance and treatment: A dilacerated crown may be an aesthetic problem. Often the surface of a dilacerated crown is irregular, leading to a highly plaque-retentive surface. Extraction or endodontic treatment may be difficult in the case of a dilacerated root, hence the need for radiography before extraction of any tooth. Severely dilacerated teeth may be unable to erupt (Figure 6.17).

Dens invaginatus (*dens in dente*, 'tooth within a tooth')

Dens in dente is an uncommon tooth anomaly, with only a few cases described in the veterinary literature. It represents an invagination of enamel and dentine from the tooth surface. This invagination can be superficial (crown) to deep (crown and root). The aetiology of the condition is unknown. In humans, the mild form is fairly common (up to 5%). The clinical significance of *dens in dente* depends on the severity of the lesion, varying from higher caries susceptibility to pulpal necrosis and periapical inflammation.

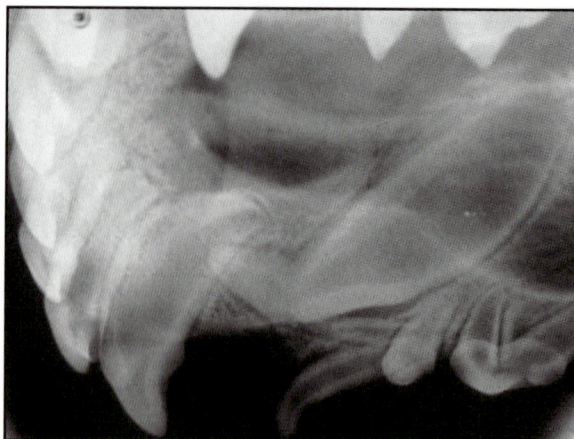

6.17 Dilaceration of the crown of the left upper canine tooth. Due to the position of the angulated crown tip, the tooth was unable to erupt. © Leen Verhaert.

Supernumerary roots

Accessory tooth roots can be seen in dogs and cats. In the dog, the upper third premolar is most commonly involved (Figure 6.18). In the cat, accessory tooth roots are seen most frequently in the upper second (9%) and third (10%) premolars (Verstraete and Terpak, 1997). Radiographic recognition of supernumerary roots is very important when endodontic treatment or extraction of the involved tooth is necessary.

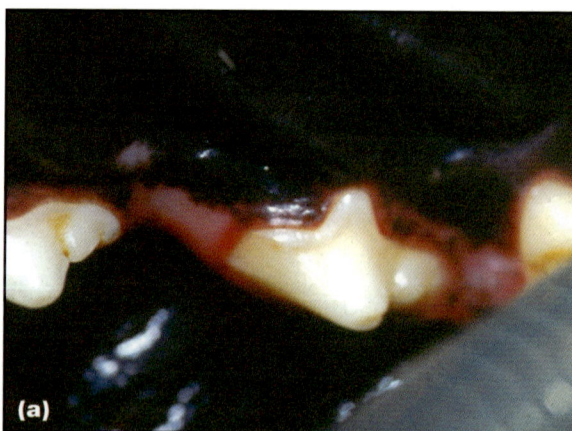

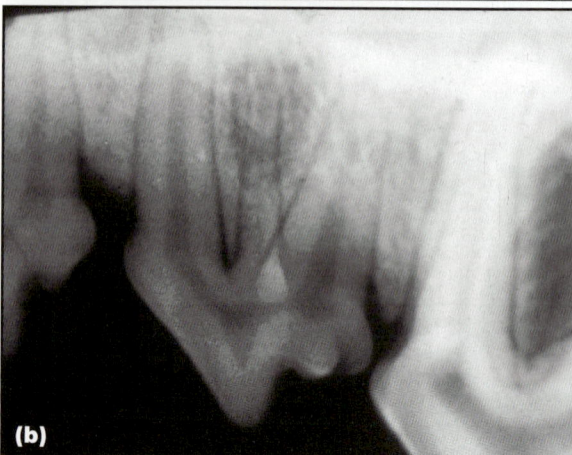

6.18 Upper third premolar in a dog with a supernumerary (palatal) root. **(a)** Clinical view. **(b)** Radiographic view. © Leen Verhaert.

Enamel pearls (enamel drops)

Enamel pearls are small foci of excessive enamel on the surface of the tooth apical to the cementoenamel junction. They occur most frequently in the bifurcation or trifurcation area of the tooth. Occasionally the enamel pearl is supported by dentine, and very rarely a pulp horn extends into it. Clinically these are only significant when located in a periodontally diseased area, since there is no periodontal attachment to enamel pearls.

Other shape defects

Other defects may regularly be seen. The clinical importance of any defect varies from insignificant and mainly cosmetic, to extremely significant leading to pulp necrosis and tooth abscess. Since developmental dental disturbances are regularly seen, and may very well be hardly recognizable during clinical examination, radiographs in dentistry are of utmost importance. Only radiographs will inform the clinician of the true nature of the tooth and its root.

Structural defects in the enamel

Amelogenesis imperfecta

Amelogenesis imperfecta is a hereditary form of enamel defect that affects both dentitions. The incidence in dogs and cats is unknown. Three types have been described in human dentistry: enamel hypoplasia, enamel hypocalcification and enamel hypomaturation. In the hypoplastic type, teeth erupt with insufficient amounts of enamel, ranging from pits and grooves in the surface to complete absence or aplasia of enamel. In the hypocalcified type, the enamel is present but it is soft and friable so that it fractures and wears readily. The teeth tend to darken with age due to exogenous staining.

Genetic factors act more or less strongly throughout the whole duration of amelogenesis. Characteristically, therefore, all the teeth may be affected and defects involve a large part of the enamel, or are randomly distributed throughout the enamel. In contrast, exogenous factors affecting enamel formation

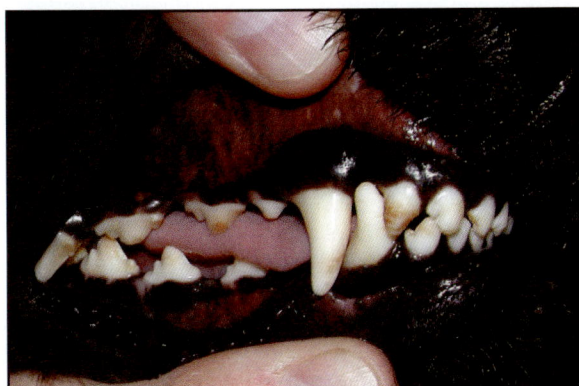

6.19 Standard Poodle with enamel defects on all teeth. Although enamel is present, it is soft and friable. It takes up pigments (brown discoloration) and chips off readily with normal mastication (crown tip has lost the enamel on several teeth). In this animal, histological examination of the deciduous teeth was indicative of amelogenesis imperfecta. Three other related Standard Poodles were presented with similar defects. © Leen Verhaert.

tend to act only for a short time and leave a pattern of defects only in that part of the enamel formed during the course of the disease.

A form of amelogenesis imperfecta was strongly suspected in a series of four related Standard Poodles (Verhaert, 2002) (Figure 6.19).

Environmental: hypoplasia, hypocalcification and hypomaturation

Environmental enamel defects are a common structural defect seen in dogs' teeth, but they are extremely rare in the cat. Enamel defects occur as a result of injury during the formative stage of enamel development (up to 4 months of age); once the enamel has mineralized, no such defect can be produced.

Enamel develops in two stages: a secretory stage (matrix production and early mineralization) and a maturation stage (increase in mineral content by withdrawal of water and protein). In enamel hypoplasia, the enamel is quantitatively defective (i.e. insufficient amount but with normal hardness, the disturbance affecting matrix formation). Qualitatively defective enamel (normal amount but hypomineralized, the disturbance affecting initial mineralization and maturation) is referred to as enamel hypocalcification. Some disturbances affect both matrix formation and mineralization.

The extent of the defect(s) depends on the intensity of the aetiological factor, the duration of the factor's presence and the stage at which the factor occurs during tooth development. Any serious nutritional deficiency or systemic disease is potentially capable of producing enamel dysplasia in the areas of the teeth that are being formed at that time. Aetiological factors may occur locally or systemically, and examples include:

- Vitamin deficiencies (vitamin A, vitamin D or rickets)
- Epitheliotropic viruses (e.g. distemper virus)
- Hypocalcaemia
- Excessive fluoride ingestion
- Local infection, local trauma.

Trauma to the deciduous tooth (luxation, complicated fracture with subsequent inflammation at the root apex) and imprudent extraction technique when removing a deciduous tooth in a young puppy are well known causes of localized enamel dysplasia. Sometimes no apparent cause can be identified (idiopathic).

Clinical presentation varies. In a mild form, one or a few small grooves, pits or fissures are seen on the tooth surface. In more severe generalized forms, horizontally arranged rows of deep pits may be seen across the tooth surface (Figure 6.20). In localized forms, a part of the crown may have no enamel at all, or have defective, brittle enamel (Figure 6.21ab). In all cases, tooth colour may vary from white opaque to yellow to brown. Teeth with enamel dysplasia may appear normal at the time of tooth eruption. With time they become discoloured, as the porous enamel absorbs pigments, or the defective enamel flakes off with use.

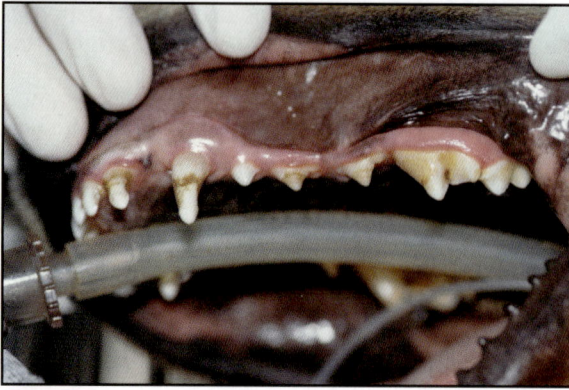

6.20 Environmental enamel dysplasia (generalized). This type of enamel dysplasia is likely to be caused by systemic factors during enamel development. © Leen Verhaert.

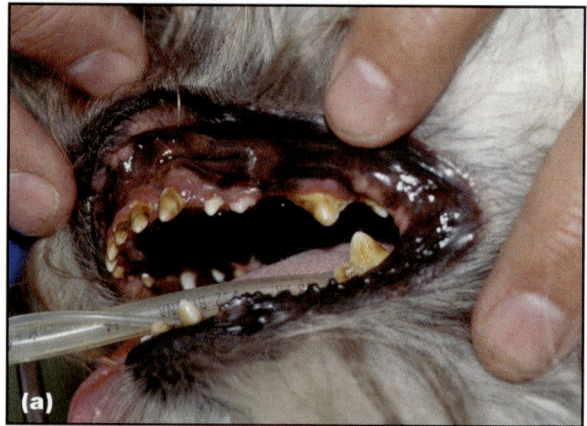

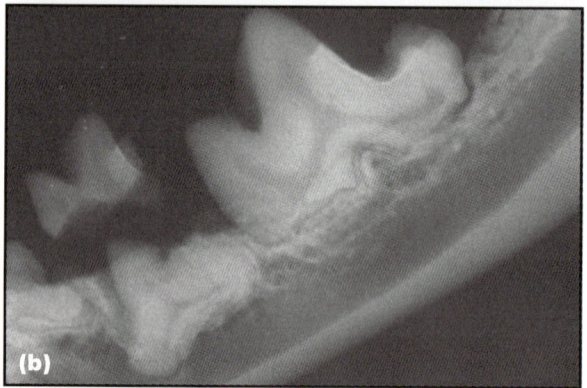

6.21 Environmental enamel dysplasia (localized). **(a)** Enamel hypoplasia. The enamel is missing at the middle third of the crown of the upper canine tooth. The enamel that is present is of normal hardness and colour. **(b)** Enamel hypocalcification. The enamel is soft and friable, takes up pigments (brown discoloration) and flakes off with normal use. © Leen Verhaert.

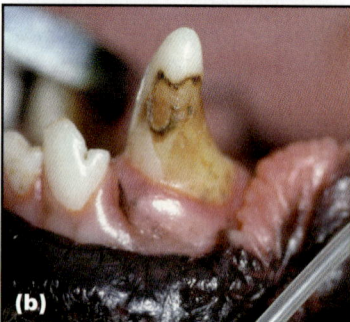

6.22 One-year-old mongrel dog with multiple developmental dental disorders as a result of distemper virus infection at the age of 6 weeks. **(a)** Generalized enamel dysplasia, with brown discoloration of most teeth and short canine tooth crowns. Note that the first premolars and persistent deciduous second premolar are unaffected, because these teeth were not actively developing enamel at the time of the systemic disease. **(b)** Radiographic appearance. Root abnormalities are obvious; the roots are short and blunt and in some teeth virtually absent. © Leen Verhaert.

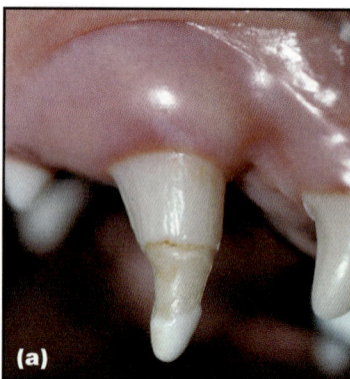

Severely affected teeth may show root abnormalities as a result of abnormalities in Hertwig's root sheath (Hertwig's root sheath comprises the cells of the inner and outer enamel epithelium and directs root formation). An example is shown in Figure 6.22, and similar cases were described by Arnbjerg (1986) and Bittegeko *et al.* (1995). All these cases were related to distemper virus infection.

Clinical significance and treatment of enamel defects

Poorly protected or exposed dentine is painful due to the existence of dentinal tubules, which contain odontoblastic processes, nerve fibrils, collagen and a complex matrix. With time, sensitivity will disappear as a result of reparative dentine laid down by a healthy pulp. However, in severe cases the pulp may become chronically inflamed from infection via the poorly protected or exposed dentine tubules and be unable to lay down reparative dentine. Periapical disease may develop.

Therefore, radiographic examination of all teeth affected by enamel defects is indicated, and should be repeated at regular intervals throughout the animal's life to detect complications such as periapical disease.

Treatment options include restoration of the defect (in localized forms) and sealing of the dentine tubules to protect the pulp. Since affected teeth have a very irregular, plaque-retentive surface, good oral home care (daily tooth brushing) is very important. Teeth affected by periapical pathology need more extensive treatment, i.e. extraction or endodontic treatment.

Topical fluoride application may be useful in cases where enamel is still present: fluoride will enhance enamel mineralization and will make it more resistant to acid dissolution. Topical fluoride application can also reduce dentine sensitivity. Care should be taken with the use of fluoride as it is toxic on ingestion. Daily use in animals (e.g. in toothpaste) is not recommended.

When scaling severely affected teeth it is safer to use hand instruments than sonic/ultrasonic equipment. Hypocalcified enamel may be so soft that it is easily removed by power scalers. Furthermore, power scalers may cause thermal damage to the less protected pulp.

Other structural defects

Very few reports exist in veterinary literature regarding dentine defects. The inherited conditions dentinogenesis imperfecta (hereditary opalescent dentine) and dentinal dysplasia are described in human literature. Dentine hypocalcification has the same causes as environmental enamel defects, and can only be detected by histological examination (presence of globular dentine).

Regional odontodysplasia affects both dentine and enamel, and has been described in the dog. One or several teeth in a localized area are affected, and are described as 'ghost teeth' (Figure 6.23). Affected teeth have an abnormal structure, with very thin enamel and dentine, which shows defective mineralization. The cause is unknown, though numerous aetiological factors have been suggested. Because of the poor quality of affected teeth, extraction is the treatment of choice.

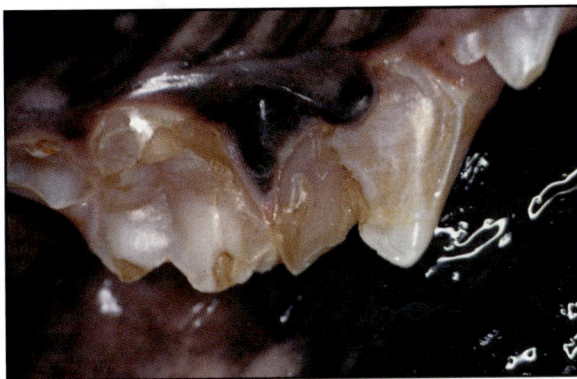

6.23 Regional odontodysplasia ('ghost teeth'). Although the shape of the teeth is normal in this case, enamel and dentine are thin and the pulp can be seen shining through. The enamel flakes off with normal mastication and the teeth fracture readily due to poor quality. Extraction of affected teeth is the treatment of choice. (Courtesy of David A. Crossley.)

Disorders of eruption and shedding

Persistent deciduous teeth

Persistent deciduous teeth, i.e. deciduous teeth that are still present when their permanent counterparts are erupting, are very common in toy and small dog breeds. The condition is likely to be inherited, at least in some breeds.

Persistent deciduous teeth are associated with permanent tooth malposition (Figure 6.24). In general, the maxillary permanent canine tooth will erupt rostrally to the deciduous canine. The mandibular permanent canine will erupt lingually to the deciduous canine. The permanent incisors will erupt lingually/palatally to the deciduous incisors.

Persistent deciduous teeth may cause or aggravate malocclusion and promote periodontal disease due to crowding, and should therefore be extracted. Whenever a deciduous and a permanent tooth of the same type are present at the same time at the same location, the deciduous tooth should be extracted as soon as possible.

Extraction of deciduous teeth should be done with extreme care, as they have long and narrow roots that

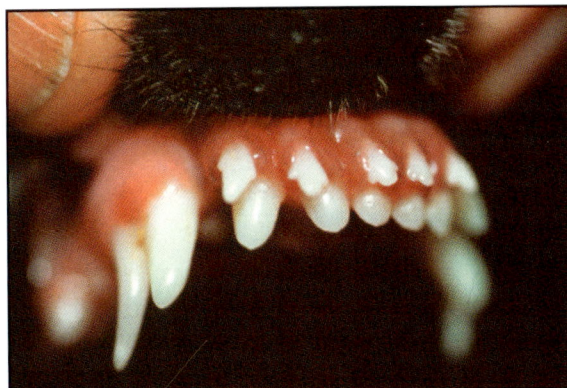

6.24 Yorkshire Terrier with persistent deciduous teeth. The permanent incisors have erupted palatally to the deciduous teeth. The permanent upper canine tooth has erupted mesially to the deciduous tooth. This particular dog had 17 persistent deciduous teeth. © Leen Verhaert.

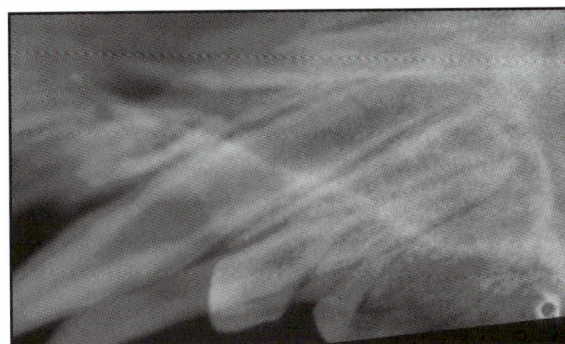

6.25 Radiographic view of a persistent maxillary deciduous canine tooth. The deciduous tooth is distal to the permanent tooth. The root is long and narrow and will fracture easily if the extraction is not done with extreme care. An open extraction technique is highly recommended. © Leen Verhaert.

fracture easily (Figure 6.25). An open (surgical) extraction technique is indicated for deciduous canine teeth (see Chapter 11).

Impacted and embedded teeth

An impacted tooth is one that fails to erupt into its normal position because of some physical barrier in the eruption path (usually another tooth). Generally this is an acquired condition but it can be genetic. Impaction can be caused by trauma or simply because the tooth's position in the alveolus is abnormal, so that it is unable to erupt into its normal position. A tooth with a severely dilacerated crown may be unable to erupt.

Embedded teeth are those that are unerupted because of some failure of the normal eruption mechanism (Figure 6.26).

Clinical significance and treatment: Impacted and embedded teeth need to be differentiated from missing teeth. Radiographs are therefore indicated when a tooth is clinically missing. Impacted teeth may cause resorption of the roots of adjacent teeth. In humans, periodic pain due to tooth impaction has been described. A dentigerous cyst may develop around the coronal portion of the tooth, and when left untreated such a cyst may become extensive, resulting in

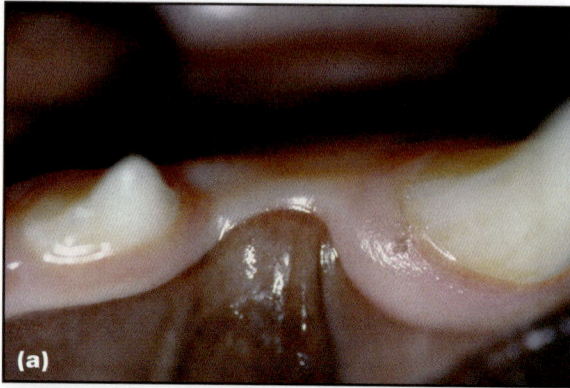

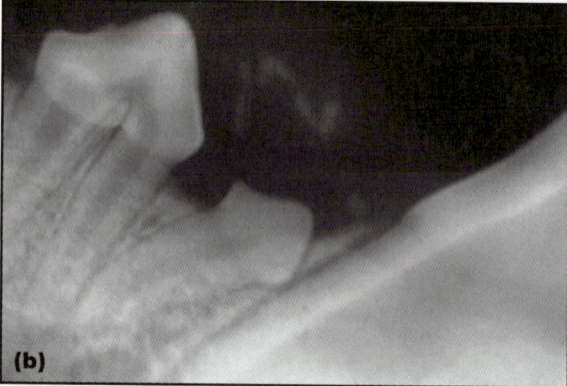

6.26 Unerupted first premolar. **(a)** The crown of the lower first premolar appears to be missing on clinical examination. **(b)** Radiographic examination shows the unerupted lower first premolar. © Leen Verhaert.

resorption of bone and tooth roots (Figure 6.27). On rare occasions, an ameloblastoma or squamous cell carcinoma may arise from the lining of a dentigerous cyst (Neville *et al.*, 2002). For these reasons, impacted and embedded teeth should be treated or at least radiographically monitored on a regular basis.

Depending on the presenting problem, treatment may consist of removing the overlying gingival tissue (operculectomy) or extraction of the tooth. When the tooth crown is covered only by gingival tissue, and no other physical barrier is present, a condition that is

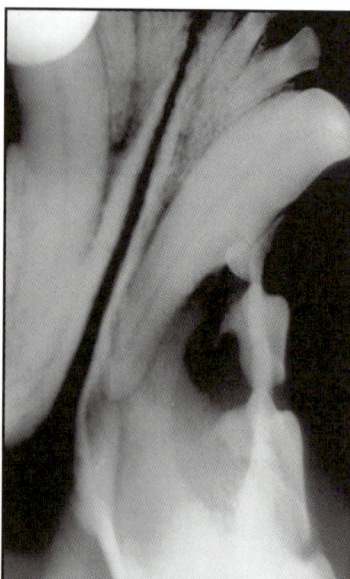

6.27 Large dentigerous cyst in a Boxer, caused by an unerupted lower first premolar. The dog was presented because of pink discoloration of the lower canine. Radiographic examination revealed extensive resorption affecting the bone and the roots of the canine and first, second and third premolar teeth.
© Leen Verhaert.

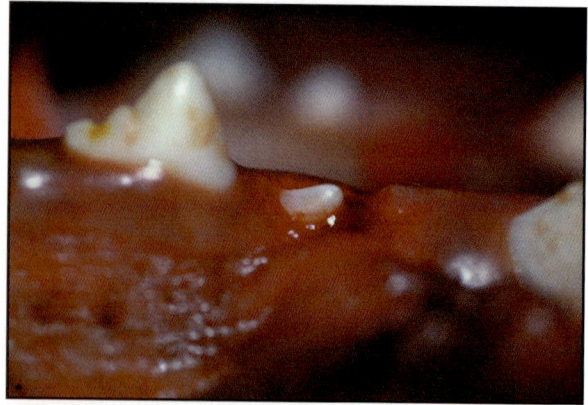

6.28 Operculectomy of a lower first premolar. An elliptical incision is made around the unerupted crown, and the overlying gingival tissue is removed. This will usually result in further eruption of the tooth. © Leen Verhaert.

often seen in unerupted first premolars, simply excising the overlying tissue will in most cases lead to eruption of the tooth (Figure 6.28). When the tooth is covered by a considerable amount of bone, or where there is crown or root deformation, extraction of the tooth is usually indicated.

Ectopic teeth

An ectopic tooth is one in an abnormal position (Figure 6.29). In some cases, this can lead to a severe malocclusion and an animal with an uncomfortable bite. In these cases, extraction is the treatment of choice.

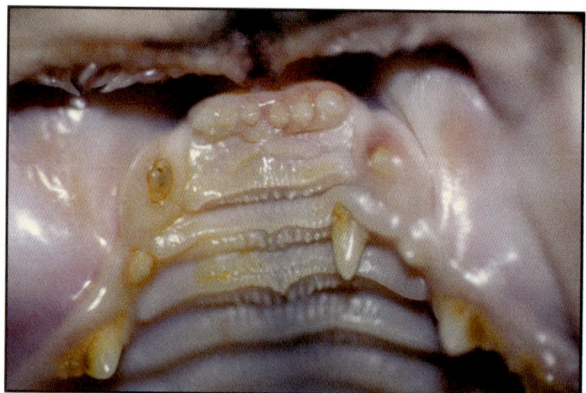

6.29 Ectopic maxillary canine tooth in a Persian cat. Note that the maxillary deciduous canines were clipped by the breeder to cover up a malocclusion. Both deciduous canine roots and the ectopic upper left permanent canine were extracted. The upper right permanent canine tooth was missing. © Leen Verhaert.

Developmental defects of the jaws

Cleft palate

Congenital cleft of the palate has been reported in both the dog and the cat and may be associated with other defects. Cleft palate is a descriptive term that refers to full-thickness longitudinal defects of the primary or secondary palate. It can be inherited or can result from an insult (nutritional, hormonal, mechanical or toxic) during the critical stage of fetal development when the

Chapter 6 Developmental oral and dental conditions

two palatine shelves fuse, thereby separating the oral and nasal cavities (in dogs 25 to 28 days gestation). A wide variety of dog and cat breeds are affected sporadically, suggesting that non-genetic causes are more common than genetic causes. Uncontrolled diabetes mellitus, folic acid deficiency and administration of certain drugs during pregnancy may result in cleft palate with or without other congenital defects. Examples of these drugs are: steroids, vitamin A, griseofulvin, antimitotic drugs (Waldron and Martin, 1991; Hennet, 1996). Broad-headed fetuses have a greater tendency to be affected by nutritional, hormonal and toxic factors. The incidence of cleft palate is higher in brachycephalic breeds, but other breeds are also affected. Inherited cleft palate has been reported in many breeds, including English Bulldog, Brittany Spaniel, Australian Shepherd Dog, Shih Tzu and Bernese Mountain Dog (Cooper and Mattern, 1971; Sponenberg and Bowling, 1985; Padgett *et al.*, 1986; Richtsmeier *et al.*, 1994).

Cleft primary palate

The primary palate consists of the lip and incisive bones. Incomplete closure of the primary palate is a primary cleft or cleft lip, and is obvious at birth as an abnormal fissure in the upper lip (harelip). Affected animals must be examined for coexisting clefts of the secondary palate.

Cleft primary palate is a rare anomaly, usually presenting as a unilateral fissure, and rarely results in clinical signs but is rather a cosmetic anomaly. The very uncommon complete bilateral clefts of the primary palate do lead to problems in suckling, and repair in these cases is necessary.

The objective in repair of primary clefts is closure of the cleft lip and the nasal floor. The lip closure is allowed to heal completely before the cleft between the incisive bones is repaired. Surgical repair requires complex three-dimensional flap construction and is best referred to a surgeon familiar with reconstructive and advanced oral surgery.

Cleft secondary palate

A secondary cleft involves the hard and soft palate (Figure 6.30). It is more common than a primary cleft

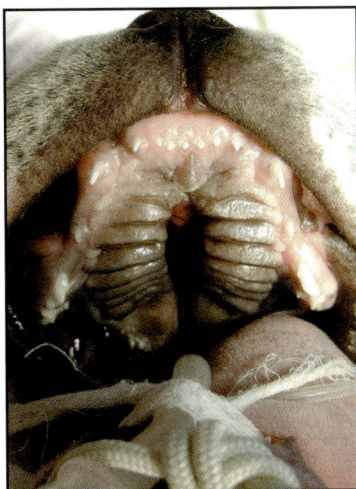

6.30

Cleft secondary palate in an English Bulldog aged 14 weeks. The dog was of normal size for his age and was in good condition, but suffered from bilateral nasal discharge that would not respond to antibiotic treatment. On intraoral inspection, a wide midline cleft was seen in the hard and soft palate. © Leen Verhaert.

palate. Hard palate defects are typically midline, except rostrally at the level of the palatine fissure when combined with a primary cleft. Hard palate defects are usually associated with midline soft palate defects. Clefts confined to the soft palate may be midline, unilateral or bilateral.

Congenital hard and/or soft palate defects permit entry of food and fluid into the nasal cavity, resulting in direct irritation of the nasal mucosa and secondary rhinitis, nasal discharge, and a high risk of possibly fatal aspiration pneumonia.

Most animals with a cleft of the hard palate are diagnosed early in life. If a cleft is present, normal suckling is difficult, and during nursing sneezing, coughing and nasal reflux may be observed. Affected animals usually show signs of poor growth. In most cases the breeder will elect for euthanasia of an affected animal. When cleft palate is diagnosed, and the owner wants surgical repair, tube feeding several times daily should be performed to avoid recurrent aspiration pneumonia until the animal reaches a suitable age and size for anaesthesia and surgical repair. Most procedures are performed in animals at 2–4 months of age. Before surgical correction, the owner should be informed of a possible heritability factor and should be advised not to breed from the affected animal.

Clefts of the caudal soft palate are generally well tolerated, and are often diagnosed later in life. Clinical signs include chronic rhinitis, cough and slower growth. Clefts of the entire soft palate allow food and fluid to enter the nasal cavity, leading to signs similar to those seen with hard palate defects.

Bilateral absence of part of the soft palate is a rare but severe deformity, clinically presenting as a short palate with a pseudo uvula in the midline.

Animals with congenital palatal defects should be examined carefully, since occasionally other defects can be detected. Animals with congenital defects of the secondary palate may show radiographic signs of otitis media, although clinical signs of ear disease (deafness) have only been reported in one cat (Gregory, 2000).

General principles of repair: Surgery should be carefully planned, since the first attempt at closure has the best chance of success. The owner must be informed that several surgical procedures may be necessary to close the defect fully. Surgery should not be attempted by inexperienced surgeons, and patients with palatal clefts should be referred to someone familiar with oral surgical procedures. General principles of repair include:

- Gentle tissue handling. Tissue desiccation must be avoided, it should not be crushed, and the use of electrosurgical equipment should be avoided
- Covering flaps should be large compared with the size of the defect, to minimize tension on the suture line and permit overlapping of tissues
- Connective tissue and accompanying vessels need to stay attached to the flap, to ensure viability
- Cleanly incised edges of tissue should be

apposed. Flaps sutured to intact epithelial surfaces will not heal (this is very important, as it is often the cause of oral wound dehiscence)
- Where possible, suture lines should not lie over the defect
- Fine synthetic, preferably monofilament, absorbable suture material (4/0 or 5/0) works best in the oral cavity. Stainless steel wire should be avoided since it may severely traumatize the tongue
- If previous surgery has been performed, several weeks (six or more) should be allowed between procedures to permit revascularization of tissue
- Pain control is of the utmost importance, particularly if large areas of denuded bone are exposed and left to granulate.

Midline cleft of the hard palate: Several techniques have been described for repair. The most widely used are the bi-pedicle advancement technique (modified Von Langenbeck) and an overlapping mucoperiosteal flap technique described by Harvey (1987).

For the *bi-pedicle advancement technique*: four full-thickness incisions are made in the palatal mucosa, one on each side of the cleft and another along the palatal aspect of each dental arch. The muco-

periosteal flap is freed from the underlying bone with a periosteal elevator. Care should be taken to avoid severing the major palatine artery. The two bi-pedicle flaps are sutured together in the midline in a simple interrupted pattern. Clefts of up to 35% of the width of the palate can be closed with this technique. Modifications include a split flap procedure (leaving the lateral half of the palatine bone covered with periosteum) and a two-layer closure, but these are beyond the scope of this chapter. In all bi-pedicle advancement flap techniques, sutures lie over the defect, and the sutures may not be completely tension free, resulting in wound breakdown.

In the *overlapping flap technique* (Figure 6.31): the incisions made in the palatal mucosa are asymmetrical. On one side of the defect, an incision is made palatal to the dental arch, and a flap is raised that remains attached to the edge of the palatal defect. The major palatine artery must remain attached to the flap. On the other side of the defect, an incision is made to the bone at the edge of the cleft and the tissue is again freed with a periosteal elevator. The incisions extend to the junction of the hard and soft palate. The first flap is flipped over to go underneath the second flap (the inverted flap is sandwiched between the bony palate and the palatal periosteum). Both are then kept in apposition using

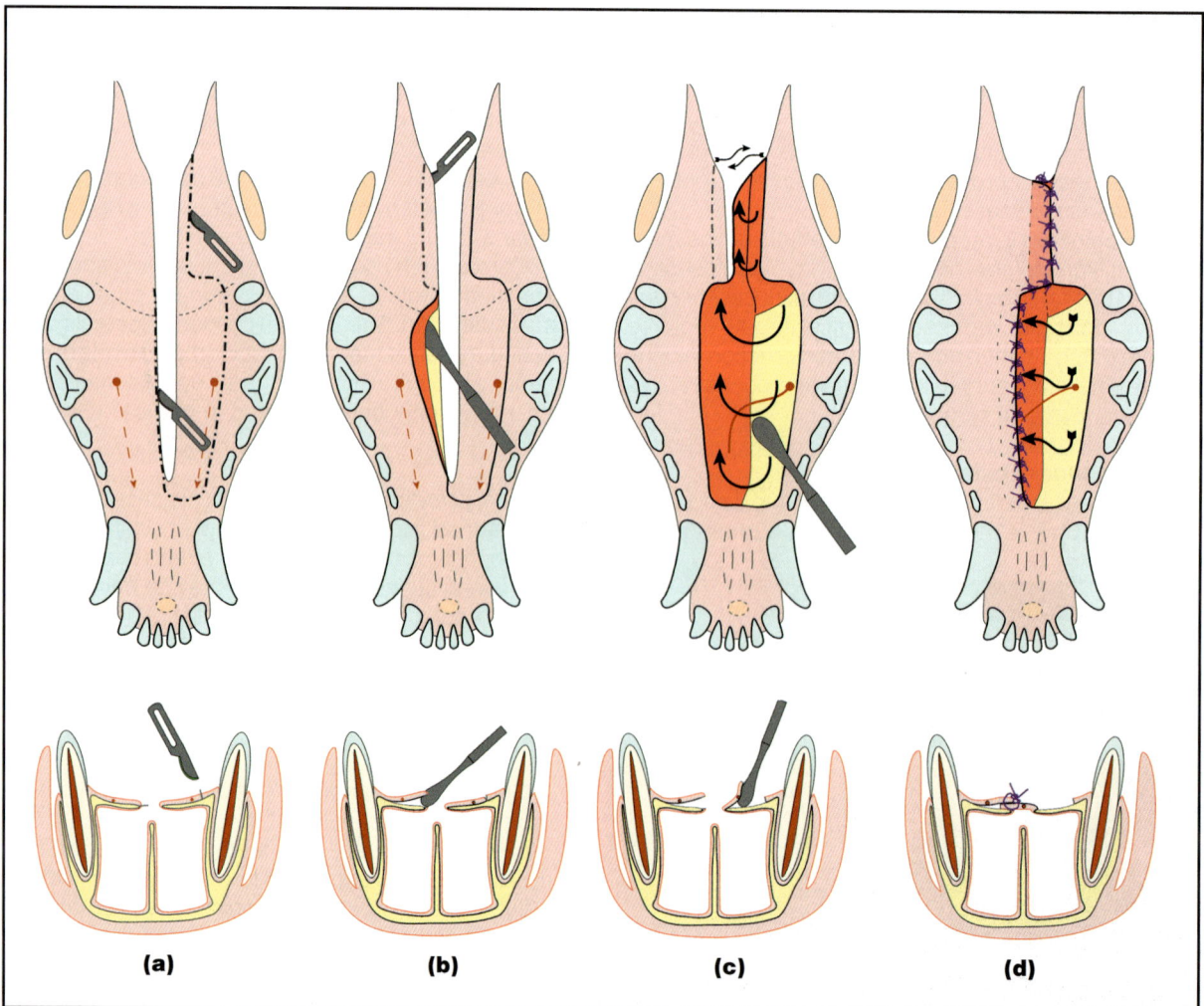

(a)   **(b)**   **(c)**   **(d)**

6.31 Overlapping flap technique for midline cleft palate repair. **(a)** Incisions to create flaps. **(b)** Periosteal elevator is used to raise the flaps. **(c)** One flap is turned and laid under the other. **(d)** The flaps are sutured together.

horizontal mattress and simple interrupted sutures. A major advantage of this technique is that the sutures are not lying over the defect, and that a wide area of connective tissue contact is provided without tension. Severe jaw growth retardation (both length and width) has been reported when large areas of denuded bone are left to granulate (due to contraction of the collagen in the granulation tissue), especially in very young animals with wide defects.

Midline soft palate defects: In many cases, a simple appositional flap technique can be used if the defect is not too wide. Incisions are made in the medial edges of the soft palate defect and each is divided to form two soft tissue flaps. Nasal and oral flaps are closed as separate layers. Where possible, apposition of the palatine muscles is advised, to have a functional soft palate. Wider defects require releasing incisions and suturing of the palatine muscles as a separate layer to relieve tension on the suture line.

Unilateral soft palate defects: The simple flap technique as described for midline soft palate defects is usually unsuccessful for unilateral defects, and more elaborate flap techniques may be needed. Buccal mucosal flaps (Sager and Nefen, 1998) or soft palate and pharyngeal mucosal flaps (Nelson, 2003) can be used to close such defects, but a description of the techniques is beyond the scope of this chapter. The same techniques can be used to close bilateral soft palate defects, but when the defect is large, wound breakdown is common. Furthermore, muscle function will not be restored and the healed soft palate may not function as a sphincter.

Postoperative considerations: Postoperative pain control is extremely important, especially when large areas of denuded bone exist. A pain-free animal will eat more readily, feel more comfortable and, without stress, the wounds will heal much quicker.

Soft, non-sticky food, such as small pieces of meat, should be fed in the postoperative period (two weeks). Chewing on hard objects should be prevented. For the first few days postoperatively an Elizabethan collar is advised, to prevent pawing at the mouth. Healing should be evaluated after two weeks.

With very large defects, placing an oesophago-stomy tube is advisable, although in most cases this is not necessary.

Complications of palatal surgery: Usually, there is considerable haemorrhage during palatal surgery as a result of the rich blood supply to the oral tissues. Periodic pressure is usually sufficient to obtain haemostasis. In areas to be sutured, use of electrocautery is contraindicated since it will interfere with healing.

Wound dehiscence is the most common complication following surgery. Tension on the suture line and use of electrocautery will predispose to dehiscence. A common location for wound breakdown is in the area of the incisive papilla. Small rostral defects may not cause clinical signs and therefore may not need any further surgery. Larger or more caudal defects will need clo-sure once the full extent of dehiscence is known and the tissues have revascularized (several weeks later).

The pharynx may be occluded due to postoperative swelling of the soft palate or blood clots; therefore animals undergoing this type of surgery need to be carefully monitored during recovery.

Temporomandibular joint dysplasia

Temporomandibular joint (TMJ) dysplasia has been reported in many breeds, but Irish Setters and Bassett Hounds seem to be over-represented in the literature. Dysplasia of the TMJ can result in joint laxity and shifting of the mandible and locking of the mandibular coronoid process outside the zygomatic arch, especially in animals with a relatively narrow maxilla. The patient is presented with the mouth locked open, with a lateral shift of the mandible to one side and a visible protrusion of the coronoid process in the area of the zygomatic arch. The open-mouth jaw locking may correct spontaneously, or the coronoid process may need to be manipulated back into place. Treatment of recurrent jaw-locking episodes is usually by resection of the rostroventral part of the zygomatic arch, sometimes combined with coronoid process reduction.

TMJ dysplasia is a common asymptomatic condition in Cavalier King Charles Spaniels and should be regarded as a normal anatomical variation in this breed (Dickie *et al.*, 2002).

Craniomandibular osteopathy

Craniomandibular osteopathy (CMO) is an uncommon non-neoplastic proliferative bone disease, primarily affecting the bones of the head and occasionally the long bones. Bones commonly involved include the parietal and occipital bones, the mandibular rami and tympanic bullae. In large-breed dogs, the lesions are usually confined to the mandible. The lesions are usually bilateral and symmetrical. The disease is self-limiting and occurs in young dogs 3–8 months of age. It is most often seen in West Highland White, Cairn, Scottish and other terriers, but the disease has been documented in other breeds, including the Shetland Sheepdog, Labrador and Golden Retriever, Great Dane, Dobermann, Boxer, German Shepherd Dog, Bullmastiff, Pyrenean Mountain Dog, English Bulldog, Irish Setter and Border Collie.

The aetiology of this syndrome is unknown. An autosomal recessive mode of inheritance is known in West Highland White Terriers, and there may be a hereditary predisposition in Scottish Terriers. Sporadic occurrence in unrelated breeds suggests that aetiological factors other than genetics must be involved. Aetiological factors that have been suggested are viral infection (canine distemper virus) and bacterial infection (*Escherichia coli*). In a report on 12 Irish Setters with canine leucocyte adhesion deficiency, seven had signs consistent with CMO, suggesting that impaired immunity may be a possible factor in some cases of CMO (Trowald-Wigh *et al.*, 2000).

Clinical signs

Clinical signs usually relate to persistent or intermittent pain associated with opening of the mouth and intermittent episodes of fever. Signs that may be seen are depression, hypersalivation and dysphagia. The mandibular thickening is palpable as a firm, painful, usually bilaterally symmetrical swelling (Figure 6.32a). If the angular process of the mandible and the tympanic bulla are involved, jaw movement is diminished and temporal and masseter muscle atrophy may be evident. Once skeletal maturity is reached, the abnormal bone growth stops, often regresses and may recede completely.

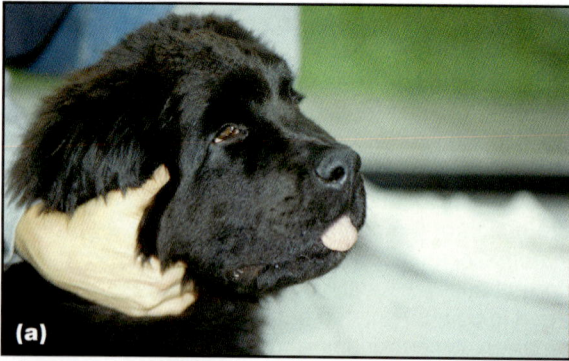

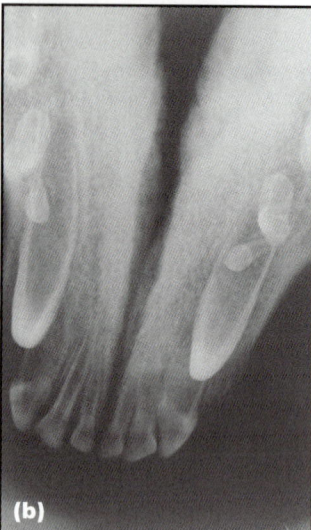

6.32

Craniomandibular osteopathy in a Newfoundland.
(a) This dog was presented with intermittent episodes of fever, depression and dysphagia. A firm, painful, bilateral mandibular thickening was palpable and resulted in the typical 'lion jaw' appearance.
(b) Radiographic appearance, showing dense osseous proliferations from the periosteal surfaces of the mandibles. © Leen Verhaert.

Diagnosis
Diagnosis is based on clinical signs, physical findings, radiography and histopathology.

On radiography, dense osseous proliferations projecting from the periosteal surfaces of the affected bones can be seen (Figure 6.32b). In severe cases, the angular process of the mandible may fuse with the tympanic bulla and mechanically obstruct jaw motion or lead to a bony fusion of the TMJ. The histopathological appearance is similar to that of osteitis deformans or Paget's disease in humans. There is a generalized thickening of bony trabeculae. A typical mosaic pattern due to well demarcated cement lines is seen between newly and previously deposited lamellar bone. Inflammatory cells may or may not be observed (Alexander, 1983).

Prognosis and treatment
Prognosis largely depends on which bones are involved and to what degree. Extensive involvement of the tympanic bullae, or bony fusion of the TMJ, may warrant euthanasia.

Treatment is aimed at reducing pain and inflammation, and providing nutritional support if needed. When the therapeutic response to non-steroidal anti-inflammatory drugs is poor, corticosteroids may be used. Signs may wax and wane spontaneously; therefore, treatment responses are not always easy to assess. Surgical treatment (excision of the proliferation) has led to reappearance of the proliferations within a few weeks, and is therefore not useful.

Fibrous osteodystrophy in the young dog ('rubber jaw')
Dogs with congenital renal dysplasia will show features of secondary hyperparathyroidism that can be noticed first in the jaws. Affected animals often present with facial swelling and poor growth.

The jaws are thickened and have a rubbery consistency on firm palpation. The teeth are mobile and the oral mucosa may be ulcerated (Figure 6.33a). On radiography, loss of bone density of the maxillary and mandibular bones is obvious, with loss of the normal trabecular bone structure. Loss of the lamina dura is evident, with the teeth appearing to float in fibrous tissue (Figure 6.33b). Prognosis is extremely poor.

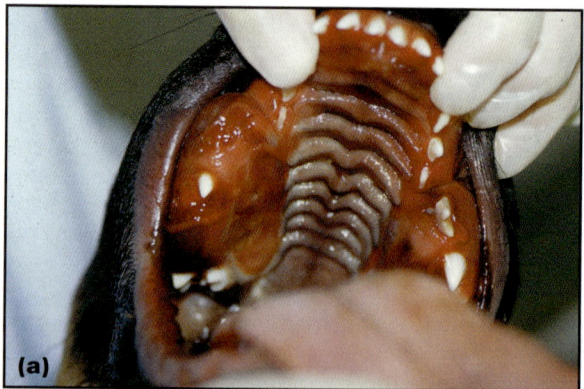

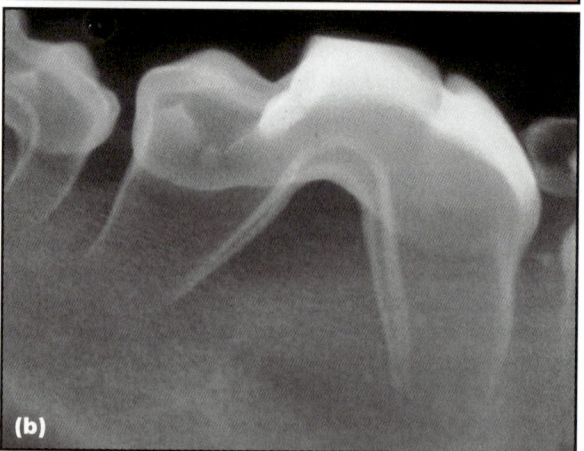

6.33 'Rubber jaw' in a 5-month-old Bull Mastiff with congenital renal dysplasia (post-mortem photographs). **(a)** Clinical findings. The jaws are thickened and have a rubbery consistency on palpation. The teeth are mobile and the oral mucosa may be ulcerated, as is obvious in this picture. **(b)** Radiographic findings. Loss of normal trabecular bone structure and loss of lamina dura dentis. The teeth seem to float in fibrous tissue. Interestingly, histological examination failed to show any abnormalities of the teeth and periodontal ligament. © Leen Verhaert.

References and further reading

Alexander JW (1983) Selected skeletal dysplasias: craniomandibular osteopathy, multiple cartilaginous exostoses and hypertrophic osteodystrophy. *Veterinary Clinics of North America: Small Animal Practice* **13**, 55–70

Arnbjerg J (1986) Schmelz- und Wurzelhypoplasien nach Staupe. *Kleintierpraxis* **31**, 323–326

Bittegeko SBPR, Arnbjerg J, Nkya R and Tevik A (1995) Multiple dental developmental abnormalities following Canine Distemper infection. *Journal of Small Animal Practice* **31**, 42–45

Cooper HK Jr and Mattern GW (1971) Genetic studies of cleft lip and palate in dogs. *Birth Defects Original Article Series* **7**, 98–100

Dickie AM, Schwarz T and Sullivan M (2002) Temporomandibular joint morphology in Cavalier King Charles Spaniels. *Veterinary Radiology and Ultrasound* **43**, 260–266

Gioso MA (2001) Mandible and mandibular first molar tooth measurements in dogs: relationship of radiographic height to body weight. *Journal of Veterinary Dentistry* **18**, 65–68

Gorrel C (2004) Occlusion and malocclusion. In: *Veterinary Dentistry for the General Practitioner*, ed. C Gorrel, pp. 35–46. Saunders, Edinburgh

Gorrel C (2004) Common oral conditions. In: *Veterinary Dentistry for the General Practitioner*, ed. C Gorrel, pp. 69–85. Saunders, Edinburgh

Gregory SP (2000) Middle ear disease associated with congenital palatine defects in seven dogs and one cat. *Journal of Small Animal Practice* **41**, 398–401

Harvey CE (1987) Palate defects in dogs and cats. *Compendium on Continuing Education for the Practicing Veterinarian* **9**, 404–418

Harvey CE and Emily PP (1993) Occlusion, occlusive abnormalities, and orthodontic treatment. In: *Small Animal Dentistry*, ed. CE Harvey and P Emily, pp 266–296. Mosby, St Louis

Hennet P (1996) Anomalies du développement du palais et des lèvres. *Le Point Vétérinaire* **28**(185), 1677–1681

Hennet P (2003) Orthodontics. In: *Textbook of Small Animal Surgery*, 3rd edn, ed. D Slatter, pp. 2686–2695. WB Saunders, Philadelphia

Huchkowsky SL (2002) Craniomandibular osteopathy in a bullmastiff. *Canadian Veterinary Journal* **43**, 883–885

Nelson AW (2003) Cleft palate. In: *Textbook of Small Animal Surgery*, 3rd edn, ed. D Slatter, pp. 814–823. WB Saunders, Philadelphia

Neville BW, Damm DD, Allen CM and Bouquot JE (2002) Odontogenic cysts and tumours. In: *Oral and Maxillofacial Pathology, 2nd edn*, ed. BW Neville *et al.*, pp. 589–609. WB Saunders, Philadelphia

Nik Noriah Nik-Hussein and Zubaidah Abdul Majid (1996) Dental anomalies in the primary dentition: distribution and correlation with the permanent dentition. *Journal of Clinical Pediatric Dentistry* **21**, 15–19

Padgett GA, Bell TG and Patterson WR (1986) Genetic disorders affecting reproduction and periparturient care. *Veterinary Clinics of North America: Small Animal Practice* **16**, 577–586

Regezi JA and Sciubba J (1993) Abnormalities of teeth. In: *Oral Pathology: Clinical–Pathologic Correlations, 2nd edn*, ed. JA Regezi *et al.*, pp. 494–501. WB Saunders, Philadelphia

Reiter AM (2004) Symphysiotomy, symphysiectomy, and intermandibular arthrodesis in a cat with open-mouth jaw locking – case report and literature review. *Journal of Veterinary Dentistry* **21**, 147–158

Richtsmeier JT, Sack GH, Grausz HM and Cork LC (1994) Cleft palate with autosomal recessive transmission in Brittany spaniels. *Cleft Palate Craniofacial Journal* **31**, 364–371

Sager M and Nefen S (1998) Use of buccal mucosal flaps for the correction of congenital soft palate defects in three dogs. *Veterinary Surgery* **27**, 358–363

Shipp AD and Fahrenkrug P (1992) Orthodontics. In: *Practitioner's Guide to Veterinary Dentistry*, ed. AD Shipp, pp. 117–147. Dr Shipp's Laboratories, Beverly Hills

Sponenberg DP and Bowling AT (1985) Heritable syndrome of skeletal defects in a family of Australian shepherd dogs. *Journal of Heredity* **76**, 393–394

Trope M and Chivian N (1994) Root resorption. In: *Pathways of the Pulp, 6th edn*, ed. S Cohen and C Burns, pp. 486–512. Mosby, St Louis

Trowald-Wigh G, Ekman S, Hansson K, Hedhammar A and Hard af Segerstad C (2000) Clinical, radiological and pathological features of 12 Irish Setters with canine leucocyte adhesion deficiency. *Journal of Small Animal Practice* **41**, 211–217

Verhaert L (1999) A removable orthodontic device for the treatment of lingually displaced mandibular canine teeth in young dogs. *Journal of Veterinary Dentistry* **16**, 69–75

Verhaert L (2002) Suspected amelogenesis imperfecta in a Standard Poodle. *Proceedings of the 16th Annual Veterinary Dental Forum*, Savannah.

Verstraete FJM (2003) Oral pathology. In: *Textbook of Small Animal Surgery, 3rd edn*, ed. D Slatter, pp. 2638–2651. WB Saunders, Philadelphia

Verstraete FJM and Terpak CH (1997) Anatomical variations in the dentition of the domestic cat. *Journal of Veterinary Dentistry* **14**, 137–140

Waldron DR and Martin RA (1991) Cleft palate repair. *Problems in Veterinary Medicine* **3**, 142–152

Watson ADJ, Adams WM and Thomas CB (1995) Craniomandibular osteopathy in dogs. *Compendium on Continuing Education for the Practicing Veterinarian* **17**, 911–922

7

Canine infectious, inflammatory and immune-mediated oral conditions

Anthony Caiafa

This chapter covers the infectious, inflammatory and immune-mediated conditions that affect the oral cavity of dogs. They include:

- Periodontal disease: aetiology, pathogenesis, diagnosis, management and prevention
- Other oral diseases associated with periodontal disease
- Dental caries, including aetiopathogenesis, diagnosis and management
- Immune-mediated diseases involving the oral cavity and muscles of mastication, e.g. systemic lupus erythematosis, pemphigus, bullous pemphigoid and masticatory muscle myositis
- Other infectious diseases of the oral cavity, including bacterial, fungal, parasitic and viral diseases
- Salivary gland disease.

Periodontal disease

Introduction

Periodontal diseases (PDs) are plaque-induced diseases of the supporting structures of teeth. The two main forms of PD are gingivitis (the reversible inflammation of the gingiva) and periodontitis (the inflammation and irreversible destruction of the tooth's supporting structures, namely the gingiva, the periodontal ligament (PDL), cementum and alveolar bone). Plaque accumulation leads to gingival inflammation (gingivitis). Gingivitis always precedes periodontitis, but gingivitis does not always progress to periodontitis.

The oral mucosa is unique in that it is made up of an ectodermal lining, which is pierced by the teeth; as a result the dentogingival margin represents a weak area in the oral mucosa's protective and defensive roles (Figure 7.1).

Incidence

PD is arguably the most common disease in small animal practice today (University of Minnesota, 1996; Harvey, 1998). A large proportion of adult dogs and cats have some degree of PD. The disease is so common that clinicians should always examine the oral cavity thoroughly as part of any routine health assessment.

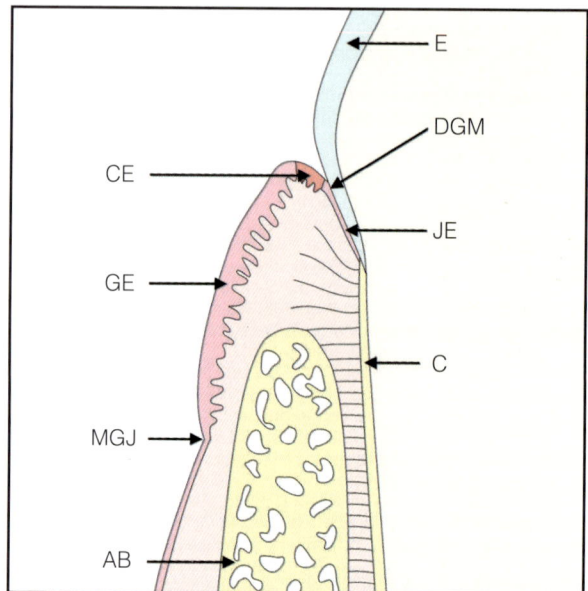

7.1 The normal relationship of tooth to periodontium. AB = Alveolar bone; C = Cementum; CE = Crevicular epithelium; DGM = Dentogingival margin; E = Enamel; GE = Gingival epithelium; JE = Junctional epithelium; MGJ = Mucogingival junction.

Aetiology and natural progression

PD initiation and progression occurs due to complex interactions between oral bacteria and both the host's immune system and periodontium (Figure 7.2).

Primary factors

Bacteria are the primary aetiological factor that initiates PD. Gingivitis occurs in the presence of both Gram-positive and Gram-negative aerobic and anaerobic bacteria. Periodontitis is initiated by the presence of mainly Gram-negative anaerobic bacteria. Bacteria and bacterial products, including toxins, stimulate the host defences to initiate both innate and humoral immune responses. It is important to understand that this subsequent host response with the release of cytokines and other inflammatory mediators causes the direct loss of gingival connective tissue, PDL, cementum and alveolar bone.

Secondary factors

Local secondary factors that predispose to the initiation and contribute to the rate of progression of the disease process include calculus, tooth crowding

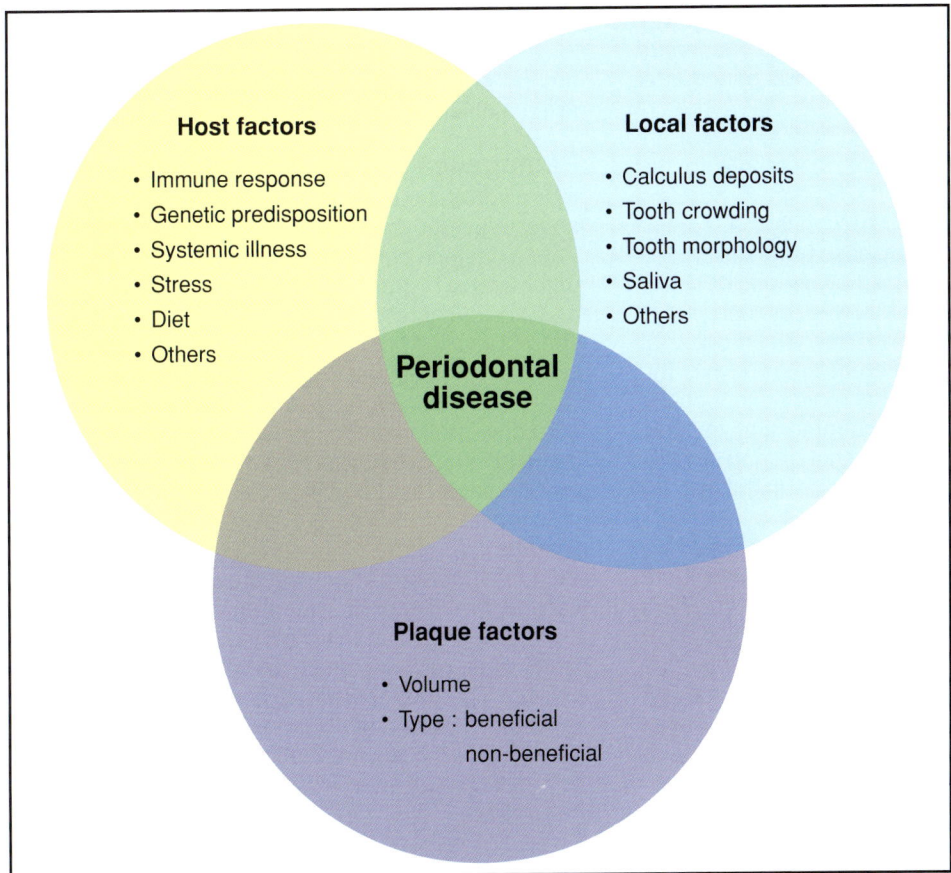

Host factors

- Immune response
- Genetic predisposition
- Systemic illness
- Stress
- Diet
- Others

Local factors

- Calculus deposits
- Tooth crowding
- Tooth morphology
- Saliva
- Others

Periodontal disease

Plaque factors

- Volume
- Type : beneficial
          non-beneficial

(especially in small breeds; Figure 7.3), tooth morphology, supernumerary teeth, mouth breathing (dries the mucosal surface) and salivary gland dysfunction with subsequent decreased saliva flow (saliva flow aids in the clearance of unattached oral bacteria) as well as the loss of antimicrobials, including immunoglobulin A (IgA), found in the saliva.

Systemic secondary factors favouring the development and progression of periodontitis include: illnesses, such as renal failure and diabetes mellitus; inherited diseases, such as cyclic neutropenia in collies; immunopathies; and nutritional imbalances. In humans, smoking is a major risk factor for the develop-

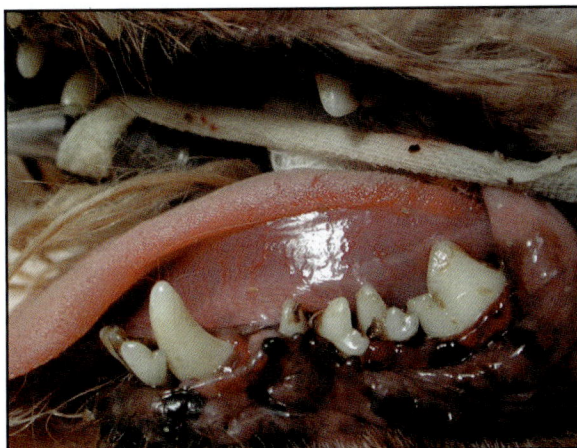

7.3 Local secondary predisposing factor; tooth crowding (mandibular premolars) in a small-breed dog.

ment and progression of periodontitis. Other factors such as psychological stress (reduces immune system function) and occasionally poor diet can affect the host's protective mechanisms, which in turn can aggrevate PD. A plaque retentive diet (i.e. food that is sticky) can also influence disease progression in dogs. These secondary factors contribute to the overall severity of the disease.

Genetic predisposition

Genetic predispostion is seen as a risk factor for periodontitis based on studies in humans (Nares, 2003). The host's immune response to periodontal pathogens can be a major contributing factor to PD progression. Genetic differences in the expression of inflammatory cytokines (inflammatory mediators), especially interleukin-1 (IL-1), has been investigated in humans. It has been shown that people carrying the IL-1 genotype are at increased risk of developing periodontitis (Korman et al., 1997). This risk increases dramatically if that person smokes cigarettes. In dogs, it is suspected that certain breeds (e.g. Greyhounds, Maltese dogs) are more susceptible to an aggressive form of periodontitis. Genetic tests using interleukin expression are now being developed to determine whether certain breeds of dogs have increased susceptibility to periodontitis.

Disease progression

The bacteria that initiate PD reside within the gingival sulcus. Bacterial reservoirs can also be found on the tongue, tonsils and oral mucosa, as well as in calculus, cementum defects and other areas of the oral cavity and face (e.g. lip-fold dermatitis). These reservoirs may assist in the recolonization of treated periodontal pockets.

Bacteria, their byproducts and toxins, as well as the host's own defence systems, contribute to the initiation and continuation of PD. Studies in humans have shown that periodontitis has neither a 'continuous' nor a 'linear' pattern of disease progression. PD is a disease that is characterized by periods of active tissue destruction ('bursts') followed by periods of quiescence (Socransky *et al.,* 1984). It can occur at different locations and at different times within the mouth (random burst theory of chronic periodontitis). Socransky *et al.* (1984) demonstrated that multiple sites showed breakdown within a short period of time, followed by periods of remission that might last for months or even years.

There can be varying grades of periodontitis within the same mouth, or even involving the same tooth (Figure 7.4). In humans, periodontitis tends to affect posterior teeth (particularly the molars) more than anterior teeth (i.e. incisors, canines). This may be due in part to the greater difficulty in performing oral hygiene on posterior teeth as well as the more complex root morphology of multi-rooted teeth, especially molar teeth.

In one study of 162 randomly selected dogs submitted for necropsy (Hamp *et al.,* 1997) the caudal maxillary and mandibular premolars and molars were the teeth most frequently periodontally affected by periodontitis. Alveolar bone loss was more severe in the maxilla, while corresponding bone loss in the mandible was often related to increasing age.

In dogs and cats, there is an increase in the severity of PD with increasing age and a decrease in the severity of disease with increasing body weight, with smaller dog breeds being at particular risk of developing PD (Harvey *et al.,* 1994). The increased risk of disease in small dogs may be related to less alveolar bone supporting the teeth and tooth crowding, resulting in plaque traps.

The buccal surfaces of the teeth seem to be more affected than the lingual surfaces (the tongue aids in the mechanical cleaning of the lingual surfaces). Untreated periodontitis in humans can progress at the rate

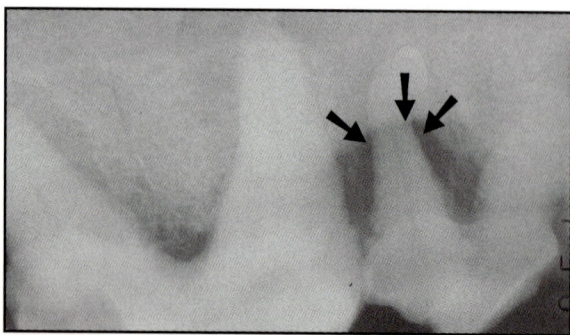

7.4 Differences in the degree of periodontitis involving the same tooth. Radiograph of the maxillary third and fourth premolars in a dog. Note the severe bone loss involving the distal root of the third premolar (arrowed) with moderate bone loss around the mesial root.

of 0.2 mm attachment loss (AL) per year (Loe *et al.,*1978). At the present time, the rate of progress of untreated PD in dogs is unknown. Untreated periodontitis may ultimately lead to loss of the affected tooth.

Pathogenesis

PD requires the presence of bacteria. Dogs and cats have over 300 bacterial species in the oral cavity. These bacteria colonize the surfaces of the teeth and other areas of the mouth, forming biofilms or communities of bacteria known as plaque. Plaque biofilms interact with the host with the normal outcome being to constrain the bacteria in a state of commensal equilibrium (i.e. beneficial plaque). This state of equilibrium or harmony prevents the growth of more pathogenic bacteria within the biofilm. However, if this host–bacteria equilibrium is disturbed it can lead to disease.

Plaque

Plaque forms soon after teeth erupt into the mouth and very quickly after professional scaling and polishing or tooth brushing. The initial phase of plaque formation starts when bacteria attach to the tooth surface via the pellicle. The tooth pellicle is a glycoprotein layer derived from saliva, crevicular fluid and cell debris. The pellicle is firmly attached to the tooth surface and can reform within minutes following brushing or mechanical scaling.

Bacteria attach to this sticky pellicle and through it to the tooth surface via specific mechanisms. Initially, the colonizing bacteria are predominantly Gram-positive microorganisms, such as *Actinomyces* and *Streptococcus.* These early colonizers attach supragingivally and begin a process of multiplication and maturation. Bacteria produce a glycocalyx (glycopolysaccharide) that allows them to adhere to each other and to the tooth surface. This binding allows the bacteria to eventually form colonies or biofilms, which protect as well as nourish the bacteria and aid in their survival.

As the plaque matures, a shift from beneficial predominantly Gram-positive facultative flora to a disease-related predominantly Gram-negative motile anaerobic flora occurs. This shift is associated with the initiation of gingivitis and, if plaque is left undisturbed, in some animals progression to periodontitis. In a study in humans (Saini *et al.,* 2003) samples taken from the gingival sulcus showed that the ratio of aerobic and facultative anaerobic bacteria to anaerobic bacteria decreased as lesions progressed from healthy gingiva to gingivitis to periodontitis. Large numbers of anaerobes were isolated from cases of periodontitis.

Specific plaque hypothesis: Periodontitis is often associated with specific microorganisms, which are seen in higher numbers in disease than in health (specific plaque hypothesis). The specific plaque hypothesis (Loesche, 1976) states that periodontitis results from the action of one or several specific pathogenic species, whose numbers increase in disease.

In humans, it is currently thought that between 10 and 15 periodontal pathogens are involved in the pathogenic process of chronic periodontitis.

Biofilms: Periodontal pathogens multiply within complex biofilm structures. Bacterial biofilms are ecological communities of bacteria, which provide micro-environments with differing pH and oxygen levels; there is also metabolic cooperation with exchange of metabolites to aid growth. Some organisms in the biofilm may protect other key organisms from antimicrobial attack. These organisms can produce an exopolysaccharide matrix for mutual protection from host defences and systemic as well as locally delivered antimicrobials.

Antimicrobial penetration into bacterial biofilms is more difficult compared with the antimicrobial effect on planktonic bacteria. Studies have shown that even with the use of higher concentrations (well above the minimum inhibitory concentration) of antimicrobials, such as clindamycin hydrochloride and doxycycline, the mature biofilm can still survive (Eick *et al.,* 2004; Walker *et al.,* 2004). However, an *in vitro* study has shown that certain antimicrobials (e.g. clindamycin hydrochloride) can at least suppress biofilm formation (Ichimiya *et al.*, 1994).

Biofilms can occur both supra- and subgingivally, as well as in other organs of the body. In humans, supragingival plaque is often seen as a thin white film covering the teeth. Once attached, plaque can only be removed from the tooth surface by mechanical means, i.e. tooth brushing or abrasive diets. Undisturbed plaque left in contact with the gingiva for some time initiates an inflammatory response within the gingiva. This results in swelling and lifting of the gingiva away from the tooth, and the development of periodontal pockets (pseudopockets) without AL (*chronic marginal gingivitis*).

Gingivitis

Chronic marginal gingivitis is defined as inflammation of the marginal gingival tissues and is characterized by redness, swelling and bleeding. Gingivitis can occur within days of plaque accumulation but, if treated correctly, is reversible and gingival health is quickly restored (Loe *et al.*, 1965). However, if the plaque is left to mature further, chronic gingivitis ensues (Figure 7.5) and the plaque eventually penetrates into the gingival sulcus. The bacterial composition of the plaque changes to a predominantly Gram-negative anaerobic motile flora. This flora is responsible for the initiation of periodontitis.

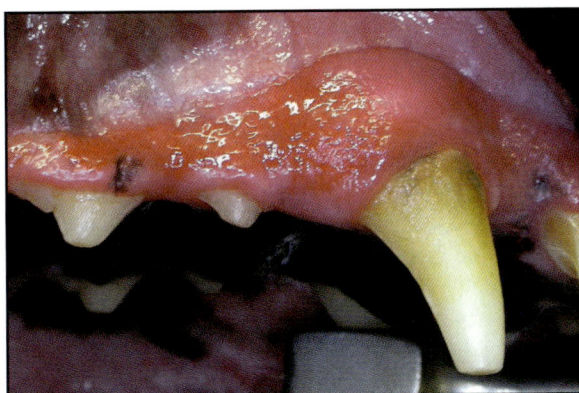

7.5 Signs of gingival inflammation include swelling, redness and loss of gingival contour. Gingivitis involving the maxillary canine, first and second premolars. (Courtesy of W. Fitzgerald.)

Periodontitis

The principal bacteria incriminated in PD in dogs are the obligate anaerobes: *Porphyromonas* spp., including *P. gingivalis, P. salivosa, P. gulae* and *P. denticanis; Fusobacterium; Prevotella*; and the highly motile anaerobic spirochaetes (Hardham *et al.,* 2005a). The bacteria and their toxins penetrate the sulcular (crevicular) and junctional epithelium and initiate an acute, then chronic, inflammatory response by the body. The end result of this process is periodontal soft tissue damage and alveolar bone resorption. This leads to AL (periodontal pocketing and gingival recession) as well as to tooth mobility and in some cases tooth loss. Pocket formation, when it occurs, results from bacteria-induced inflammation and eventual destruction of the supporting structures of the tooth.

In summary, virulent bacteria and a susceptible host are necessary for disease to occur. If either one is absent, disease will not occur.

Histopathogenesis and immunology

The histopathogenesis of PD can be divided into four stages (Page and Schroeder, 1976; Soames and Southam, 1995) (Figure 7.6):

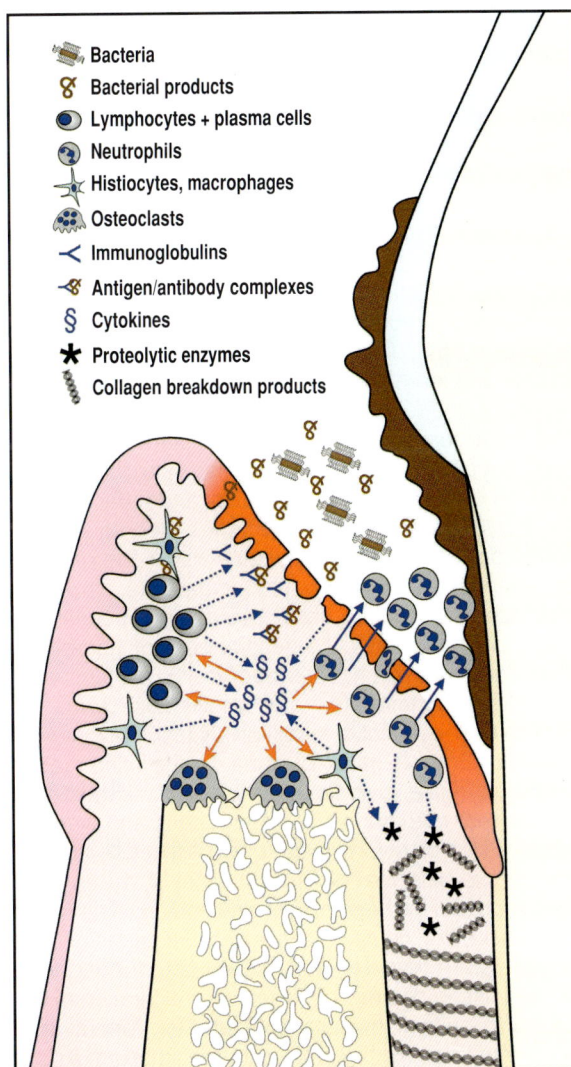

Bacteria
Bacterial products
Lymphocytes + plasma cells
Neutrophils
Histiocytes, macrophages
Osteoclasts
Immunoglobulins
Antigen/antibody complexes
Cytokines
Proteolytic enzymes
Collagen breakdown products

7.6 Histopathogenesis of periodontal disease.

1. The initial lesion (gingivitis).
2. The early lesion (gingivitis).
3. The established lesion (chronic gingivitis).
4. The advanced lesion (periodontitis).

Gingiva in health: The marginal gingiva forms a firm collar around the tooth. It is covered by keratinized stratified squamous epithelium, which has a rapid cell turnover, thus allowing the gingiva to remain healthy and functional whilst withstanding the everyday rigours of normal masticatory activity. Sulcular epithelium, non-keratinized stratified squamous epithelium, lines the gingival sulcus. It continues on to the junctional epithelium, where the epithelial cells have spaces between them (that widen in disease) and attach to each other via specialized structures called desmosomes. Junctional epithelial cells adjacent to the tooth surface attach to the tooth via hemi-desmosomes (tonofilaments radiating from the cell).

The initial lesion: The initial lesion of gingivitis can start up to 4 days following the onset of plaque accumulation. A mixture of Gram-positive and Gram-negative rods and cocci (non-specific plaque) induce vasculitis of small blood vessels in the gingiva. Bacteria and their products, including lipopolysaccharides (endotoxins derived from the cell membrane of Gram-negative bacteria) penetrate the sulcular and junctional epithelium and gain access to the connective tissue. There is essentially an acute inflammatory response and loss of integrity of the junctional epithelium.

Due to increased vascular permeability (in response to chemotactic factors) there is an exudation of inflammatory cells (mainly polymorphonuclear (PMN) cells) and protein-rich fluids (including immunoglobulins and complement) into the gingival connective tissue and gingival sulcus. This causes swelling of the gingival tissues and increased flow of crevicular fluid.

The early lesion: The early lesion starts between 4 and 7 days following the onset of plaque accumulation. There is overlap between the initial and early lesions. The inflammatory reaction becomes chronic and expands both laterally and apically within the gingiva. Collagenases produced by plaque bacteria, as well as proteases from PMN cells, destroy the connective tissue of the gingiva. Large numbers of fibroblasts show degenerative changes (apoptosis). The junctional epithelial attachment to the enamel is destroyed.

The development of subgingival plaque favours the growth of Gram-negative bacteria. As the inflammation becomes more chronic, there is an infiltration of monocytes, macrophages, plasma cells and lymphocytes into the gingival tissues. There is a dense infiltrate of lymphoid cells (mainly T-lymphocytes) in the connective tissue and the beginning of a cell-mediated immune response. The complement and prostaglandin (PG) pathways are triggered and this leads to further host-derived tissue destruction. There is proliferation of the junctional epithelium basal cells and the formation of small rete ridges in the oral sulcular epithelium. As the tissue destruction continues, there is collagen loss in the connective tissue apical to the junctional epithelium.

The established lesion: Two or three weeks following plaque accumulation, the established lesion evolves from the early lesion. There is continuation of the chronic inflammatory response with cell death, damage to connective tissue and further growth of subgingival plaque. The established lesion can continue for a long time without progressing to periodontitis.

The junctional epithelium detaches from the enamel, resulting in widening of the gingival sulcus. The altered junctional epithelium becomes pocket epithelium without, at this point, apical migration. The pocket epithelium can be thickened in places, but ulcerated and thin in other areas. The thin ulcerated pocket epithelium bleeds easily. There is a shift in the inflammatory cell make-up from lymphocytes to plasma cells and the production of large amounts of immunoglobulins in the connective tissue and gingival sulcus. At this point, the process is still reversible.

The advanced lesion: The cause of the shift from reversible to irreversible change is not known, but is thought to be related to an increase in plasma cells within the connective tissue. This lesion is characterized by the loss of the connective tissue attachment to the tooth root. There is loss of alveolar bone and pocket formation (periodontitis).

Plasma cells dominate the infiltrate at all stages of the advanced lesion. The bacterial biofilm changes to a predominantly Gram-negative anaerobic flora. There is destruction of the supra-alveolar gingival fibres and these fibres lose their attachment to the cementum. Following this, cementoblasts start to die and with this there is migration of the apical junctional epithelial cells further along the root surface, which progressively deepens the pocket. As the disease extends apically, there is destruction of the PDL cells and fibres. The production of large quantities of IL-1, tumour necrosis factor, matrix metalloproteinases (MMPs) and PGE_2 derived from the host cells, as well as cells of the immune system, inhibit collagen production. They also stimulate osteoclasts to destroy alveolar marginal bone, and, clinically, pocketing and AL is detected. There are periods of remission and healing, with repair interspersed with periods of active disease and continuation of AL.

Types of attachment loss

AL refers to the loss of periodontal attachment surrounding the tooth. AL is measured from a fixed landmark on the tooth, usually the cementoenamel junction, to the depth of the periodontal pocket. AL can be associated with vertical or horizontal alveolar bone loss, with or without gingival recession.

Vertical alveolar bone loss: Alveolar bone loss can be vertical and lead to infrabony (intrabony or subalveolar margin) pockets, where there is some marginal alveolar bone coronal to the apical extent of the pocket (Figure 7.7). Infrabony pockets can be further classified as one-, two- or three-walled pocket defects (Figure 7.8) depending on how many bony walls surround the affected root surface. In humans, vertical bone loss often occurs around the molars due to the thicker cortical plates surrounding these teeth.

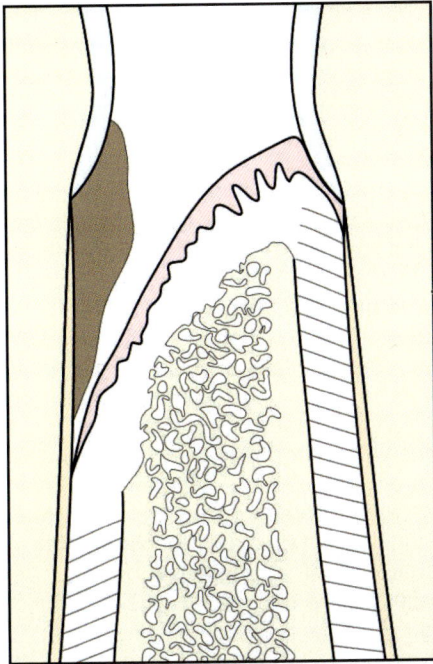

7.7 Infrabony pocket. Note the vertical (angular) pattern of bone loss.

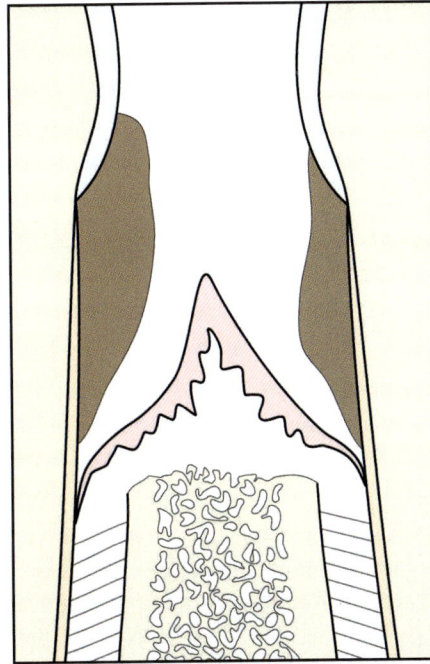

7.9 Suprabony pocket. Note the horizontal pattern of bone loss.

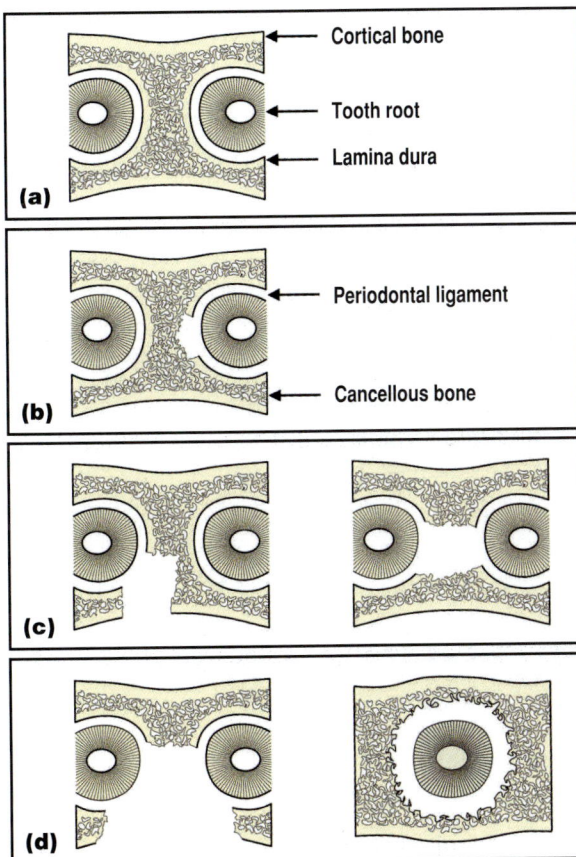

7.8 Infrabony pocket types. **(a)** Normal; **(b)** 3-walled; **(c)** 2-walled; **(d)** 1-walled.

Horizontal alveolar bone loss: Bone loss can also be horizontal and cause suprabony (supra-alveolar margin) pockets (Figure 7.9) with the level of the marginal alveolar bone being apical to the bottom of the pocket. In humans, horizontal bone loss occurs more often around incisor teeth, due to a narrower bony septum.

Gingival recession: Gingival recession can occur with or without pocket formation. Recession is associated with AL. The amount of recession is usually measured from the cementoenamel junction of the tooth to the level of the free gingival margin. AL is the sum of the gingival recession and probing depth measurements.

Gingival hyperplasia: Gingival hyperplasia (Figure 7.10) can lead to increased probing depths, often without AL (so called pseudo-pockets). There is gingival enlargement coronally. Aetiologies include inflammatory mediated causes, familial (Boxers), drug-induced (ciclosporin, diphenylhydantoin) and idiopathic causes.

Gingival hyperplasia may predispose the animal to PD due to increased plaque accumulation and greater difficulty in plaque removal. It is advised that the affected areas be radiographed to look for evidence of alveolar bone loss. Excised gingival tissue should be submitted for histopathological examination to rule out neoplasia.

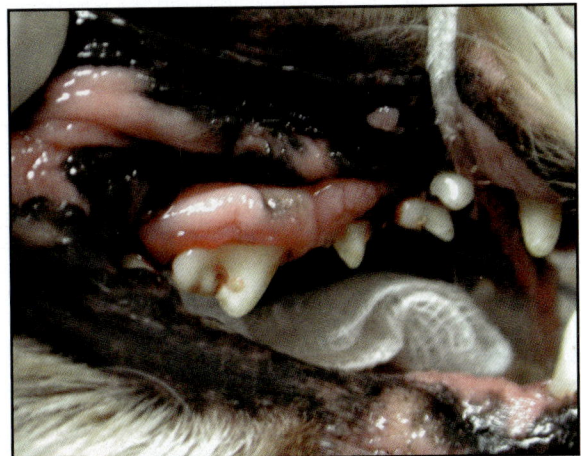

7.10 Gingival hyperplasia in a Cavalier King Charles Spaniel.

Systemic inflammation

PD is not only a localized disease but can also result in a systemic bacteraemia and release of inflammatory mediators. This may lead to organ dysfunction in humans. Systemic markers of inflammation, such as C-reactive protein, have been shown to be elevated in the serum of patients with periodontitis (Ebersole *et al.*, 1997). Serum C-reactive protein levels were also frequently elevated in patients with cardiovascular disease.

A recent study conducted in 38 dogs (Rawlinson *et al.*, 2005) looked at the association between the concentration of systemic inflammatory parameters (including serum C-reactive protein, urine protein:creatinine ratio, blood pressure, microalbuminuria) and severity of PD and then, after appropriate treatment of the PD, the changes in these systemic parameters. The study showed that increases in the concentration of systemic inflammatory markers were positively correlated to the severity of PD. After periodontal therapy, there was a significant decrease in the concentration of some of these inflammatory markers. The study showed that PD leads to systemic inflammation that is significantly reduced with appropriate periodontal therapy. Rawlinson *et al.* (2005) concluded that further research was required to fully understand the significance of these changes. In humans, the association between PD and systemic disease is currently the subject of much research.

Calculus

Bacterial plaque is often attached to calculus. Calculus is mineralized plaque (Figure 7.11) and in itself does not initiate PD. However, it does provide a roughened surface for plaque to adhere to, as well as interfering with home care and plaque removal. Therefore, calculus indirectly contributes to the pathogenic process.

A recent study (Tan *et al.*, 2004) considered a possible direct contribution of calculus to the PD pathogenic process. This study demonstrated viable aerobic and anaerobic bacteria living in cavities and lacunae within supragingival calculus of human subjects. The study concluded that this may be clinically important, because incomplete removal of supragingival calculus may act as a reservoir for periodontal pathogens.

Supragingival calculus formation begins with the precipitation of minerals from saliva. The precipitation of minerals from crevicular fluid initiates the formation of subgingival calculus. Calculus tends to form in layers and frequently food debris is embedded between these layers. In dogs, it often consists of a mixture of calcium carbonate and calcium phosphate.

Once formed, calculus is difficult to remove with conventional home oral hygiene practices (i.e. tooth brushing) and its removal necessitates professional scaling under general anaesthesia. Saliva contains phosphoproteins, which normally prevent the formation of calculus on teeth. Plaque bacteria, however, produce proteases that break down these phosphoproteins, allowing the mineralization of plaque. Thus, the greatest quantities of supragingival calculus are often found closest to the duct openings of the major salivary glands.

In humans, calculus can begin to form within 48 hours of plaque accumulation, but more commonly forms in 2–4 weeks on undisturbed plaque. Subgingival calculus can form on the dentine and cementum, as well as on cemental defects along the root surface. Exposed furcation sites can also accumulate calculus. This can complicate calculus removal when performing root surface debridement.

Clinical signs

One of the most common signs of PD is halitosis (oral malodour). Oral bacteria, especially anaerobic bacteria, produce volatile sulphur compounds (VSCs) that lead to oral malodour. VSCs are also toxic to mucosal epithelium and contribute to periodontal breakdown.

Other symptoms can include excessive salivation, blood in the saliva, dysphagia, oral mucosal ulceration, pain on chewing and lethargy (Figure 7.12). However, dogs with PD often show few or no symptoms until the disease is well advanced. This may contribute to the late presentation of these dogs to the veterinary practice, making management of their disease more difficult.

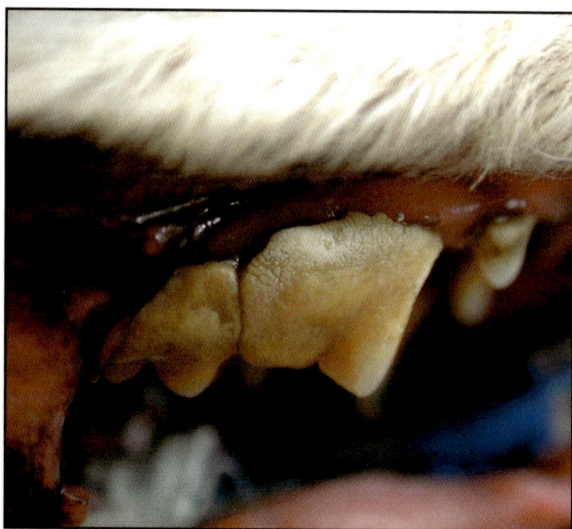

7.11 Heavy calculus formation around the maxillary fourth premolar and first molar.

Halitosis (oral malodour)
Difficulty eating
Pain on eating
Excessive salivation, blood-tinged saliva
Variable amounts of plaque and calculus
Inflamed, bleeding gingiva
Gingival ulceration
Purulent discharge from periodontal pocket
Loss of normal gingival contour
Gingival recession
Furcation exposure
Tooth mobility
Lethargy

7.12 Clinical signs and symptoms associated with periodontal disease.

Diagnosis

A systematic approach is necessary when assessing and recording the extent of PD in the dog. This should always include a thorough clinical examination of other organ systems before the oral examination begins.

The oral examination will include inspection and palpation of the extraoral structures, including the face, lips, muscles of mastication, temporomandibular joints (TMJs), salivary glands, lymph nodes, maxillae and mandibles, looking for swelling, atrophy or assymetry. Inspection of the intraoral structures should follow, including the hard and soft tissues with the focus on the dentition, gingiva, mucosa, tongue, tonsils and occlusion. On visual inspection, a dog with periodontitis may show evidence of gingival swelling, redness and altered gingival contour around the teeth. There may also be areas with gingival recession, furcation exposures (in multi-rooted teeth) or purulent discharge from periodontal pockets. There can be variable amounts of plaque and calculus present, although as a general rule, the more plaque and calculus covering the tooth surface, the more severe the disease in susceptible animals.

In humans, specific tests have been developed to measure markers of inflammation within the gingival crevicular fluid (GCF) and serum of patients with periodontitis. PGE_2 levels may be elevated in the GCF of patients with periodontitis (Nelson *et al.*, 1992). In this study, an automated enzyme immunoassay to measure PGE_2 in GCF from humans and a dog model was developed as an indicator of PD. The study showed that raised PGE_2 in GCF correlated well with increased pocket depth and gingival bleeding scores.

PD often affects the mouth uniformly, with the extent of disease being similar on both sides of the mouth, but sometimes to differing degrees of severity. However, if the disease presentation is not uniform or presents as a localized lesion, other causes such as immunopathy or neoplasia need to be ruled out.

Oral pathology, such as fractured teeth, may lead to altered chewing patterns with a subsequent increase in plaque, calculus and periodontitis on the affected side. The contralateral side often has clean teeth with healthy gingiva. The presence and extent of plaque and calculus accumulation should be noted. The use of a plaque disclosing dye on the teeth will demonstrate to the owner the extent of the problem.

A thorough periodontal examination can only be performed with the dog under general anaesthesia. Because periodontitis usually worsens with increasing age, periodontal therapy is often performed on middle-aged to geriatric patients under general anaesthesia. It is therefore important to carry out an anaesthetic risk assessment (see Chapter 3) prior to embarking on what can often be a lengthy procedure.

Grading periodontal disease

There are a number of methods of grading the severity of the disease. However, it must be remembered that different degrees of severity can all occur in the same mouth or even at different sites around the same tooth. Grading is based on the extent of AL as measured with a periodontal probe (Figure 7.13).

AL is indicative of the periodontal destruction that

Disease extent	Grade of PD	Periodontal health	Plaque and calculus	Radiographic findings	Prognosis
Healthy gingiva	0	Normal firm gingiva with gingival contour well adapted to tooth. Stippled coral pink or pigmented gingiva. No abnormal tooth mobility. No bleeding on probing (BOP)	Very little	No radiographic evidence of attachment loss (AL). Normal alveolar marginal bone with presence of crestal lamina dura	Excellent
Established gingivitis	I	Redness and swelling of gingival margin. Gingiva starting to pull away from tooth. Pseudo-pockets may be present. BOP	Variable amounts	No radiographic evidence of AL	Reversible
Mild periodontitis	II	As above, loss of gingival contour: ± furcation involvement; ± gingival recession/pocketing; ± tooth mobility. BOP	Variable amounts; usually heavier than for established gingivitis	Rounding of marginal bone <25% AL	Irreversible, but controllable
Moderate periodontitis	III	As above. BOP (active disease). Furcation involvement. Tooth mobility present	Variable amounts; usually heavier than for mild periodontitis	Horizontal or vertical bone loss 25–50% AL	Irreversible, but controllable
Severe periodontitis	IV	As above. Furcation involvement: ± purulent discharge from pockets; ± spontaneous gingival bleeding; ± periodontal abscess formation. Tooth mobility more prominent	Variable amounts; usually heavier than for moderate periodontitis	Horizontal or vertical bone loss >50% AL	Irreversible, but controllable. Some extractions inevitable

7.13 Periodontal disease grading system.

occurs due to the effects of both bacterial toxins and the host's own defence system. The disease often progresses in stages over a long period of time (Figure 7.14). However, if untreated, the natural progression of the disease can lead to tooth loss.

Treatment of gingivitis

Gingivitis is usually caused by the build-up of undisturbed plaque (non-specific plaque) around the tooth. The aim of treating gingivitis is to restore the affected gingival tissues to clinical health, by the thorough removal of plaque, and then to maintain gingival health, thereby preventing progression to periodontitis. This can often be simply accomplished by instigating such measures as home care (e.g. daily tooth brushing) with periodic professional assessment and treatment to maintain gingival health.

Treatment of periodontitis

There are two main modes of treatment for periodontitis:

- Non-surgical periodontal therapy
- Periodontal surgery.

The ultimate goal of periodontal therapy is to pro-vide treatment that will arrest disease progression and give long-term stability by preventing further tissue destruction at those sites already affected, whilst also preventing disease at unaffected sites. Effective control of periodontitis depends upon the identification and treatment of the bacterial infection and subsequent prevention of its recurrence.

Plaque removal is essential in preventing and controlling periodontitis. Plaque removal can be accomplished by a combination of mechanical and chemical plaque reduction techniques, dietary manipulation and regular professional periodontal therapy. However, the removal of supragingival plaque has little effect on established subgingival plaque. Pockets deeper than 3 mm in dogs may require root debridement (closed or non-surgical). A decision regarding open root debridement (requiring periodontal surgery) would depend on the response of the periodontium to closed root debridement.

After the initial periodontal assessment, a treatment plan should be formulated that addresses the patient's disease and the owner's concerns. The plan should include ongoing monitoring and, if necessary, alterations to the periodontal management, which may include more advanced periodontal therapy. However,

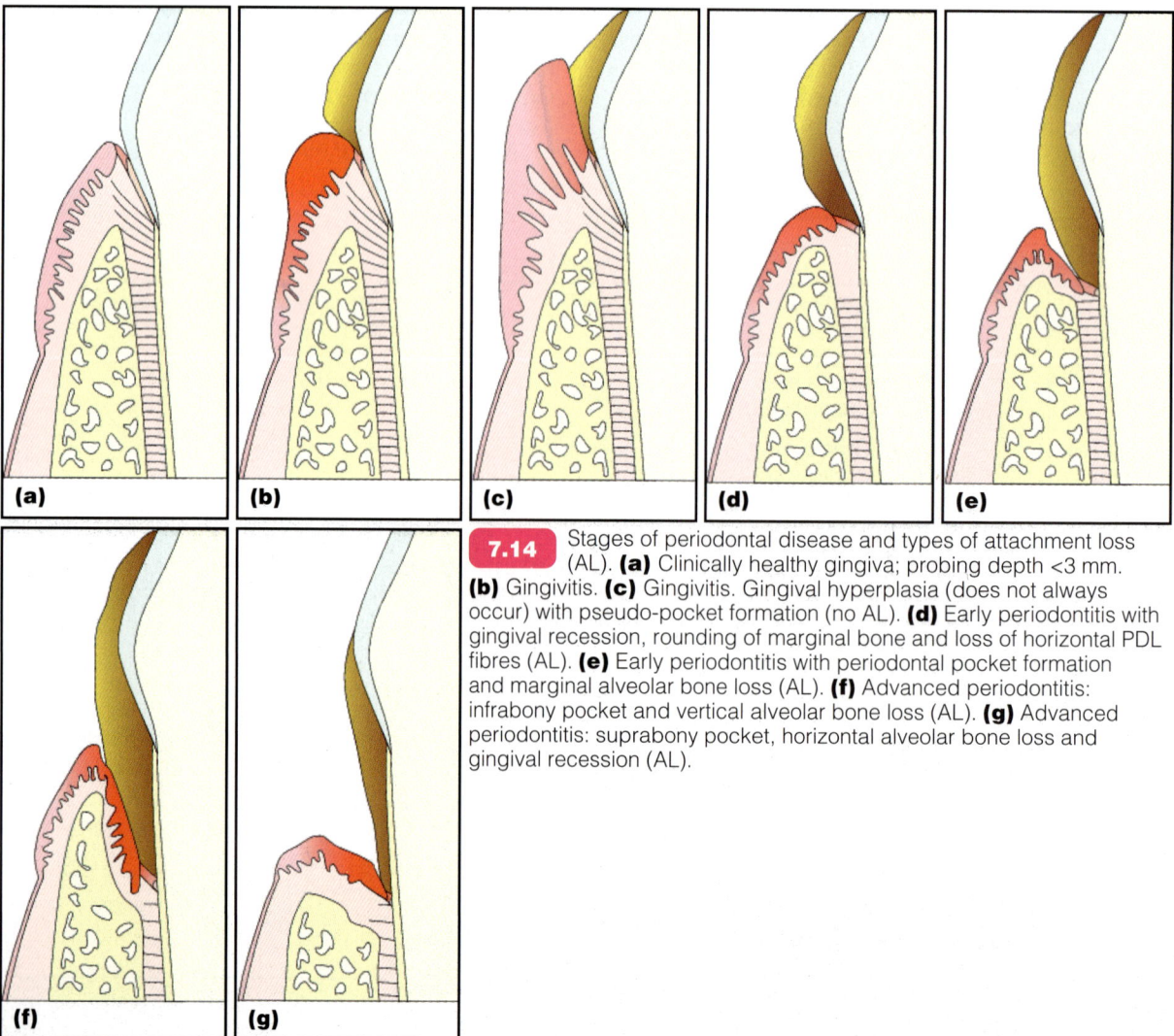

7.14 Stages of periodontal disease and types of attachment loss (AL). **(a)** Clinically healthy gingiva; probing depth <3 mm. **(b)** Gingivitis. **(c)** Gingivitis. Gingival hyperplasia (does not always occur) with pseudo-pocket formation (no AL). **(d)** Early periodontitis with gingival recession, rounding of marginal bone and loss of horizontal PDL fibres (AL). **(e)** Early periodontitis with periodontal pocket formation and marginal alveolar bone loss (AL). **(f)** Advanced periodontitis: infrabony pocket and vertical alveolar bone loss (AL). **(g)** Advanced periodontitis: suprabony pocket, horizontal alveolar bone loss and gingival recession (AL).

no treatment plan can be formulated without a detailed discussion of home care and plaque control with the owner. Home care and the continued removal of plaque remains the cornerstone of PD prevention and control (see 'Home care advice').

Non-surgical periodontal therapy

Non-surgical periodontal therapy involves scaling and closed root debridement under general anaesthesia. It is always the first line treatment for managing PD. No matter whether non-surgical or surgical periodontal therapy is performed, there are a number of steps involved in managing PD.

The steps involved in non-surgical periodontal therapy are:

1. Periodontal probing and charting.
2. Oral radiography.
3. Recording of all findings and development of a treatment plan.
4. Gross removal of supragingival plaque and calculus.
5. Supra- and subgingival tooth debridement.
6. Polishing.
7. Sulcular lavage.
8. Antimicrobial treatments (where indicated).
9. Home care advice and PD prevention.
10. Recall and review.

Periodontal probing and charting: Periodontitis is a disease of the periodontium and involves the loss of periodontal attachment to the tooth. The only way to assess the extent of the disease is to assess the loss of periodontal attachment (by probing and radiography) and to record the information.

Periodontal probing with a blunt-ended probe (see Chapter 5) measures the depth of the gingival sulcus or pocket, and provides a practical way of assessing periodontal health or disease. Normal sulcus depth in the dog is <3 mm. The probe is held in a modified pen grip with a finger rest, and is placed parallel to the long axis of the tooth (Figure 7.15). With light pressure the probe is gently walked around the tooth to measure

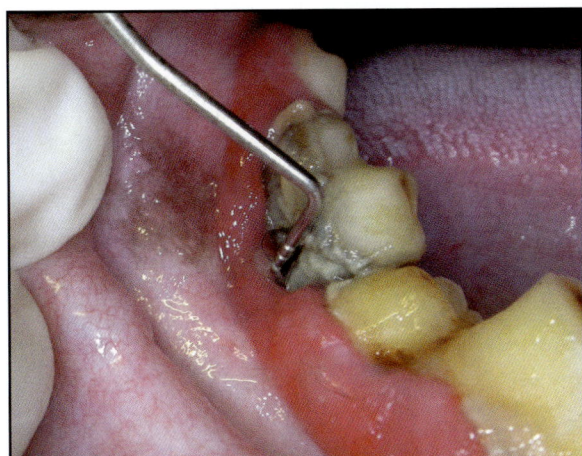

7.15 Measuring attachment loss with a periodontal probe. An 8 mm periodontal pocket was found in the mid-buccal area of the mesial root of the mandibular second molar. (Courtesy of W. Fitzgerald.)

pocket depth.

Pocket depth is measured from the free gingival margin to the base of the pocket. This measurement is recorded to the nearest millimetre. If gingival recession is present, the periodontal probe can also be used to measure this recession. The measurement (to the nearest mm) is taken from the cementoenamel junction to the free gingival margin. Where recession is present, the addition of the recession and pocket measurements gives the AL measurement for that particular tooth surface. Bleeding on probing (BOP) can also be noted at this time as it is a sign of inflammation at that site.

In humans, the severity of periodontitis is based on a number of findings including: tooth mobility, BOP, AL, furcation involvement, purulent discharge from pockets and tooth pain associated with percussion or thermal sensitivity testing. A prognosis is then assigned to each tooth.

As well as the periodontal probe, the dental explorer is a useful tool when examining teeth for pulpal exposures, external resorptive lesions, furcation involvement and dental caries. It can also be used post-root debridement to assess for the presence of residual calculus. A dental mirror may also aid in examining the palatal and lingual surfaces of teeth.

All findings should be recorded on a dental chart (see Chapters 2 and 5). Missing, rotated and fractured teeth, probing depths (up to 6 points per tooth), gingival recession and hyperplasia, mobility, furcation involvement and other oral pathology can all be recorded on a dental chart. Charting not only records the current state of the dentition and soft tissues of the oral cavity, allowing the formulation of a treatment plan, but also provides a permanent record for future comparisons.

Patient positioning is important when carrying out a thorough oral examination under general anaesthesia. The author prefers the dog to be in left lateral and then right lateral recumbency for examination and treatment, but other positions such as dorsal recumbency may be preferred. The gold standard for airway protection is a cuffed endotracheal (ET) tube. The author also places gauze packs into the back of the mouth to prevent calculus and other debris from entering the oropharynx, larynx and trachea (see Chapter 3).

Oral radiography: Oral radiography is a useful diagnostic tool for assessing periodontitis. Oral radiographs demonstrate alveolar bone height and in cases of periodontitis will show generalized horizontal and localized vertical alveolar bone loss. Radiographs can be taken prior to treatment and at regular intervals afterwards to monitor disease control or progression.

In the healthy human periodontium, the alveolar marginal bone should be about 2 mm from the cemento-enamel junction (Hausmann *et al.*, 1991).

Most dogs with periodontitis show a horizontal type of bone loss (Figure 7.16), although vertical or angular bone loss (Figure 7.17) occur frequently, especially palatally to the maxillary canine tooth.

Radiographic signs of periodontitis include resorption of the alveolar margin, widening of the PDL space, loss of lamina dura (cortical bone of the

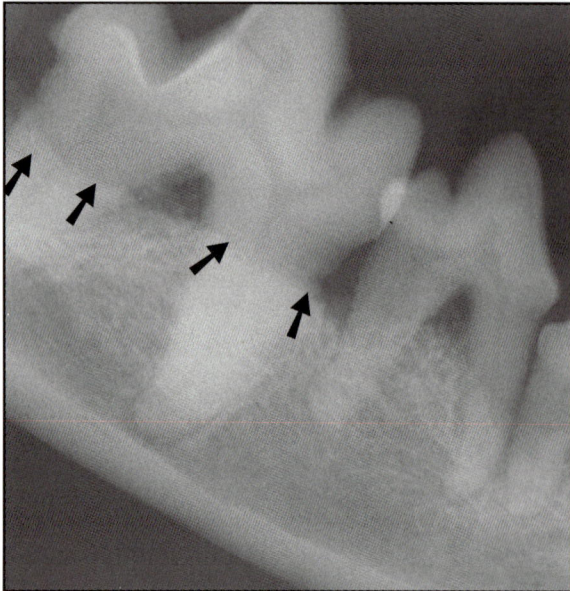

7.16 Horizontal bone loss (arrowed) around the distal root of the mandibular fourth premolar and the mesial and distal roots of the first molar. Clinical examination revealed furcation grade 2 on both of these teeth. (Courtesy of W. Fitzgerald.)

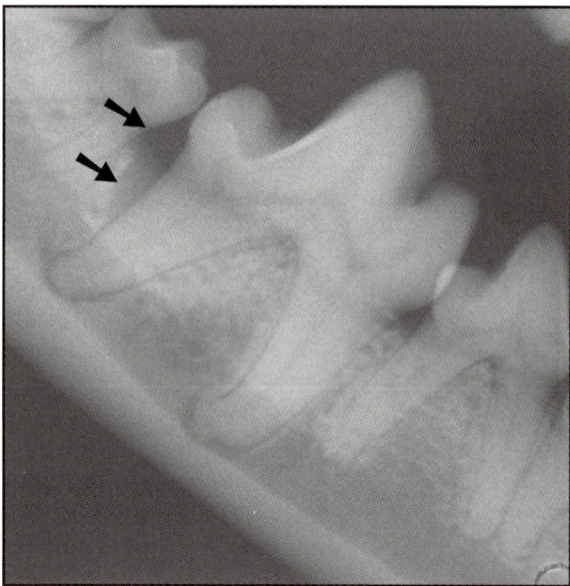

7.17 Vertical bone loss (arrowed) around the distal root of the mandibular first molar. Widening of the PDL space around the mesial and distal root apices is often a normal radiographic finding.

alveolus) and alveolar bone destruction. Radiographs can also reveal subgingival calculus deposits, as well as showing other forms of pathology (such as periapical lesions) and tumours of both soft and hard tissues.

Prior to treating periodontitis, a full-mouth radiographic examination is recommended. This not only provides a base level assessment of disease but can also aid in the detection of other pathology that may not be clinically evident during the oral examination. The advent of digital radiography has further enhanced the use of radiography in the monitoring of periodontal treatment success or failure (digital subtraction radiography).

Recording and treatment planning: The periodontal probing depths are recorded on a dental chart along with any other abnormalities. The dental chart is an important document that is a permanent record of the state of the dentition and soft tissues at a given point in time. Because PD is a chronic disease, the chart offers the clinician the ability to compare records from previous charting(s) and thus assess the success or failure of treatment. The record is also a medico-legal document a copy of which can be given to the owner or forwarded to a specialist when referral is considered.

After all abnormalities, including gingival recession and hyperplasia, BOP, mobility, suppuration, furcation involvement, probing depths and loss of attachment, have been recorded, a treatment plan can be formulated. A number of factors need to be considered when formulating a treatment plan. Some of the more important factors to consider include:

- The ability or inability of the owners to comply with home care will have a major influence on the clinician's decision-making. However, the initiation of home care may be easier to perform for both patient and owner following the initial periodontal therapy. If, after the initial therapy and subsequent gingival healing, home care is ineffective or lacking, the clinician will need to consider more aggressive periodontal therapies, including more frequent professional interventions
- The extent and severity of the disease, based on periodontal probing and radiographs
- The strategic value of teeth and preserving functional units, e.g. the maxillary and mandibular canine teeth and the maxillary fourth premolar and mandibular first molar
- The decision to refer: for those patients requiring more advanced periodontal therapy, including periodontal surgery with or without local delivery of antimicrobials (perioceutics).

It should be remembered that the primary role of treatment is to remove plaque, disrupt the subgingival biofilm, promote healing and to formulate an ongoing treatment plan that will prevent or slow down plaque reformation.

Gross removal of supragingival plaque and calculus: Prior to periodontal therapy, the oral cavity should be flushed with a dilute solution of chlorhexidine gluconate (0.12–0.2%). This will help reduce the bacterial aerosol that occurs during mechanical scaling. The removal of gross calculus, with instruments such as calculus removers (Figure 7.18), allows speedier removal of smaller deposits by mechanical or hand scalers.

WARNING
Care should be taken when using calculus removers so as not to cause iatrogenic damage to the teeth or soft tissues.

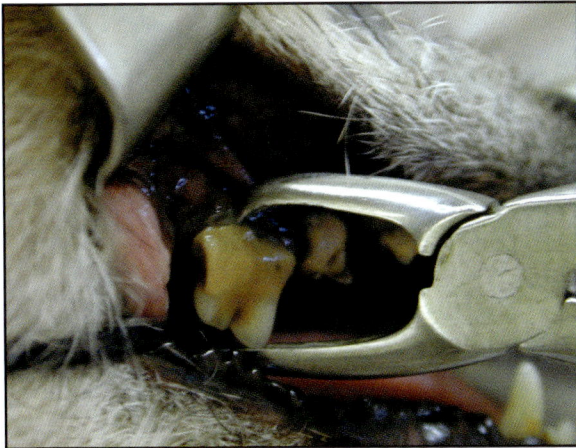

7.18 Calculus remover applied to the maxillary fourth premolar. Care must be taken not to fracture the crown when removing the calculus. (Courtesy of D. Clarke.)

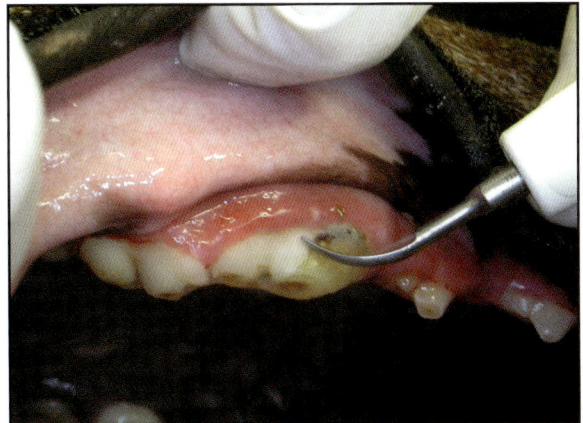

7.19 Piezoelectric scaler: using the side of the instrument tip. This dog had moderate generalized abrasion. Tertiary dentine is visible on some teeth and must be distinguished from pulp exposure and caries.

Supra- and subgingival debridement: The removal of supra- and subgingival plaque and calculus is achieved by a combination of mechanical scaling, hand scaling and polishing.

Mechanical scaling: There are two forms of mechanical (power driven) scalers:

• Sonic
• Ultrasonic.

Sonic scalers are air turbine units that operate between 3000 and 8000 cycles per second (cps). They are used less often in veterinary dentistry than ultrasonic scalers due mainly to their expense and their slowness in removing plaque and calculus. However, one of the benefits of using sonic scalers is lower heat production, thus reducing the chance of iatrogenic thermal injury to the pulp.

Ultrasonic scalers include magnetostrictive and piezoelectric scalers. The magnetostrictive ultrasonic scaler is the most widely used and consists of a metal stack or ferrite rod, which vibrates under the influence of an electromagnetic field. Magnetostrictive instruments operate between 18000 and 45000 cps. When an electric current is applied to a wire coil in the handpiece, an electromagnetic field is created around the stack or rod, causing it to constrict. An alternating current causes an alternating electromagnetic field, resulting in tip vibration. The tip movement of magnetostrictive scalers ranges from linear to elliptical or circular, depending on the type of unit and the shape and length of the tip. Magnetostrictive tip movement allows for activation of all surfaces of the tip at once. Usually it is preferred that the side of the tip is used against the tooth to minimize heat concentration and help prevent iatrogenic thermal damage to the pulp. A water spray is essential to dissipate heat as well as to produce cavitational activity. This cavitation effect disrupts bacterial cell walls and can operate slightly beyond the reach of the tip (a benefit when used in deep pockets).

The other form of ultrasonic scaler is the piezoelectric scaler (Figure 7.19). The piezoelectric scaler has crystals within the handpiece that undergo dimensional change. The piezoelectric unit operates at 25000–50000 cps with a linear tip movement; and only two sides of the tip are active (Drisko, 2000).

Scalers should be held so that the long axis of the scaler tip is parallel with the tooth surface; this prevents the concentration of heat in one area or gouging and scratching of the tooth. Mechanical scalers should be used with a continuous motion and for no longer than 15 seconds at a time on any one tooth. Light strokes with minimal pressure should be employed. The use of the modified pen grip with finger rests is recommended (Figure 7.20). The fine aerosol that develops with the use of mechanical scalers is laden with bacteria. It is recommended that facemasks and protective eyewear be worn at all times to protect the operator and assistant (see Chapter 4).

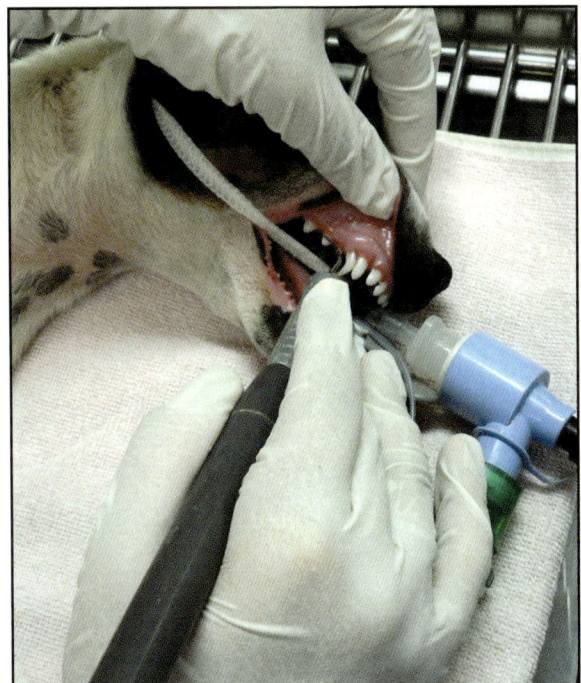

7.20 Use of the modified pen grip to hold the scaler handle. Note the persistent 504 in this dog.

Mechanical scalers may also be used subgingivally, as long as they are used with a reduced power setting, for short periods of time and with adequate water cooling. There are a number of slimline scaler tips with design features enabling the water coolant to get to the entire tip, even when inserted into the periodontal pocket. The operator still needs to be cautious when using these subgingival scaler tips to prevent iatrogenic thermal damage to the tooth. The tips of piezo-electric scalers tend not to generate as much heat as those of magnetostrictive scalers, because they do not generate a magnetic field. They may be used subgingivally with due care. There are also mechanical scalers available that can deliver chlorhexidene gluconate as the coolant, although the benefit of this form of delivery is debatable.

Hand scaling: Following mechanical scaling, sharp hand scalers are used to remove any remaining plaque or calculus.

The *H6–H7 sickle scaler* is ideal for supragingival calculus removal. It is often used to remove large heavy deposits, thus improving access to the subgingival area for other instruments. It has a flat blade cut at 90 degrees to the shank. Both sides of the blade have cutting edges. In cross-section, the blade of a scaler is triangular, whereas a curette is semicircular.

Curettes are used for supra- and subgingival scaling. Curettes come in a number of different types (curettes used in human dentistry can be of a universal or site-specific type). Gracey curettes (e.g. Gracey 7/8) are a popular choice for subgingival scaling and root debridement (i.e. the effective removal of plaque and calculus with minimal damage to the root surface). Curettes remove plaque as well as calculus.

Gracey curettes have the cutting edge at the lower aspect of the blade. If the curette is held vertically and viewed side on, the cutting edge of the blade is the lowest part of the blade. Most Gracey curettes are manufactured so that the face of the blade is offset at about 70 degrees to the lower shank. To avoid damaging the gingival tissues when entering the pocket, the working end of the curette is introduced with the face of the blade 'closed' or flattened against the tooth surface.

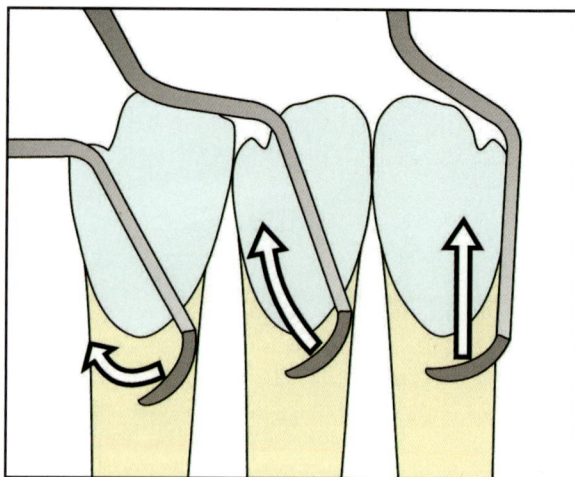

7.22 Use of curette subgingivally with overlapping horizontal, oblique and vertical working strokes to thoroughly remove root surface debris.

The blade of a Gracey curette is correctly adapted when the lower cutting edge is against the tooth and the terminal shank is parallel to the tooth surface being scaled (Figure 7.21). While maintaining the shank parallel to the tooth surface, a series of overlapping pull strokes (Figure 7.22) are performed to clean the entire root surface. The minimum number of strokes necessary to give a clean root surface is recommended to prevent iatrogenic damage to the root surface.

Studies (Hughes and Smales, 1986; Nyman *et al.*, 1986) have shown that it is neither necessary nor desirable to aggresively plane the surface of the root, as it removes too much healthy tooth structure and increases the risk of recession and root exposure (this results in tooth sensitivity in humans). Overzealous root planing can also remove important proteins, such as bone morphogenic protein, and slow down fibrous reattachment to the root.

Endotoxins (lipopolysaccharides) from Gram-negative bacteria are present on the cementum surface only, and not within the cementum and dentine of the root as previously thought. The removal of diseased cementum or dentine is not necessary to achieve periodontal healing. Therefore, it may be counter-

7.21 **(a)** The working end of the curette is inserted into the gingival sulcus with the face of the blade 'closed' and the cutting edge of the instrument against the root surface. **(b)** The working end of the curette is 'opened' so that the lower shank of the instrument is parallel to the tooth surface. **(c)** Curette in the 'active' position; the cutting edge is against the tooth allowing the implementation of short pulling strokes (working strokes).

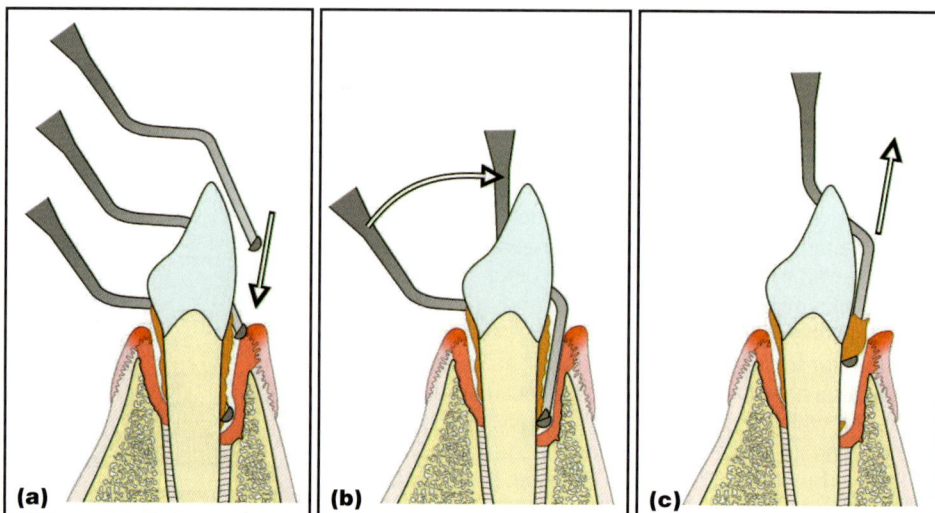

productive for the future periodontal health of the tooth to vigorously perform root planing (Hughes *et al.,* 1988; Cadosch *et al.,* 2003).

It is important to ascertain the thoroughness of subgingival scaling by exploring the tooth surface with a dental explorer. The explorer can be used to detect remaining deposits within the gingival pocket and re-scaling will be necessary if deposits remain. With any form of hand scaling, the instruments must be sharp. Therefore, in order to get the best results, it is important to sharpen the instruments following the manufacturer's instructions before and during the hand scaling procedure if necessary.

Future advancements: Erbium: YAG-laser radiation has been shown experimentally to aid in calculus removal and the destruction of subgingival perio-pathogens. However, the risk of pulpal necrosis through thermal injury is real. Further research is continuing concerning the use of lasers in the management of PD.

Ultrasonic scalers that are capable of analysing the tooth surface for the presence of plaque and calculus are now available for human periodontal treatment. Through a visual display, these mechanical instruments inform the operator of residual plaque and calculus on the tooth surface, thus improving sub-gingival plaque and calculus removal.

Polishing: After scaling and root surface debridement have been performed, polishing of the tooth surface is carried out with the use of a slow speed handpiece, prophy head, polishing cup and polishing paste. The paste is available in varying degrees of abrasiveness.

The main aims of polishing are to smooth over any scratches that may have been created during scaling, and to remove any residual plaque and stain. Care should be taken to avoid spending long periods of time polishing a single tooth as there is a risk of iatrogenic thermal injury to the pulp. The cup should rotate at <1000 rpm and there must always be sufficient polishing paste on the polishing cup. The polishing cup can also be 'flared' for polishing subgingivally to remove residual plaque (Figure 7.23).

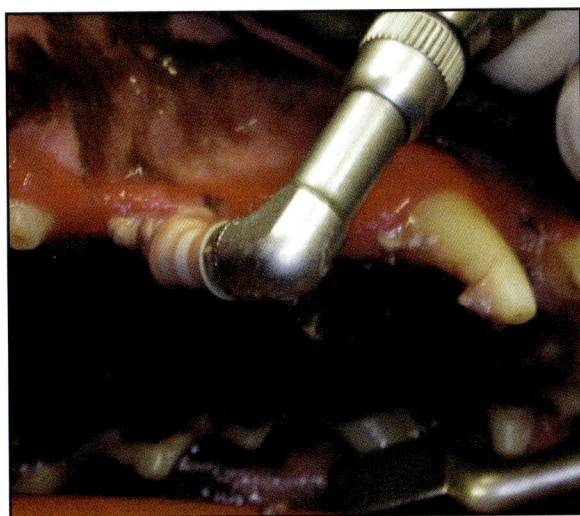

7.23 Polishing teeth. The polishing cup is gently flared to polish subgingivally.

Sulcular lavage: It has been shown, through a number of studies in humans, that sulcular lavage is unnecessary. The flow of gingival fluid as well as bleeding from the sulcus is enough to dislodge any unattached debris. However, if required, the removal of 'prophy' paste and other debris can be done with the gentle use of the air/water spray on the three-in-one syringe or with a blunt-ended needle and syringe.

Antimicrobial treatments: Bacteraemia may occur during any periodontal procedure. This bacteraemia may last about 20 minutes, but in the healthy animal bacteria are quickly cleared by the reticuloendothelial (monocyte:macrophage) system. There is usually no need to place the dog on a course of antimicrobials prior to the procedure (see Antimicrobial therapy).

Chlorhexidine gluconate can be used as a long-term chemical plaque retardant in the dog. It is a broad spectrum antimicrobial with excellent efficacy in the oral cavity. Bacterial resistance to chlorhexidine is unlikely, as opposed to potential resistance associated with systemically or locally delivered antimicrobials. It does, however, require sufficient contact time with the oral tissues to be effective, but it has good substantivity (persistence of action) and binds to hard as well as soft tissues of the oral cavity.

Chlorhexidine has a somewhat unpleasant taste, can alter taste perception and sometimes may irritate mucosal surfaces. If used continuously for more than a few weeks, it can also stain teeth and may precipitate calculus formation. In established periodontitis, chlorhexidine will not penetrate deep into the periodontal pocket and so will have no effect on deep subgingival periodontal pathogens.

Systemic antimicrobials may be necessary as a short-term adjunct to scaling and root debridement. A more detailed discussion follows later in the chapter. Locally delivered antimicrobials (perioceutics) can be used in the management of deeper periodontal pockets.

Home care advice and PD prevention: Home care refers to the procedures that owners can perform at home to retard the accumulation of dental plaque and thus prevent or stabilize PD. This is an integral part of the dental 'prophylaxis' because without it the plaque and calculus will quickly reform.

The main goal of home care is the daily removal of plaque. Home care, however, cannot successfully remove dental plaque once it has mineralized into calculus, nor can home care alone manage those dogs with established periodontitis. Home care needs to be individually tailored to the prevention and control of the animal's disease with reference to the ability and compliance of the owner to instigate plaque control. For home care to work, therefore, not only is firm and continuing commitment needed from the owner, but also advice from the veterinary surgeon that is seen to be practical and realistic. Unwilling owners or unco-operative pets make for an unrewarding exercise.

The periodic disturbance of subgingival plaque and the removal of plaque from areas that cannot be accessed by home care (i.e. furcation sites) should be performed on a regular basis by the clinician. The frequency of this professional intervention will be dictated by the stability of the periodontium as assessed by oral examination and by the level of plaque control achieved at home.

Home care products: There are a large number of home care products available to the pet owner. The gold standard for plaque removal and for the prevention of PD still remains daily tooth brushing (Figure 7.24). Without this, plaque accumulation is inevitable. Chemical agents, such as chlorhexidine gluconate, have also been shown to help prevent gingivitis in dogs.

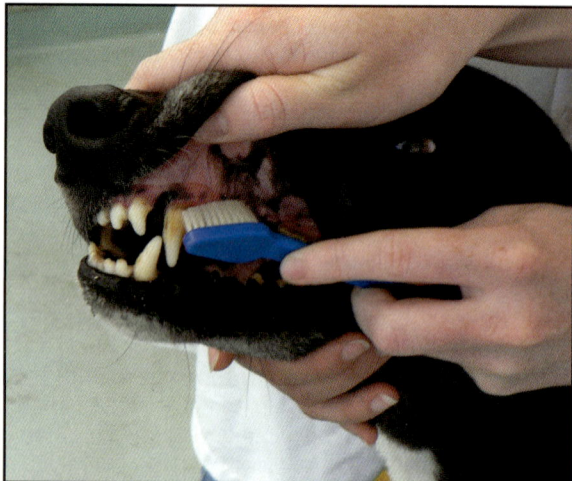

7.24 Daily tooth brushing.

The use of flavoured 'dog' dentifrices may make the brushing experience more enjoyable for the animal. All owners should be offered a demonstration of the tooth brushing technique (modified Bass method) and ideally, the owner should then be observed performing the brushing technique on their pet. A brush with filaments of medium stiffness is used with the modified Bass method. For the maxillary teeth, the tooth brush filaments are angled dorsally at 45 degrees and the tooth brush moved across the teeth in a circular motion, concentrating on the tooth/gingival margin. For the mandibular teeth the bristles are angled ventrally at 45 degrees and the same circular action used (Figure 7.25). Pet tooth brushes must be replaced regularly as worn brushes are ineffective. Power driven tooth brushes use an oscillating action.

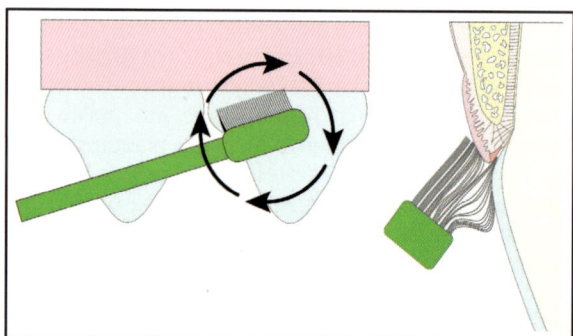

7.25 Modified Bass technique. The tooth brush head is angled at 45 degrees and used in a circular motion.

Diet: The use of dietary texture to control plaque accumulation is an important part of PD prevention, especially when tooth brushing compliance by pet owners is low. However, with established periodontitis, the effects of 'dental' diets and chews in controlling the disease is unknown. Soluble zinc salts have been used in a number of home care products for their antibacterial properties. Zinc salts may also be effective in controlling oral malodour (VSC) by binding to sulphur and forming insoluble compounds that emit little odour.

Polyphosphates, such as hexametaphosphate, have been incorporated into foods and other home care products because of their ability to bind to salivary calcium. This binding helps prevent the formation of calculus, although there is no effect on plaque formation. A recent study (Roudebush *et al.,* 2005) reviewed home care products based on current evidence-based veterinary dentistry. The study made a number of recommendations regarding home care products that are used to prevent PD in both dogs and cats. The study showed that for dental home care to control plaque accumulation and gingivitis in dogs, the highest quality of evidence existed for tooth brushing, chlorhexidine, dental foods with textural characteristics, proprietary dental treats and short-term use of dental sealants. Furthermore, tooth brushing, dental foods with textural characteristics, dental foods or treats with polyphosphates and proprietary rawhide chews were recommended for the control of calculus formation in dogs. The study concluded that other home care dental products used in dogs that were supported by a lower quality of evidence should not be recommended without further published studies.

In 1997 the Veterinary Oral Health Council (VOHC) was established to offer a seal of acceptance to those oral hygiene products and foods that were shown in controlled studies to retard plaque and calculus. Today, the VOHC Seal of Acceptance system for plaque and tartar control products is endorsed by a number of Veterinary Dental Organisations throughout the world. A list of endorsed products can be found on the VOHC website (www.vohc.org).

Recall and review: The clinician should schedule recalls based on the severity of the disease. A review of home care compliance, including dietary management, should be carried out on a regular basis. If the motivated owner is having difficulty implementing home care recommendations, the clinician should be prepared to offer alternatives including more frequent professional interventions.

The reinforcement of daily tooth brushing combined with practical demonstrations of brushing technique should be included in the recall process. Since the advent of power driven tooth brushes in human oral care, the use of these brushes as pet home care tools is on the increase.

Client education and motivation remain an integral part of PD prevention and control. It is also important to establish the time intervals between professional scaling and cleaning, based on the success or failure of past treatments.

Periodontal surgery

Periodontal surgery is performed for a number of reasons, including:

- The removal of plaque and calculus by direct visualization of the root surface
- The reduction of pocket depth
- Crown lengthening
- Periodontium regenerating techniques.

Periodontal surgery should not be the first line treatment in managing PD. Before periodontal surgery is considered, factors such as the cooperation of the patient, the commitment and the ability of the owner to perform home care (including daily tooth brushing), the cost of the procedure and the aesthetic and functional importance of the tooth or teeth requiring periodontal surgery should all be evaluated by the clinician.

Non-surgical therapy or closed scaling and root planing is always performed prior to surgical treatment of periodontitis. Non-surgical therapy will always provide some benefit. However, surgery is indicated where non-surgical methods fail to control the disease (Wang and Greenwell, 2001). Surgery should be reserved for deep pockets (>4 mm) that have not responded to closed debridement and then only after further periodontal assessments, including dental radiography, have been carried out.

Periodontal surgery can:

- Provide direct access to enable thorough cleaning of the root surface
- Provide a more accurate determination of prognosis for a tooth as a result of direct visualization of its bony support
- Aid in home care, as a result of periodontal pocket depth reduction
- Lengthen the clinical crown (crown lengthening) to aid in the placement of a restoration
- Regain lost periodontium using regenerative approaches (guided tissue regeneration, GTR).

Periodontal surgery, especially those modalities involving pocket depth reduction, represents an effort to decrease the subgingival microbial load and to prevent recurrence of periodontal breakdown. The three main surgical procedures are:

- Procedures to restore tissue attachment
- Resective procedures
- Grafting and regeneration procedures.

Types of periodontal surgery:

Procedures to restore tissue attachment: Subgingival curettage includes the removal of the diseased gingival pocket epithelium. Closed debridement techniques may also inadvertently remove pocket epithelium.

Open flap debridement allows visual access to the root surface for root surface debridement and the removal of very little pocket epithelium. It involves an intrasulcular incision from the free gingival margin down to the bone. The flap allows intimate postopera-

tive contact between the gingival connective tissue and the root surface. Its drawbacks include an inability to achieve pocket elimination and the formation of a long junctional epithelium (LJE), although LJE is still considered a favourable and stable outcome.

Resective procedures (pocket elimination procedures): Gingivectomy: The aim is to excise excessive gingival tissue in cases of pseudo-pocket formation, as seen in gingival hyperplasia in Boxers. Gingivectomy may also be performed to correct gingival deformities or in some cases of crown lengthening, being careful to maintain some attached gingiva (Figure 7.26).

Apically repositioned flap: This is defined as the apical displacement of the entire mucogingival unit. It involves pocket elimination. It does preserve and retain all of the attached gingiva. It also allows access to the root surface, including furcation areas, for instrumentation and osseous surgery. It is often indicated in crown lengthening cases with deep suprabony or infrabony pocketing. Pocket reduction makes home care simpler, thus facilitating better plaque control (Figure 7.27).

Osseous resection: This is defined as the reshaping of alveolar bone to achieve a physiological contour. It is often used in crown lengthening techniques and when carrying out an apically repositioned flap procedure. Referral of advanced or non-responsive periodontitis cases requiring osseous resection to a specialist may be required.

Grafting and guided tissue regeneration: These specialized techniques are aimed at correcting excessive soft tissue or alveolar bone loss. Free gingival grafts can be used to replace lost attached gingiva. The grafts are harvested from other areas with sufficient attached gingiva. Sliding pedicle grafts can be used to cover exposed root surfaces. Newer alloplastic products, including synthetic bone graft materials (Consil® Dental), can be used to fill infrabony defects resulting from periodontitis. They appear to have an osteoconductive function, promoting osteoblast activity around the ceramic particles. Osseous repair or regeneration has been found to occur when Bioglass® was placed for alveolar ridge maintenance following extraction and treatment of infrabony osseous defects (DeForge,1997).

However, there are a number of controlled studies demonstrating that synthetic ceramic particles may actually interfere with bone formation (Slotte and Lundgren, 1999; Stavropoulos et al., 2003). In these studies, histological analysis showed bioactive glass particles embedded in a sea of connective tissue. In another study performed on dogs (Plotzke et al., 1993) the authors came to the conclusion that 'in the treatment of Class II furcations in dogs, the alloplastic particles were well tolerated but encapsulated by connective tissue fibres. Thus, it did not promote regeneration and did not resorb'. At the present time, the use of osteoconductive products alone as a scaffold for ingrowth of bone progenitor cells seems to be clinically unpredictable, where sometimes bone is found in intimate contact with the product and at other times the product is surrounded by fibrous tissue. Whether this is

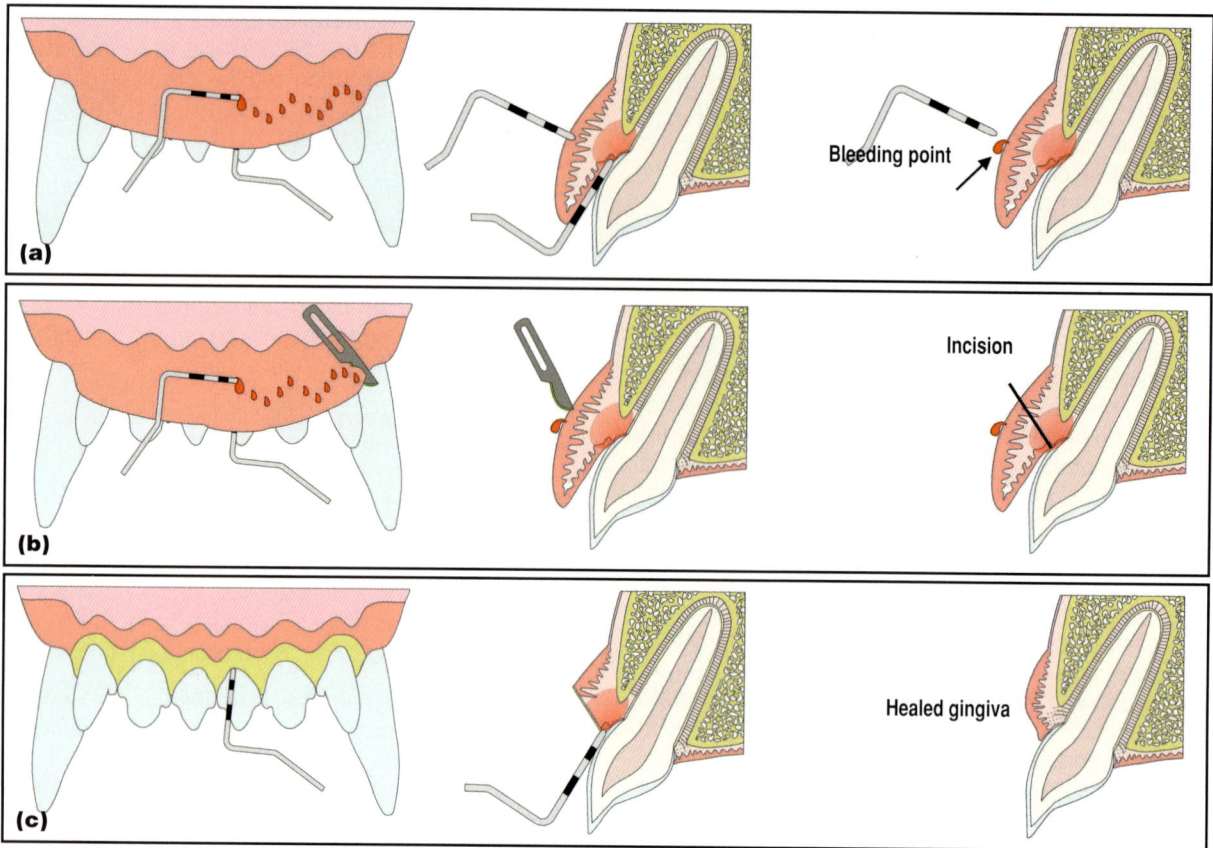

7.26   Gingivectomy. **(a)** Pocket depth is measured and the apical limit of the pocket marked at several points with the periodontal probe to create a number of bleeding points. **(b)** The row of bleeding points is a guide to the line of incision. With the blade angled at 45 degrees, the incision is made apical to the line of bleeding points so that the blade contacts tooth at the bottom of the pocket. This approach offers a good gingival contour around the tooth post-healing. **(c)** Post-gingivectomy and healing; the pocket is eliminated.

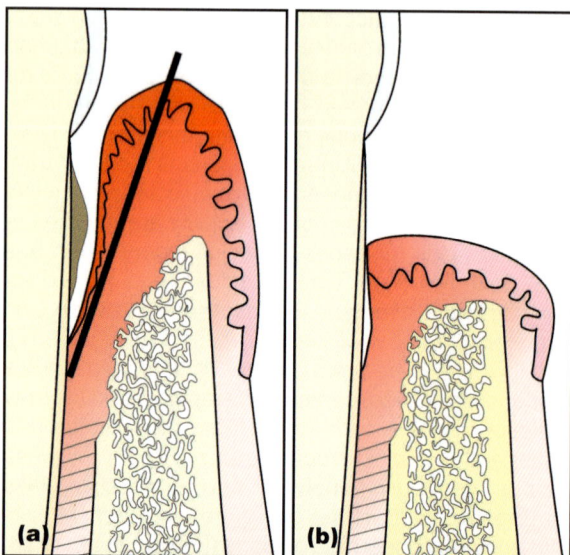

7.27   Apically repositioned flap. **(a)** An incision (black line) is made directly into the pocket, to the depth of the pocket, whilst preserving gingival tissue. A full-thickness flap is then freed from its attachment to the periosteum. **(b)** After removing all calculus and root debris, the flap is repositioned apically, until its edge just covers the bone margin. The flap is then sutured in this new position. The pocket has been eliminated. Osteoplasty may be performed at the same time.

clinically relevant is uncertain. The use of resorbable or non-resorbable membranes to regenerate the structures of the periodontium has been used on occasions to manage teeth with pocketing and severe AL. GTR promotes the ingress of the PDL, while acting as a barrier to epithelial down growth into the pocket. This allows the establishment of all the components of the periodontium (PDL, alveolar bone, cementum, gingival connective tissue and gingival epithelium). However, GTR can have variable results and may not always offer a predictable outcome. Meticulous home care is critical to the success of GTR procedures.

In the future, the use of the bioactive products, such as bone morphogenic protein (BMP), to regenerate the components of the periodontium may replace other methods of regeneration.

Some of the complications that can be seen post-surgical periodontal therapy include pain, swelling, blood loss, infection and root sensitivity (more often seen in humans). Other potential but rare risks include sloughing of the mucoperiosteal flap, root resorption and ankylosis.

Complications associated with periodontitis

Complications due to periodontitis can be divided into local and systemic. *Local complications* include periodontal abscess (see later), osteomyelitis, local lymphadenopathy, immunopathies, periodontic–endodontic lesions and oronasal fistula formation (see later).

Systemic complications associated with periodontitis may occur and there is an enormous amount of research in humans looking at the association between periodontitis and systemic disease. However, proving the link between cause and effect of chronic diseases, such as PD, is not an easy task. It has long been recognized that certain systemic diseases, such as poorly controlled diabetes mellitus, influence the initiation and progression of periodontitis in humans (Grossi and Genco, 1998) and the same may be true in animals. The reverse, namely periodontitis being a risk factor for other organ disease, is now being considered a possibility.

This two-way relationship between periodontitis and systemic disease, which has previously rarely been considered, has resulted in the phrase *periodontal medicine* (Offenbacher, 1996). This is a broad term that defines a rapidly developing branch of periodontology, which focuses on the emerging relationship between periodontal health or disease and systemic health or disease. A causal link is still difficult to prove and intervention studies are required.

It is now accepted that dental or oral surgery procedures, periodontal probing, tooth brushing and mastication cause transient bacteraemias, which, in the healthy patient, are quickly cleared by the reticuloendothelial system (Harari *et al.*, 1993; Nieves *et al.*, 1997). Research suggests that inflammatory mediators and bacterial toxins (especially endotoxins) can also be released from the periodontal pocket into the circulation. The contribution of oral bacteria (within periodontal pockets) to bacterial endocarditis has been acknowledged for decades. The need for antimicrobial prophylaxis for those patients with circulatory disturbances within the heart and its major vessels is recognized in both human and veterinary dental fields.

Research has shown a link between periodontitis and cardiovascular disease, as well as pre-term low birth weight babies in humans (Offenbacher *et al.*, 1996). In animals these links are difficult to establish and there is little evidence in the veterinary literature to support a link between periodontitis and organ dysfunction. However, the similar nature of periodontal disease initiation and progression in humans and dogs supports a possible link between PD and organ dysfunction in dogs (DeBowes *et al.*, 1996).

Antimicrobial (adjunctive) therapy in the management of periodontitis

Antimicrobials (including antiseptics and antibiotics) are commonly used in the management of periodontitis in veterinary dentistry. Antimicrobial usage has often been based on the belief that because PD is caused by a bacterial infection, and antimicrobials kill or control the growth of bacteria, antimicrobials should play an integral part in the treatment of this infection. Often the choice of antimicrobial is decided on empirical grounds with no culture and sensitivity/antibiogram testing carried out. However, the management of PD is quite different from the treatment of most bacterial infections for a number of reasons.

The bacterial flora present in the oral cavity is always heterogenous and relatively complex and often varies from animal to animal. The presence or absence of a single bacterial species cannot be directly correlated with disease presence or its absence. In addition, PD is often asymptomatic in its earlier stages. Furthermore, the host response itself contributes to disease progression. Before prescribing antimicrobials, the clinician must consider such issues as choice of antimicrobial, dosing regimen, length of treatment, evaluation of treatment outcome and short- and long-term benefits from adjunctive antibiotic therapy.

Sometimes, the clinician must resist pressure from owners to prescribe antimicrobials without any other periodontal therapy. It is the author's opinion that the use of antimicrobials without periodontal debridement is unacceptable practice, based on the difficulty of antimicrobial penetration into the plaque biofilm, unless that biofilm has been disrupted by mechanical debridement. Rational prescribing of antibiotics would include the selection of the antimicrobial with the narrowest spectrum of activity against known periodontal pathogens, the fewest side effects and the use of so-called 'first line antimicrobials', saving other agents for when resistance is encountered.

Antimicrobials, such as amoxicillin–clavulanate, clindamycin hydrochloride and metronidazole seem to be particularly effective against periodontal pathogens, based on pharmacokinetic and clinical studies (Sarkiala and Harvey, 1993). Topical chlorhexidine gluconate is also very effective against plaque bacteria and can be used after more complex periodontal therapies, where tooth brushing initially may be uncomfortable for the animal.

Locally delivered antimicrobials have been used in periodontal therapy for a number of years. Doxycycline used as a sustained release polymer is registered for use in dogs. It is mainly used in deep periodontal pockets (>4 mm) as adjunctive therapy to closed root debridement. It is particularly useful in the infrabony pocket associated with the palatal surface of the maxillary canine tooth. Doxycycline gel should only be applied to teeth that have been cleaned and polished.

Doxycycline gel is a two syringe system: syringe A contains the polymer delivery system and syringe B contains the doxycycline. The syringe contents are thoroughly mixed and, using a blunt canula, introduced into the periodontal pocket, filling the pocket to the gingival margin. A few drops of water are applied over the site to cause the gel to polymerize. Doxycycline gel can remain in the periodontal pocket for several weeks. The teeth should not be brushed for two weeks following placement of the gel.

The development of other local antimicrobial delivery systems may in future reduce the adjunctive use of systemic antimicrobials, whilst improving the successful management of PD.

The *benefits* of short-term antimicrobial adjunctive therapy include:

- The reduced need for surgical or open periodontal debridement
- A reduction in periodontal pathogens, including bacterial reservoirs on the tongue and other oral soft tissues (systemic antimicrobials only)

• Moderate short-term improvement in periodontal probing depths when compared with root debridement alone.

Adjunctive therapy may also lengthen the time intervals between professional scaling. Prophylactic antimicrobial usage is important when performing periodontal debridement on those animals with heart disease, those that are immunocompromised or severely debilitated with organ failure, or those suffering from metabolic disease. The consequences of bacteraemia and organ seeding are relevant in these animals.

The *disadvantages* of antimicrobials include:

• Cost (especially locally delivered antimicrobials)
• Poor owner compliance (systemic antimicrobials only)
• Possible bacterial drug resistance (short- or long-term)
• Gastrointestinal irritation (systemic antimicrobials)
• Superinfections.

The long-term benefit of antimicrobial usage in PD is currently not proven. Recently, studies in humans have been carried out into the long-term use of subantimicrobial dose doxycycline (SDD) at 20 mg total dose twice daily as an adjunct to root debridement (Ciancio and Ashley, 1998; Choi *et al.*, 2004). The use of doxycycline in this way is related to the drug's anticollagenase activity, rather than any antimicrobial effect. The drug is being used in this way to modify the host's potentially destructive inflammatory response to periodontal pathogens. These studies have shown statistically significant improvements in periodontal attachment (pocket reduction) when compared with scaling and root planing alone. However, there is uncertainty as to how SDD therapy can be combined with other treatment modalities such as periodontal surgery or locally delivered antimicrobials. Futhermore, the duration of treatment with SDD is uncertain and it is unknown what risks are involved with the long-term use of the drug.

Clindamycin hydrochloride has been used in a 'pulse therapy' regime (5.5 mg/kg q12h for the first 5 days of every month) in the management of chronic PD in dogs. At present, there are no published data to support this therapeutic regimen.

Summary: Periodontal treatment aims at restoring a microbial flora compatible with periodontal health. Veterinary dental studies have shown only short-term benefits from antimicrobial usage. The long-term usage of antimicrobials in the management of PD cannot be encouraged due to unproven benefits and possible side effects.

Both systemically and locally delivered antimicrobials (when combined with mechanical debridement) should be considered for otherwise healthy patients that have severe chronic periodontitis, an acute periodontal infection, are undergoing periodontal surgery or who fail to respond to conventional root debridement. Their usage should only be for the short-term, particularly following periodontal surgery, where

home care may be delayed to allow for uninterrupted wound healing. Animals that have PD and impaired host defences will also benefit from antimicrobial therapy in the short-term.

Vaccination against periodontal pathogens

Currently, there are studies (Hardham *et al.*, 2005b) being performed on a possible vaccine against one of the bacterial pathogens associated with periodontitis. A monovalent canine PD vaccine made of inactivated, whole-cell bacterin preparations of *Porphyromonas gulae* has shown significantly reduced alveolar bone loss in a mouse model challenged with various PD pathogens. The initial results are encouraging, but it must be remembered that PD is a complex disease with multiple periodontal pathogens present. This vaccine may offer another treatment option in preventing the progression of periodontitis in animals.

Other oral diseases associated with periodontitis

Periodontal destruction can lead to other oral diseases that are associated with periodontitis. Extensive loss of supporting bone can lead to such conditions as:

• Chronic oronasal communication (e.g. fistula)
• Acute oronasal communication (e.g. periodontal abscess)
• Periodontic–endodontic lesions.

In some dogs, the greatest amount of tissue destruction seen with periodontitis is not caused solely by the periodontal pathogens themselves, but by the host's own immune response to the pathogens. This can lead to excessive amounts of tissue inflammation, ulceration and destruction.

Oronasal fistula

This is a chronic condition where, because of advanced periodontitis, there is destruction of the palatal alveolar bone plate surrounding a maxillary tooth. The most common locations for an oronasal fistula are the palatal aspect of the maxillary canine tooth (Figure 7.28) or the alveolus after the loss of a periodontally

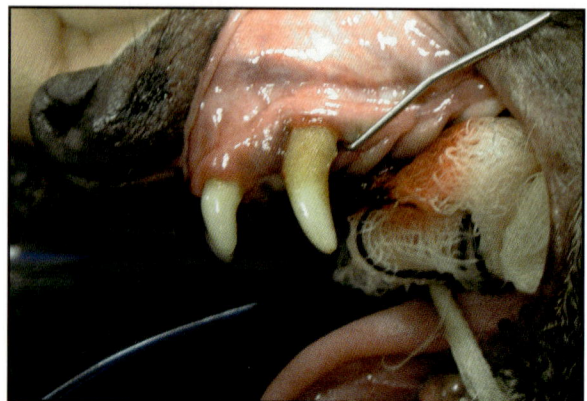

7.28 Oronasal fistula. Deep pocketing (>10 mm) on the distopalatal surface of a maxillary canine tooth in an Italian Greyhound.

compromised canine tooth; although they can be associated with other teeth.

Dogs with dolichocephalic head types (e.g. Whippets, Italian Greyhounds, Dachshunds) seem to be more at risk of developing a fistula. Dogs may present with a history of sneezing sometimes with nasal haemorrhage or mucopurulent discharge.

The condition may be unilateral or bilateral. It can also occur as an iatrogenic complication (oronasal communication) post-extraction of a periodontally involved maxillary canine tooth. Diagnosis is confirmed by demonstrating deep pocketing palatally to the maxillary canine tooth, and nasal bleeding after periodontal probing of the pocket. Another technique, favoured by the author to aid in diagnosis, is to hold the nose in a dependent position and place the flexible outer sheath of an intravenous catheter attached to a syringe containing saline into the palatal periodontal pocket. The tip of the catheter should be at the depth of the periodontal pocket. Gentle finger pressure is applied to the free gingival margin on the palatal side to create a seal and the saline gently injected into the pocket. If there is a communication or fistula present, saline will be seen dripping out of the ipsilateral nostril. The opposite side should also be checked for a possible fistula.

Oronasal fistulas should be treated by extracting the offending tooth and closing the fistula with a mucoperiosteal flap (single or double flap technique). The patient should be placed on a course of antimicrobials (clindamycin hydrochloride is a good choice), including a 3–5 day course prior to surgery to help resolve the chronic infection associated with the fistula. This provides healthier gingiva for suturing and therefore improves healing.

Periodontal abscess

Periodontal abscesses can be an acute exacerbation of chronic PD. They often occur in deep pockets, where there is entrapment of bacteria, foreign bodies (including hair) and other debris. They can also be associated with an iatrogenic complication post-scaling due to incomplete debridement to the depth of the periodontal pocket with subsequent healing above the non-debrided area. This traps bacteria or calculus deep in the pocket and an abscess may occur. This can result in rapid and extensive bone loss.

The treatment of periodontal abscesses often involves the alleviation of pain, the establishment of drainage either through the pocket or via periodontal flap surgery, the removal of plaque, calculus and other debris via root debridement, and the control of spread of the infection with or without the use of antimicrobials.

Periodontic–endodontic lesions

Periodontic–endodontic lesions occur when periodontal pathogens gain access to the endodontic system of the tooth either via lateral canals, accessory canals or through the apex of the tooth. This leads to pulpal inflammation and eventual pulpal necrosis and can be seen on periapical radiographs (Figure 7.29) as a radiolucency extending along the length of the root to the apical area of the tooth. Treatment of choice in these cases is root canal therapy together with the appropriate periodontal therapy. The affected root can

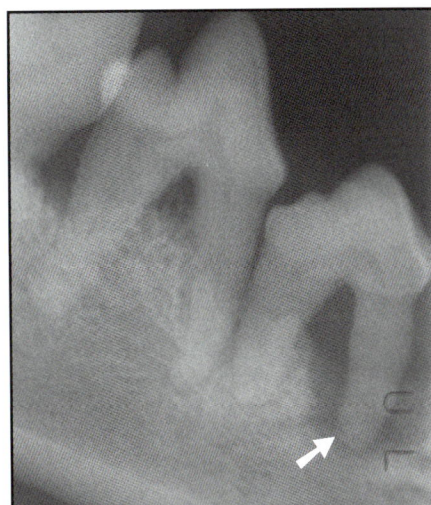

7.29 Periodontic–endodontic lesion (arrowed) involving the mesial root of the mandibular third premolar.

also be resected with periodontal therapy and restoration performed on the remaining periodontally sound crown:root segment. Prognosis in these cases is guarded.

Stomatitis

Chronic ulcerative paradental stomatitis

Chronic ulcerative paradental stomatitis (CUPS) is characterized by severe ulceration often on the buccal mucosa overlying the teeth. It is most commonly seen on the buccal mucosa overlying the maxillary canine tooth (Figure 7.30) and fourth premolar but also can be seen on the lateral border of the tongue (where it touches the lingual surface of mandibular teeth). Often, severe ulcerations are associated with gingival recession. As with any ulceration, these lesions can be very painful. Symptoms may include severe halitosis, hypersalivation, pain during mastication and general malaise. On clinical examination there may be mandibular lymphadenopathy and sometimes lip-fold dermatitis due to the excessive salivation. There are often heavy accumulations of plaque associated with local or sometimes more generalized mucosal ulceration and inflammation. Usually there is concurrent generalized periodontitis. The aetiology of this condition is not

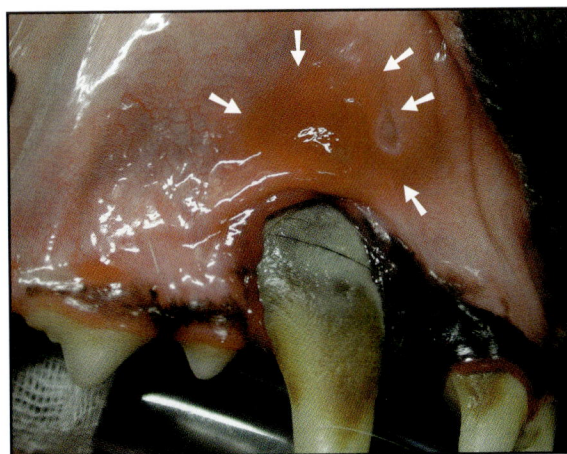

7.30 CUPS lesion in the labial mucosa (arrowed) adjacent to the maxillary canine tooth. Note the gingival recession and heavy calculus deposits on the root surface.

known, but some veterinary dentists believe that it is related to an abnormal host response to antigenic stimulation from plaque bacteria.

Immune-mediated disease and other immuno-pathies should be ruled out, especially when dealing with multiple oral ulcerations. Blood examination and biopsy may be necessary to rule out other causes. Culture and sensitivity/antibiogram tests may be required to aid diagnosis and specific treatment.

Treatment of this disease can be difficult. These dogs have very painful mouths and home care is difficult to initiate until the ulceration has subsided. Clients need to be informed of the chronic nature of the disease. After professional scaling and root debridement is performed, meticulous home care is initiated. The use of antimicrobials is warranted, especially during the healing phase where home care may be difficult, although the benefits of long-term antimicrobial 'pulse therapy' is unknown.

Due to the painful nature of this condition, the use of analgesics is recommended. Glucocorticoids, especially oral prednisolone, have also been used to suppress the marked inflammation associated with this condition. Non-steroidal anti-inflammatory drugs (NSAIDs) and steroids should not be given concurrently. However, even after conservative management with home care and medications, a number of these cases may need to be managed with extraction of the offending tooth or teeth.

Ulcerative stomatitis

A familial ulcerative stomatitis can occur in Maltese dogs, Cavalier King Charles Spaniels and other breeds of dog. Dogs affected with this type of stomatitis have very painful mouths (Figure 7.31) with severe halitosis and drooling of saliva. There is often secondary lip-fold dermatitis due to the excessive salivation that accompanies this condition. There may also be ulcerations on the tongue margins. The mandibular lymph nodes may be enlarged. Biopsy is usually necessary to rule out other diseases such as pemphigus or other immunopathies.

Treatment involves thorough professional scaling and root debridement, extraction of severely periodontally compromised teeth and meticulous home care by the

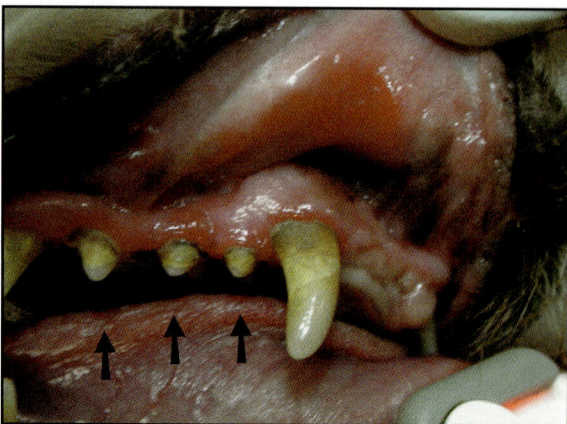

7.31 Ulcerative stomatitis in a Maltese dog, showing ulceration on the lateral border of the tongue (arrowed).

owner. Antimicrobials, such as amoxicillin–clavulanate, clindamycin hydrochloride, metronidazole and tetra-cyclines have been used to help manage this disease. The use of corticosteroids at anti-inflammatory doses may also be warranted, especially in the early management of the disease to suppress the inflammation and host response. Antimicrobial 'pulse therapy' (clindamycin hydrochloride or doxycycline hydrochloride) has also been used in the treatment of this disease with mixed results. Caudal or total tooth extractions may sometimes be necessary to manage the disease.

Necrotizing stomatitis

Necrotizing stomatitis (acute ulcerative stomatitis) is sometimes referred to as 'trench mouth' in humans, acute necrotizing ulcerative gingivitis (ANUG) or Vincent's gingivitis. In dogs, the disease starts with acute onset of a very painful mouth and difficulty with eating, as well as marked halitosis and salivation. Clinical signs include gingivitis often with a necrotic pseudo-membrane attached to the gingival tissues. Ulceration and bleeding of the gingiva are also seen.

The disease is thought to be caused by opportunistic invasion of the mucosa by organisms from the normal oral flora, including *Fusobacterium* and spirochaetes. The disease may occur in dogs with reduced host resistance, which allows bacterial invasion. Risk factors in humans include poor oral hygiene, stress, smoking or HIV infection.

Treatment is based on clinical signs and impression smears revealing large numbers of spirochaetes. Most dogs respond well to treatment with antimicrobials such as amoxicillin, amoxicillin–clavulanate or metronidazole. Owners should be advised to increase the level of home care for their pet.

Uraemic stomatitis

Uraemic stomatitis occurs as a result of uraemia associated with renal disease. Signs include severe halitosis, stomatitis and ulcerations of the oral mucosa. The margins of the tongue can also be affected and these may undergo necrosis. These lesions are thought to result from bacterial degradation of urea to form ammonia, together with dehydration and drying of the oral mucosa. Diagnosis is based on clinical signs and tests for renal disease. Treatment involves the management of the renal disease, including dietary modification and a reduction in blood urea levels.

Canine eosinophilic granuloma

Canine eosinophilic granulomas can occur in the oral cavity as ulcerative plaques. They can occur on the soft palate, under the tongue or involve other areas of oral mucosa. Cavalier King Charles Spaniels have been reported to have lesions on the soft palate or near the tonsillar crypts (Scott *et al.*, 2001). Proliferative eosinophilic lesions of the tongue can also occur in young Siberian Husky dogs. The cause is unknown, although a familial link is suspected (Guilford *et al.*, 1979). Diagnosis of eosinophilic granuloma is based on results of a biopsy, and treatment involves the use of oral glucocorticoids. Recurrence requires further treatment with glucocorticoids.

Dental caries

The incidence of dental caries is relatively low in dogs when compared with humans. In one study involving 435 dogs seen at a veterinary dental referral practice, only 23 (5.3%) had one or more carious lesions (Hale, 1998). Dental caries can occur in any breed or size of dog.

Dogs fed a diet high in fermentable carbohydrates or simple sugars, and dogs suffering from salivary gland dysfunction (illness, medications, head or neck radiation) or dehydration (reduced saliva flow), may be at greater risk of developing dental caries. Some of the reasons offered to explain the low prevalence of dental caries in carnivores include:

- Few cariogenic bacteria in the normal oral flora
- High salivary pH, which acts to neutralize acid produced by bacteria
- Tooth surfaces that are not conducive to food stagnation or impaction
- Diets that are generally low in fermentable carbohydrates
- Lower frequency of food intake compared with humans.

The tooth surfaces that are commonly affected by dental caries include the pit and fissure occlusal surfaces of molar teeth (especially the maxillary first molar), and less commonly, the smooth surfaces of teeth and the root surface.

Aetiopathogenesis

Dental caries is a plaque-induced demineralization of the calcified tissues of the teeth caused by the action of cariogenic bacteria on fermentable dietary carbohydrates. The acid produced by these bacteria demineralizes the mineral portion of the enamel and dentine with the eventual destruction of the organic material (dentine is 20% organic by weight). This allows bacterial ingress into the tooth. The cariogenic bacteria enter the dentine and dentinal tubules through the amelodentinal junction and there is lateral spread of the carious process along the amelodentinal junction, further undermining the enamel. This undermining of the enamel leads to collapse of the enamel prisms and cavitation. Once in dentine, the bacterial proteases cause further tissue damage in addition to that caused by acid production.

The outcome of this bacterial and bacterial toxin invasion into dentine is initially a reversible inflammation of the pulp (acute or chronic), which may cause tooth pain and thermal sensitivity. The pulpal response to injury is to lay down reactive secondary dentine. This non-tubular form of dentine acts as a barrier to slow the progress of bacteria and their toxins.

However, in progressing lesions the pulpal defences are overwhelmed by the advancing bacteria. Eventually the bacteria reach the pulp and this can lead to an irreversible inflammation and eventually to pulpal necrosis. Following irreversible pulpitis and pulpal necrosis, bacteria and bacterial toxins reach the apical portion of the root canal system, which results in apical periodontitis (seen as a periapical radiolucency on a radiograph). Acute apical periodontitis can cause a periapical abscess with associated severe oral pain and swelling. Chronic apical periodontitis can lead to a periapical granuloma or, if long-standing, a radicular cyst. Apical periodontitis can also occur following trauma to the tooth with or without a pulp exposure.

Dental caries is a disease caused by multiple factors. For caries to develop all four of the following are required:

- Susceptible tooth surface
- A fermentable carbohydrate source
- Cariogenic bacteria
- Time.

Some plaque bacteria (including *Streptococcus* and *Lactobacillus*) can ferment carbohydrate substrate, including glucose and sucrose, to produce acid (mainly lactic acid) as a byproduct of bacterial metabolism. The acid causes the plaque pH to fall to a point where demineralization of the tooth surface occurs. This is known as the critical pH. In humans, the critical threshold at which dissolution of enamel commences is pH 5.5. Dentine begins to dissolve at values below pH 6.4.

The occlusal surfaces of molar teeth in dogs (especially maxillary molars) are particularly susceptible to caries due in part to the stagnation of food substrate in occlusal pits and fissures. This allows cariogenic bacteria more time to ferment substrates.

Disease progression

Dental caries is not a disease process that follows a linear pattern. Demineralization of the enamel and the loss of calcium and phosphate from the hydroxyapatite crystal can be followed by a process of remineralization. Early enamel demineralization appears as a white spot or area. At this point, given the right environment, the carious lesion is reversible and can remineralize. During remineralization, calcium and phosphate are redeposited into the demineralized enamel crystal with the minerals coming from saliva or from other external sources. The remineralizing lesion may also pick up stains from dietary substrates, resulting in the remineralized lesion becoming brown or black in colour. These lesions are termed arrested caries and they should be differentiated from tooth staining, as staining also appears as a discoloration on the tooth surface (Figure 7.32).

Saliva is a crucial substance that offers physical, chemical and antibacterial properties. Water is the physical component of saliva that dilutes bacterial acids and washes away both bacteria and food substrate. The chemical component of saliva contains minerals such as calcium and phosphates which remineralize tooth structure attacked by acid, as well as buffers such as proteins and bicarbonate which can neutralize bacterial acid products. These minerals also buffer proteins and bases, such as bicarbonate, which helps to buffer any acid attack. The antibacterial component of saliva includes immunoglobulins and lysosymes that attack oral bacteria. If the carious process continues, eventually the enamel will cavitate and a hole will form. At this

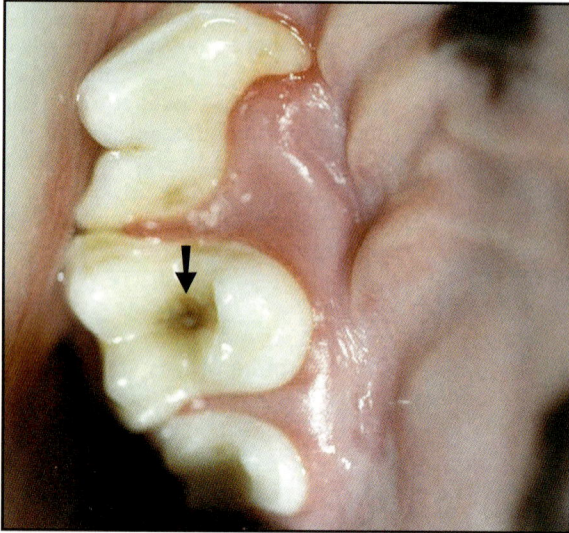

7.32 Arrested dental caries (arrowed) on the occlusal surface of the maxillary first molar. To be certain that the dental caries has arrested, *gentle* probing of the occlusal pit with a sickle explorer is recommended. In arrested caries the explorer will not engage the suspect lesion. (Courtesy of C. Tutt.)

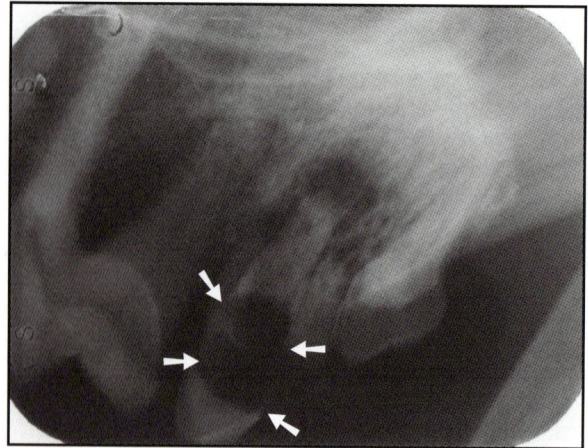

7.33 Periapical radiograph. Dental caries involving the maxillary first molar (note the large radiolucent area in the crown of the tooth; arrowed). Note also the periapical radiolucency. (Courtesy of W. Fitzgerald.)

point the process is irreversible and tooth structure has been lost. A restoration is required to replace lost tooth structure.

Diagnosis

Dental caries may be difficult to diagnose in its early stages. The diagnosis of caries requires good lighting and a clean dry tooth. Inspection of the tooth surface may reveal a 'white spot', suggesting incipient caries, or in more advanced lesions a brownish or grey discoloration may be seen under an intact enamel surface. The overt carious lesion presents with cavitation of the tooth surface.

A sharp dental explorer may be used to *gently* probe for defects in the tooth surface. The explorer will tend to stick when removed from a cavitated carious lesion (due to softened dentine). Radiographs of the affected tooth may reveal a radiolucency within the tooth or, in the case of occlusal caries, a radiolucent area below the occlusal surface. Radiographs of less advanced carious lesions may be more difficult to interpret. Radiographs often will underestimate the extent of the carious lesion (a loss of approximately 40% of the mineral content of the tooth is required before a radiolucency is observed on radiograph).

Long-standing carious lesions may lead to pulpal inflammation and eventually pulpal necrosis. Any clinical or radiographic evidence (Figure 7.33) of pulpal disease indicates that either specialist root canal (endodontic) therapy or extraction of the affected tooth will be required.

Treatment

Dental caries requires a thorough assessment to determine the underlying cause of the disease in order to allow institution of the appropriate treatment. Diet should be assessed as well as investigating other causes, such as salivary gland dysfunction. The anatomical

structure of the tooth can also be a risk factor for dental caries. Occlusal surfaces with deep pits and fissures can predispose the dog to caries. The disease in these cases is often bilateral.

In non-cavitated white spot lesions restorative intervention is not usually required and remineralization of these early lesions is often possible via dietary advice and plaque control. Regular review is essential to monitor the status of the demineralized lesion. Non-cavitated brown-grey lesions require restorative intervention.

In cavitated lesions, where there is no endodontic involvement, restoration of the lost tooth structure is required. This involves removal of diseased enamel and dentine and the placement of a restorative dental material, such as glass ionomer or composite resin. If there is extensive loss of tooth structure, restoration of the tooth may not be feasible and extraction would be required. When dealing with root caries, the management of any concurrent PD is essential. The use of topical fluorides is common in humans but not normally advised in dogs and cats due to the toxicity effects of long-term ingestion in these animals.

Immune-mediated diseases involving the oral cavity

Systemic lupus erythematosus

Systemic lupus erythematosus (SLE) is a rare disease in the dog. It is often difficult to diagnose due to its waxing and waning presentation. It is a multisystem disease involving the cutaneous, musculoskeletal, haematopoietic and urinary systems. Major signs include shifting leg lameness, fever, generalized lymphadenopathy, thrombocytopenia, anaemia, dermatoses and proteinuria.

Oral lesions are not common, but can include ulceration and crusting of the lips and nose and shallow ulcers on the oral soft tissues, including the mucosa and gingiva, sometimes with erythematous margins. Polymyositis may also occur, which can affect the muscles of mastication. Diagnosis requires a multitude of tests including haematology, biochemistry, urinalysis, serology (including anti-nuclear antibody (ANA) titres and LE prep-tests), lymph node, bone marrow and skin biopsies and possibly bacterial and fungal cultures.

Discoid lupus erythematosus

Discoid lupus erythematosus (DLE) is a mild variant form of SLE that affects the skin and oral cavity. It is one of the most common autoimmune skin diseases in the dog. There is often a loss of pigmentation on the nose and lips with crusting, scaling and fissuring. Photosensitivity is thought to contribute to the nasal lesions. DLE is more often seen in long nosed breeds, including German Shepherd Dogs and Rough Collies.

The oral lesions can involve the gingiva and the tongue, where inflammation and ulceration are seen. Diagnosis is based on the results of a biopsy. ANA testing is usually negative. Current treatments for DLE include topical glucocorticoids twice daily, topical sunblockers and oral vitamin E. Other immunosuppressive therapy is warranted if there is a poor response to topical treatments.

Vesiculobullous diseases

The two common vesiculobullous diseases encountered are:

- Pemphigus
- Bullous pemphigoid.

Pemphigus

Pemphigus is an autoimmune vesicular/bullous to pustular skin disease that is characterized by acantholysis or loss of adhesion between keratinocytes. Autoantibodies bind to c-adherins (cell-to-cell adhesion molecules), which leads to the disruption of intercellular adhesion just above the basal cell layer.

In dogs and cats five forms are recognized:

- Pemphigus foliaceus (PF)
- Pemphigus erythematosus (PE)
- Panepidermal pustular pemphigus (PPP)
- Pemphigus vulgaris (PV)
- Paraneoplastic pemphigus (PNP).

PV is the most common form in dogs and cats. At the time of presentation, 75–90% of dogs with PV have oral lesions and in 50% of cases oral lesions occur first. There appears to be no age, breed or sex predilection.

Mucocutaneous junctions, including the lips, are affected but the tongue and other oral mucosal surfaces can also be affected with non-healing ulceration. Oral vesicles are often fragile and rarely seen intact. The common appearance is of small irregular erosions, often with ragged edges. The erosions are superficial, tender and painful. Cutaneous lesions occur commonly in the axilla and groin. Systemic signs include anorexia, malaise and fever.

Diagnosis is based on multiple biopsy samples and direct immunofluorescence. Treatment involves the use of a range of immunosuppressive drugs (including prednisolone, ciclosporin, azathioprine and chlorambucil) sometimes alone or in combination.

Bullous pemphigoid

Bullous pemphigoid (BP) is a desquamating condition of the epithelium in which an autoimmune reaction occurs at the level of the basement membrane. It is characterized by fluid-filled vesicles that rupture and become ulcerated (Figure 7.34). Intact bullae are seen clinically. When the vesicles rupture, ulcerated areas with a well defined margin remain.

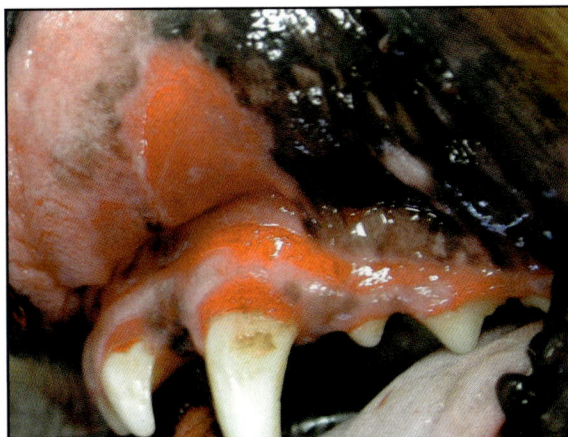

7.34 Bullous pemphigoid in a Cocker Spaniel. Note the extensive ulceration extending on to the labial mucosa.

Histologically, the tissue separation or splitting occurs at the level of the basement membrane because the targeted antigen is located in the lamina lucida of the basement membrane. IgG deposits at the basement membrane zone are common. Autoantibodies may also be detected in the serum. Serum IgG autoantibodies target the 180 kDalton epidermal protein identified as type XVII collagen in the basement membrane (Iwasaki *et al.*, 1995). Acantholysis is not seen in BP.

***Human* versus *canine* BP:** In humans BP is a relatively benign but chronic disease, often occurring on the flexural areas of the body. Mucous membranes of the oral and nasal cavities are involved in only 15–20% of patients (Ackerman, 1985). In dogs, there appears to be a breed predilection for collies, Shetland Sheepdogs and Dobermanns.

There is a disease variant of BP in humans called cicatricial pemphigoid (benign mucous membrane pemphigoid or BMMP). It affects the mucous membranes of the oral cavity and conjunctiva. Unlike BP, BMMP shows little tendency to remission and therefore often has to be treated for life. There is at present no variant form of canine BP.

Unlike the human form, canine BP has a definite predilection for mucous membranes. It also affects the skin and has a distribution similar to PV, especially the head, neck, axilla, ventral abdomen and foot pads.

Differential diagnoses and treatment: The differential diagnoses for BP include PV, SLE, toxic epidermal necrolysis, ulcerative stomatitis, drug eruptions and hidradenitis suppurativa and other causes of oral ulceration (Figure 7.35).

Periodontal disease

Malocclusion (traumatic bite)

Vitamin deficiency

Insect bites

Pemphigus vulgaris

Bullous pemphigoid

Epidermolysis bullosa acquisita

Systemic lupus erythematosus, including discoid lupus

Erythema multiforme

Toxic epidermal necrolysis

Drug eruption hypersensitivity

Hidradentis suppurativa

Vasculitis

Amyloidosis

Uraemia

Diabetes mellitus

Chronic ulcerative paradental stomatitis

Ulcerative stomatitis

Necrotizing stomatitis

Eosinophilic granuloma

Cheek chewers syndrome

Cryotherapy

Chemotherapy

Radiation therapy

Poisons and chemical irritants, including thallium

Electrical cord injury/thermal injury

Foreign bodies

Canine distemper virus infection

Candidiasis

Bacterial infections

Parasitic disease

Tumours, especially SCC, lymphoma

7.35 Differential diagnoses for oral ulceration and inflammation.

Treatment of BP normally consists of high doses of one or more immunosuppressive drugs (e.g. prednisolone, azathioprine, cyclophosphamide, chlorambucil and methotrexate) to control the condition. Reports in humans have shown some good responses to topical glucocorticoids in mild cases of bullous pemphigoid. If the canine equivalent of BP is localized to the oral cavity, topical glucocorticoids may be used alone or in combination with oral prednisolone.

Drug eruption hypersensitivity

Drug eruptions are acute hypersensitivity reactions associated with recent drug ingestion or topical drug application. In dogs, the most common drug reactions are seen with topical agents, sulphonamides (especially potentiated trimethoprim), penicillins, cephalosporin, levamisole and diethylcarbamazine (DEC).

Signs in the oral cavity may include ulceration or oedematous swelling involving the mucosa. Diagnosis is based on a history of recent drug exposure and biopsy of the affected mucosa. Withdrawal of the drug usually achieves resolution of the signs within two weeks, although in some cases lesions can persist for months.

Toxic epidermal necrolysis

Toxic epidermal necrolysis (TEN) is a rare disease involving the skin and oral mucosa. It can be associated with recent treatment with potentiated sulphonamides or beta-lactam antibiotics, although in some cases the aetiology is unknown. Signs include pyrexia, lethargy and large painful vesiculobullous lesions in the mouth. There can be epidermal eruptions sometimes involving greater than 50% of the body surface. The disease can be fatal. Treatment involves drug withdrawal, glucocorticoids, supportive therapy to prevent dehydration and the control of secondary bacterial infection.

Immune-mediated diseases affecting masticatory muscles

Masticatory muscle myositis

This is an inflammatory condition involving the muscles of mastication, namely the masseters, temporal muscles, pterygoid muscles (lateral and medial) and rostral digastric muscles. These muscles are innervated by the mandibular branch of the trigeminal nerve (CN V) (Melmed *et al.*, 2004). The limb muscles are typically spared. It was once thought to be a more localized form of polymyositis, but masticatory muscle myositis involves antibodies directed at type 2M (masticatory) fibres, which are unique to the masticatory muscles.

The condition has been historically divided into two disorders, namely eosinophilic myositis and chronic atrophic myositis, although they may represent the acute and chronic phases of the same disease. The disease can occur in any breed but mainly in younger dogs (up to 4 years old). There appears to be a predilection for large-breed dogs, including German Shepherd Dogs, Labrador and Golden Retrievers and Dobermanns, although there may be a genetic predisposition in Cavalier King Charles Spaniels.

Dogs most commonly present with jaw pain, muscle swelling involving the head or an inability to open the jaw. These signs are often seen in the acute phase of the disease. Exophthalmos may also occur in the acute phase. However, most cases present much later in the chronic or atrophic phase with masticatory muscle atrophy (Figure 7.36) and trismus. Trauma to the

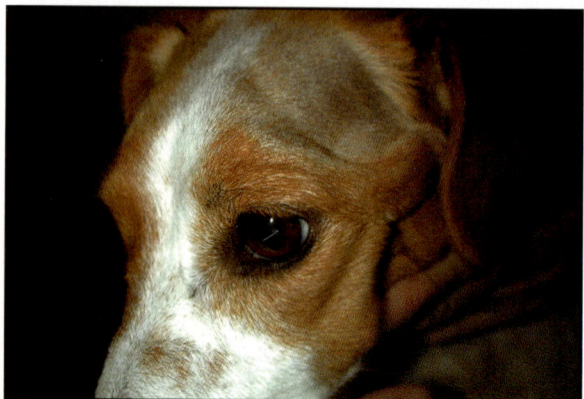

7.36 Masticatory muscle myositis with atrophy of the temporal and masseter muscles. (Courtesy of S. Holloway.)

Trauma to muscles of mastication, TMJ
TMJ dysfunction, ankylosis, luxation
Jaw fracture
Neoplasia
Acute infection involving the head
Aujeszky's disease
Systemic lupus erythematosus
Masticatory muscle myositis, other myopathies
Sialadenitis
Tetanus
Trigeminal nerve neuropathy
Foreign body
Retrobulbar abscess
Craniomandibular osteopathy
Muscular dystrophy
Radiotherapy to head and neck

7.37   Differential diagnoses for trismus.

mandible and TMJs should be ruled out as a possible cause of the trismus as well as other causes of myopathy, including infectious agents (Figure 7.37).

Diagnosis is based on a number of signs including an inability to open the jaw (trismus). Sometimes a peripheral eosinophilia is seen in the acute phase and serum creatine kinase (CK) levels may be elevated. Electromyography (EMG) is a useful diagnostic procedure to differentiate masticatory muscle myositis from other diseases, including generalized polymyositis. However, in the chronic stages of the disease EMG may be normal.

Together with clinical signs, a muscle biopsy (from the temporal muscle) and a positive blood test for circulating antibodies against masticatory muscle type 2M fibres will confirm the diagnosis. For successful treatment, the disease requires early detection and aggressive immunosuppressive therapy (prednisolone 2mg/kg p.o. q12h, and/or other immunosuppressive drugs) in the acute phase. Many cases require long-term medication to prevent relapse.

Unfortunately, cases are often presented in the chronic phase with muscle atrophy, TMJ dysfunction and muscle wasting due to an inability to maintain normal caloric intake. Procedures to improve mouth opening under general anaesthesia have been attempted, with variable success (Anderson and Harvey, 1993).

Canine polymyositis

Canine polymyositis is usually seen in large breeds of dog. Breed-associated polymyositis has been identified in Newfoundlands; they tend to be affected at a younger age than other breeds. Boxers with polymyositis may also be over-represented. The most common clinical signs in dogs with polymyositis are generalized weakness, stilted gait, dysphagia, generalized muscle atrophy, megaoesophagus and intermittent fever (Evans et al., 2004).

Megaoesophagus and dysphagia seem to be more common in Newfoundlands than other dogs affected with polymyositis. An overlap syndrome can exist where dogs with polymyositis also have masticatory myositis

and show autoantibodies against masticatory muscle type 2M fibres. Overlap can also occur with dogs affected with polymyositis and other immune-mediated connective tissue diseases such as SLE (Evans et al., 2004).

Diagnosis is based on: abnormally high serum CK concentrations; abnormal EMG; negative serological tests to rule out infectious diseases such as Toxoplasma gondii, Neospora caninum, Borrelia burgdorferi, Ehrlichia canis, Leishmania infantum and Rickettsia rickettsii. Biopsy specimens submitted for histology confirm lymphocytic infiltrates, with or without eosinophils in skeletal muscle, and necrosis of type 1 and type 2 muscle fibres. Fibrosis may also be seen. Eosinophils are more commonly seen infiltrating muscle in dogs with an inflammatory myopathy resulting from an infectious agent or in masticatory muscle myositis. Fifty percent of polymyositis cases will show positive immunofluorescence for antisarcolemmal antibodies.

Treatment for polymyositis consists of high doses of glucocorticoids, especially prednisolone.

Dermatomyositis

Dermatomyositis is a hereditary disease of the skin and muscles of young Rough Collie dogs and Shetland Sheepdogs. The condition is considered to be inherited as a dominant trait with variable expression (Hargis and Haupt, 1990; Scott et al., 2001). It is also seen in other breeds of dog, although no familial link has been proven in those breeds. Lesions first occur in dogs under six months of age. Cutaneous lesions (especially lips, face, ears, carpus, tarsus and tail) occur first and are usually followed by generalized (distal limbs) or localized muscle atrophy (particularly the muscles of mastication). If the muscles of mastication are affected, the animal may experience dysphagia.

Diagnosis is based on cutaneous and muscular disease occurring in a susceptible breed as well as biopsy of skin and muscle (Foster and Foil, 2003). Treatment consists of the use of hypoallergenic shampoos, oral vitamin E and prednisolone. Pentoxifylline can be used as a glucocorticoid-sparing drug in refractory cases.

Myositis ossificans

This is a rare condition with unknown aetiology, although trauma may initiate the focal form of the disease (Bone and McGavin, 1985). It can occur in generalized or focal forms. Focal masses may occur adjacent to the zygomatic arch, but need to be differentiated from extraskeletal osteosarcomas (Schena et al., 1989). Clinical signs of the focal form involving the zygoma area include trismus and limited mouth opening. Radiographic studies of myositis ossificans may reveal focal or multiple soft tissue radiopacities of irregular linear mineralization, along with variable periosteal reactions. Diagnosis is based on biopsy. Histopathology can reveal complete replacement of muscle by fibrous tissue and bone.

Labrador Retriever hereditary myopathy

A degenerative myopathy that is inherited as an autosomal recessive trait has been reported in

Labrador Retriever dogs in the UK and USA but has also been seen in other countries. Signs may be seen as early as six weeks or as late as seven months. Signs include muscle weakness, abnormalities of gait and posture and decreased exercise tolerance (Braund, 2005). Dogs may collapse on exertion. As the condition progresses, generalized atrophy of the skeletal muscles develops. The proximal muscles of the limbs and the muscles of the head are particularly affected and atrophy of the temporal muscles is often seen. On biopsy, alterations in fibre type percentages are a common finding. In most muscles there is a reduction in the proportion of type 2 fibres (Mehta *et al.*, 1989). There is no specific treatment for this condition.

Other infectious oral diseases

Bacterial infections

Actinomycosis

Actinomycosis may cause a localized granulomatous abscess with multiple foci of chronic suppuration involving the skin, subcutaneous tissues, lungs and bone. It is caused by the Gram-positive rods *Actinomyces viscosus* or *A. hordeovulneris,* both of which are normal inhabitants of the oral cavity of dogs.

The bacteria may cause an abscess and cellulitis involving the skin anywhere on the body, or through inhalation involve the lungs, pericardium and pleura. Infection within bone can also occur. The disease is usually initiated by a bite from another animal or foreign body penetration (e.g. grass awns). Although endogenous infection may occur, it is rare.

In humans, actinomycosis and abscessation may result from infection surrounding the mandibular third molar tooth (wisdom tooth) or extend from an infected root canal. Rarely, it can be due to animal bites (*Pasteurella* spp. may also cause an animal bite abscess in humans). The organisms may be clinically seen as 'sulphur granules' in pus and can be confirmed on the basis of Gram and acid–fast staining of smears from typical lesions. Treatment consists of surgical debridement of the abscess and prolonged antimicrobial therapy.

Nocardial stomatitis

Nocardial stomatitis is a rare infection caused by the opportunist *Nocardia* spp. *Nocardia* is a member of the family Actinomycetales, which consists of *Actinomyces*, *Nocardia*, *Mycobacterium* and *Streptomyces*.

Signs of nocardial stomatitis include reluctance to eat, pain, halitosis, hypersalivation, gingivitis and oral ulceration with areas of necrosis. The disease can resemble plaque-induced periodontitis. Lesions can also occur on the lips, buccal mucosa and soft palate, and in severe cases spread to draining lymph nodes (McKeever and Klausner, 1986). Diagnosis is based on clinical signs and culturing of a heavy growth of *Nocardia*. The organisms respond to a prolonged course of sulpha drugs continued until the lesions have completely resolved.

Fungal infections

Candidiasis is an infrequent disease of dogs, usually caused by the yeast-like fungus *Candida albicans*. It is a regular inhabitant of the gastrointestinal tract and occasionally the urinary tract. It causes an infection of the skin and mucous membrane of the gastrointestinal tract, including the mouth. The organism can multiply and cause disease in animals that are on prolonged antimicrobial therapy, immunocompromised, on immunosuppressive treatments or who have local alterations in the urinary tract environment (e.g. patients with diabetes mellitus, acidic urine, indwelling urinary catheters).

The oral form of the disease can cause white to grey ulcerative pseudomembranous lesions (thrush), sometimes extending to the oesophagus and stomach. The pseudomembrane can be wiped away (sometimes with difficulty) to reveal a bleeding base.

Diagnosis is based on deep scrapings of suspect lesions and the demonstration of the characteristic yeast-like cells and pseudohyphae in smears and wet mounts, although these are much clearer with the use of special stains, such as periodic acid–schiff (PAS) preparations. The oral form of the disease can be treated with topical antifungals such as nystatin. In humans, oral candidiasis can be associated with HIV infection.

Parasitic infections

Canine leishmaniasis

Canine leishmaniasis is a chronic parasitic infection caused by *Leishmania infantum* and *L. chagasi*. Canine leishmaniasis is transmitted by the bite of sand flies (sub-family Phlebotominae). It is endemic in the Mediterranean area and parts of the Americas and Africa (Roze, 2005). Infected dogs constitute the main reservoir of the parasite and play a key role in transmission to other mammals, including humans, where the parasite produces visceral leishmaniasis. Not all infected dogs show symptoms of the disease and asymptomatic carriers are common.

Amastigotes of the parasite multiply inside macrophages and other cells of the mononuclear family causing inflammation and immune-mediated lesions.

Clinical signs: Usual clinical signs are caused by rupture of the monocytes/macrophages, which results in IgG immune complexes forming in many organs including the spleen (causing splenomegaly), bone marrow, liver, skin (resulting in alopecia), lymph nodes (leading to generalized lymphadenopathy), intestine, eye and mucous membranes. The disease can affect the gingiva, tongue and the muscles of mastication.

Masticatory myositis and eventual atrophy of the masticatory muscles, which commonly occurs in this disease, can lead to dysphagia and weight loss. Muscle biopsy samples may show the presence of leishmanial amastigotes within macrophages and myofibres. The disease can be fatal due to renal and liver dysfunction as well as haemorrhage.

Diagnosis: The diagnosis is confirmed by demonstration of the parasite in blood smears, antibody detection by serology and polymerase chain reaction testing.

Other tests include non-specific haematological tests, which show poorly regenerative anaemia and an increase in total serum protein levels.

Treatment: Leishmaniacides, such as meglumine antimonate, and leishmaniostatics (allopurinol) are first choice drugs for treating leishmaniasis. Treatment achieves a clinical cure but not elimination of parasites, and the animals still act as carriers (Ciaramella and Corona, 2003). Repellents and insecticides (collars, shampoos and sprays) should be used to protect the dogs in those months of the year when the sand fly is active. Currently, there is research investigating the development of a vaccine for prevention of the disease.

Viral infections

Canine distemper
Canine distemper is a contagious, often fatal, multi-systemic viral disease that affects the respiratory, gastrointestinal and central nervous systems. Distemper is caused by the canine distemper virus, paramyxovirus.

Canine distemper virus is known to affect ameloblasts and odontoblasts that form enamel and dentine in the developing tooth. Puppies that survive distemper virus infection may show signs of enamel hypoplasia of their adult teeth (distemper teeth). This often presents as discoloured or pitted irregular lesions on the crowns of affected teeth. The enamel is soft and wears away quickly through normal mastication or abrasion (Figure 7.38). Permanent teeth often have

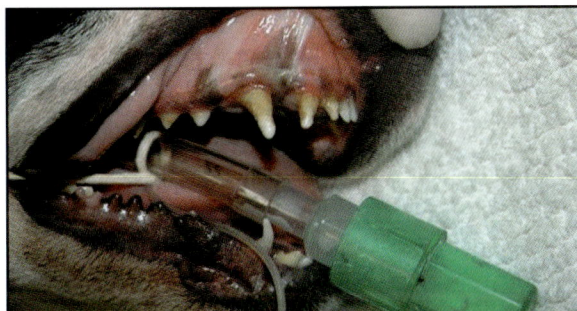

7.38 Distemper teeth. Enamel hypoplasia affecting the maxillary third incisor and canine teeth post-distemper virus infection. (Courtesy of C. Tutt.)

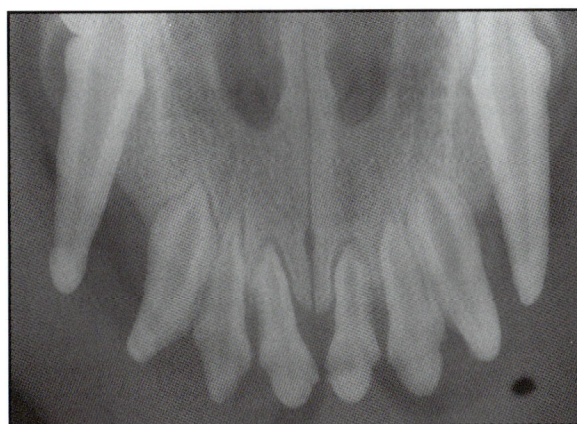

7.39 Premature closure of the apex (apexogenesis) results in abnormally shaped shorter roots.
© Cedric Tutt.

premature closure of the apex (apexogenesis) resulting in abnormally shaped shorter roots (Figure 7.39).

Distemper virus can also cause inflammation of the salivary glands (sialadenitis). Puppies may show a myoclonus (rhythmic muscle twitching) of the facial or masticatory muscles post-distemper virus infection (Fiorito, 1993). Animals that survive the initial infection may develop thickening of the nasal plane and foot pad epithelium (hard pad) at a later stage.

Canine oral papillomatosis
Numerous warts caused by the papillomavirus may occur on the mucosa of the mouth, lips, tongue, and pharynx of young dogs. Diagnosis is usually based on the characteristic appearance of a number of small to large cauliflower-like lesions involving the lips and soft tissues (Figure 7.40) of the mouth in a young dog (Nicholls *et al.*, 1999), although electron microscopy is used to reach a definitive diagnosis.

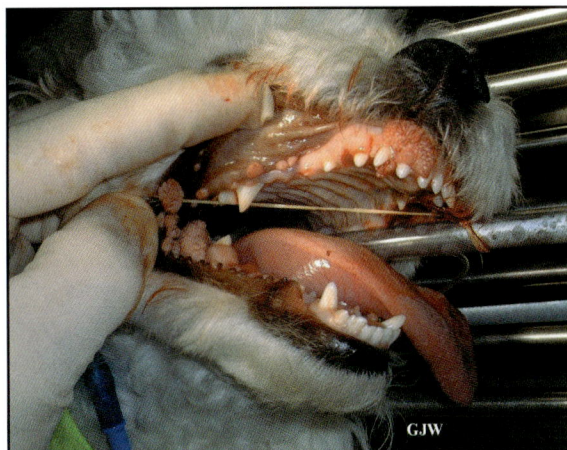

7.40 Papillomatosis. Multiple papillomas on the gingiva of a young dog. (Courtesy of G. Wilson.)

Warts usually regress spontaneously within several months and recovered dogs are immune. If owners are concerned, surgical removal of the lesions is possible, although time-consuming. Autogenous wart vaccines do not seem to be effective.

Salivary gland disease

Salivary gland diseases, although not common in dogs, include inflammatory disease, atrophy, enlargement and malignancy (see also *BSAVA Manual of Canine and Feline Head, Neck and Thoracic Surgery*). Sialocele (salivary mucocele), sialadenitis, sialolithiasis, salivary gland infarction and tumours have all been identified.

Sialocele
Sialocele is the most common salivary gland disease seen in dogs. It occurs due to leakage of saliva into the subcutaneous tissues of the ventral mandible, neck (cervical mucocele) (Figure 7.41), sublingual tissues (oral ranula) or pharyngeal tissues (pharyngeal ranula).

The sublingual salivary gland is most commonly affected and the cause is thought to be due to trauma to the gland or duct. Signs include a non-painful soft

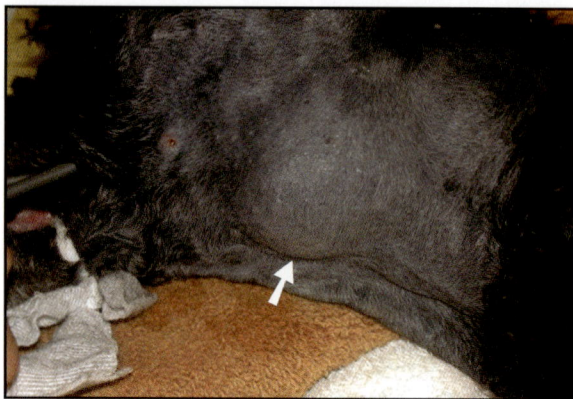

7.41 Cervical ranula. Note the saliva accumulation (arrowed) in the subcutaneous tissues of the ventral neck. (Courtesy of S. Snelling.)

swelling in the pharyngeal or neck (cervical) region. Sublingual swelling can also occur. Sometimes the swelling can become infected, especially iatrogenically after frequent needle aspirations. The swelling may also cause dysphagia or interfere with breathing if it is large.

Diagnosis is confirmed by the laboratory examination of an aspirated sample from the swelling. Treatment consists of needle aspiration of the accumulated fluid and total removal of the affected sublingual salivary gland. Due to its close proximity, the mandibular salivary gland is also removed. Bilateral removal is sometimes required for midline swellings. Marsupialization can be performed, especially for pharyngeal sialoceles.

Sialadenitis

Sialadenitis or inflammation of the salivary glands is not common. Causes may include trauma, foreign bodies or distemper virus infection. The parotid and zygomatic salivary glands are the most commonly affected. The affected gland is swollen and painful to touch. The dog may be febrile, anorexic and have trismus. Diagnosis is made on fine needle aspiration and examination. Malignancy needs to be ruled out. Treatment consists of antimicrobial therapy. Sometimes surgical drainage is required.

Sialolithiasis

Sialolithiasis or stone formation in the duct of a salivary gland is rare in dogs. It may be asymptomatic, or cause pain and swelling as a result of salivary duct obstruction. Sialography may be useful in diagnosis. Treatment consists of removal of the sialolith.

Salivary gland infarction

Salivary gland infarction is a very rare condition with unknown aetiology. It is characterized by a firm discrete swelling of salivary tissue. Biopsy specimens consistently show an abrupt interruption of blood flow to a portion of the affected gland, with resultant necrosis. It is primarily seen in the mandibular gland and it is speculated that because of the superficial location of this gland it is more subject to trauma (although the parotid gland is also superficial but infarction is

uncommon in this gland) (Spangler and Culbertson, 1991). The parotid and mandibular salivary glands are the most common glands affected by malignancy. Adenocarcinoma is the most common malignancy of salivary glands (Hammer *et al.*, 2001).

Miscellaneous

Drugs that cause xerostomia or reduced saliva flow may lead to a higher incidence of dental caries and PD. Examples of such drugs include diuretics, anticonvulsants, antihistamines and tranquillizers. Radiotherapy to the head and neck can also cause xerostomia. In humans, patients with diabetes mellitus experience alterations in salivary flow rates and in the constituents of saliva, leading to an increased incidence of oral infection (Mealey and Moritz, 2003).

A syndrome of phenobarbital-responsive sialadenosis with salivary gland enlargement has been reported in dogs and has been postulated to be a form of limbic epilepsy. Signs include pytalism, non-painful enlargement of salivary glands, especially the zygomatic and mandibular salivary glands, and episodes of gulping or retching. Response to treatment with oral phenobarbital is rapid (Boydell *et al.*, 2000).

References and further reading

Ackerman L (1985) Canine and feline pemphigus and pemphigoid – part II. Pemphigoid. *Compendium on Continuing Education for the Practicing Veterinarian* **7**(4), 281–286

Anderson J and Harvey C (1993) Masticatory muscle myositis. *Journal of Veterinary Dentistry* **10**(1), 6–8

Bone D and McGavin M (1985) Myositis ossificans in the dog: a case report and review. *Journal of the American Animal Hospital Association* **21**, 135–138

Boydell P, Pike R, Crossley D and Whitbread T (2000) Sialadenosis in dogs. *Journal of the American Veterinary Medical Association* **216**, 872–874

Braund (2005) *Clinical Neurology in Small Animals: Localization, Diagnosis and Treatment*, ed. C Vite, pp. 20–21. International Veterinary Information Service, Ithaca, New York

Cadosch J, Zimmermann U, Ruppert M, Guindy J, Case D and Zappa U (2003) Root surface debridement and endotoxin removal. *Journal of Periodontal Research* **38**, 229–236

Choi D, Moon I, Choi B, Paik J, Kim Y, Choi S and Kim C (2004) Effects of sub-antimicrobial dose doxycycline therapy on crevicular fluid MMP-8, and gingival tissue MMP-9, TIMP-1 and IL-6 levels in chronic periodontitis. *Journal of Periodontal Research* **39**(1), 20–26

Ciancio S and Ashley R (1998) Safety and efficacy of sub-antimicrobial dose doxycycline therapy in patients with adult periodontitis. *Advances in Dental Research* **12**(2), 27–31

Ciaramella P and Corona M (2003) Canine leishmaniasis: therapeutic aspects. *Compendium on Continuing Education for the Practicing Veterinarian* **25**(5), 370–375

DeBowes L, Mosier D, Logan E, Harvey C, Lowry S and Richardson D (1996) Association of periodontal disease and histologic lesions in multiple organs from 45 dogs. *Journal of Veterinary Dentistry* **13**(2), 57–60

DeForge D (1997) Evaluation of Bioglass/perioglas (consil) synthetic bone graft particulate in the dog and cat. *Journal of Veterinary Dentistry* **14**(4), 141–145

Drisko C (2000) Position paper: sonic and ultrasonic scalers in periodontics. *Journal of Periodontology* **71**, 1792–1801

Ebersole J, Machen R, Steffen M and Willmann D (1997) Systemic acute-phase reactants, C-reactive protein and haptoglobin in adult periodontitis. *Clinical Experimental Immunology* **107**(2), 347–352

Eick S, Seltmann T and Pfister W (2004) Efficacy of antibiotics to strains of periodonto-pathogenic bacteria within a single species biofilm – an *in vitro* study. *Journal of Clinical Periodontology* **31**(5), 376–383

Evans J, Levesque D and Shelton D (2004) Canine inflammatory myopathies: a clinicopathologic review of 200 cases. *Journal of Veterinary Internal Medicine* **18**, 679–691

Fiorito D (1993) Multiple oral procedures performed on a dog with distemper myoclonus. *Journal of Veterinary Dentistry* **10**(2), 10–11

Foster A and Foil C (2003) *BSAVA Manual of Small Animal Dermatology, 2nd edn*. BSAVA Publications, Gloucester

Grossi S and Genco R (1998) Periodontal disease and diabetes mellitus: a two-way relationship. *Annals of Periodontology* **3**, 51–61

Guilford W, Center S, Strombeck D, Williams D and Meyer D (1979) *Strombeck's Small Animal Gastroenterolgy, 3rd edn*. WB Saunders, Philadelphia

Hale F (1998) Dental caries in the dog. *Journal of Veterinary Dentistry* **15**(2), 79–83

Hammer A, Getsy D, Ogilvie G, Upton M, Klausner J and Kisseberth W (2001) Salivary gland neoplasia in the dog and cat: survival times and prognostic factors. *Journal of the Americal Animal Hospital Association* **37**, 478–482

Hamp S, Hamp M, Olsson S, Lindberg R and Schauman P (1997) Radiography of spontaneous periodontitis in dogs. *Journal of Periodontal Research* **32**(7), 589–597

Harari J, Besser T and Gustafson S (1993) Bacterial isolates from blood cultures of dogs undergoing dentistry. *Veterinary Surgery* **22**, 27–30

Hardham J, Dreier K, Wong J, Sfintescu C and Evans R (2005a) Pigmented anaerobic bacteria associated with canine periodontitis. *Veterinary Microbiology* **20**(106), 119–128

Hardham J, Reed M, Wong J, King K, Laurinat B, Sfintescu C and Evans R (2005b) Evaluation of a monovalent companion animal periodontal disease vaccine in an experimental mouse periodontitis model. *Vaccine* **2**, 48–56

Hargis A and Haupt K (1990) Review of familial canine dermatomyositis. *Veterinary Annals* **30**, 277–282

Harvey C (1998) Periodontal disease in dogs: etiopathogenesis, prevalence and significance. *Veterinary Clinics of North America: Small Animal Practice* **28**, 1111–1128

Harvey C, Shofer F and Laster L (1994) Association of age and body weight with periodontal disease in North American dogs. *Journal of Veterinary Dentistry* **11**, 94–105

Hausmann E, Allen K and Clerehugh V (1991) What alveolar crest level on a bite-wing radiograph represents bone loss? *Journal of Periodontology* **62**(9), 570–572

Hughes F, Anger D and Smales F (1988) Investigation of the distribution of cementum-associated lipopolysaccharides in periodontal disease by scanning electron microscope and immunohistochemistry. *Journal of Periodontal Research* **23**, 100–106

Hughes F and Smales F (1986) Immunohistochemical investigation of the presence and distribution of cementum-associated lipopolysaccharides in periodontal disease. *Journal of Periodontal Research* **21**, 660–667

Ichimiya T, Yamasaki T and Nasu M (1994) In-vitro effects of antimicrobial agents on *Pseudomonas aeruginosa* biofilm formation. *Journal of Antimicrobial Chemotherapeutics* **34**(3), 331–341

Iwasaki T, Olivry T, Lapiere J, Chan L, Peavey C, Liu Y, Jones J, Ihrke P and Woodley D (1995) Canine bullous pemphigoid (BP): identification of the 180-kDa canine BP antigen by circulating autoantibodies. *Veterinary Pathology* **32**(4), 387–393

Korman K, Crane A, Wang H, Di Giovine F, Pirk F, Wilson T, Higginbottom F, Newman M and Duff G (1997) The IL-1 genotype as a severity factor in periodontal disease. *Journal of Clinical Periodontology* **24**, 72–77

Loe H, Anerud A, Boysen H and Smith M (1978) The natural history of periodontal disease in man. The rate of periodontal destruction before 40 years of age. *Journal of Periodontology* **49**(12), 607–620

Loe H, Theilade E and Jensen S (1965) Experimental gingivitis in man. *Journal of Periodontology* **36**, 177–183

Loesche W (1976) Chemotherapy of dental plaque infections. *Oral Sciences Review* **9**, 65–107

McKeever P and Klausner J (1986) Plant awn, candidal, nocardial and necrotizing stomatitis in the dog. *Journal of the American Animal Hospital Association* **22**, 17–24

Mealey B and Moritz A (2003) Hormonal influences: effects of diabetes mellitus and endogenous female sex steroid hormones on the periodontium. *Periodontology 2000* **32**(1), 59–81

Mehta J, Braund K, McKerrell R and Toivio-Kinnucan M (1989) Analysis of muscle elements, water, and total lipids from healthy dogs and Labrador retrievers with hereditary muscular dystrophy. *American Journal of Veterinary Research* **50**, 640–644

Melmed C, Shelton G, Bergman R and Barton C (2004) Masticatory muscle myositis: pathogenesis, diagnosis and treatment. *Compendium on Continuing Education for the Practicing Veterinarian* **26**(8), 590–604

Nares S (2003) The genetic relationship to periodontal disease. *Periodontology 2000* **32**, 36–49

Nelson S, Hynd B and Pickrum H (1992) Automated enzyme immunoassay to measure prostaglandin E2 in gingival crevicular fluid. *Journal of Periodontal Research* **27**(2), 143–148

Nicholls P, Klaunberg B, Moore R, Santos E, Parry N, Gough G and Stanley M (1999) Naturally occurring, non-regressing canine oral papillomavirus infection: host immunity, virus characterization and experiemental infection. *Virology* **265**, 365–374

Nieves M, Hartwig P, Kinyon J and Riedesel D (1997) Bacterial isolates from plaque and from blood during and after routine dental procedures in dogs. *Veterinary Surgery* **26**, 26–32

Nyman S, Sarhed G, Ericsson I, Gottlow J and Karring T (1986) Role of 'diseased' root cementum in healing following treatment of periodontal disease: an experimental study in the dog. *Journal of Periodontal Research* **21**, 496–503

Offenbacher S (1996) Periodontal diseases. Pathogenesis. *Annals of Periodontology* **1**, 821–878

Offenbacher S, Katz V, Fertik G, Collins J, Boyd D, Maynor G, McKaig R and Beck J (1996) Periodontal infection as a possible risk factor for preterm low birth weight. *Journal of Periodontology* **67**, 1103–1113

Page RC and Schroeder HE (1976) Pathogenesis of inflammatory periodontal disease. A summary of current work. *Laboratory Investigation* **33**, 235–249

Plotzke A, Nasjleti C, Morrison E and Caffesse R (1993) Histologic and histometric responses to polymeric composite grafts. *Journal of Periodontology* **64**, 343–348

Rawlinson J, Goldstein R, Reiter A, Hollis N and Harvery C (2005) Tracking systemic parameters in dogs with periodonal disease. *Conference Proceedings 19th Annual Veterinary Dental Forum and World Dental Congress IX, Orlando, Florida*, pp. 49

Roudebush P, Logan E and Fraser H (2005) Evidence-based veterinary dentistry: a systematic review of homecare for prevention of periodontal disease in dogs and cats. *Journal of Veterinary Dentistry* **22**(1), 6–15

Roze M (2005) Canine leishmaniasis: a spreading disease. Diagnosis and treatment. *European Journal of Companion Animal Practice* **15**(1), 39–52

Saini S, Aparna Gupta N, Mahajan A and Arora D (2003) Microbial flora in orodental infections. *Indian Journal of Medical Microbiology* **21**(2), 111–114

Sarkiala E and Harvey C (1993) Systemic antimicrobials in the treatment of periodontitis in dogs. *Seminars in Veterinary Medicine and Surgery Small Animals* **8**(3), 197–203

Schena C, Stickle R, Dunstan R, Trapp A, Reimann K, White J, Killingsworth C and Hauptman J (1989) Extraskeletal osteosarcoma in two dogs. *Journal of the American Veterinary Medical Association* **194**, 1452–1456

Scott D, Miller W and Griffin C (2001) *Muller and Kirk's Small Animal Dermatology, 6th edn*, eds. D Scott et al., pp. 940–946. WB Saunders, Philadelphia

Slotte C and Lundgren D (1999) Augmentation of calvarial tissue using non-permeable silicone domes and bovine bone mineral. An experimental study in the rat. *Clinical Oral Implants Research* **10**, 468–476

Soames R and Southam J (1995) *Oral pathology, 2nd edn*, eds. J Soames and J Southam, pp. 96–102. Oxford University Press, Oxford

Socransky S, Haffajee A, Goodson J and Lindhe J (1984) New concepts of destructive periodontal disease. *Journal of Clinical Periodontology* **11**, 21–32

Spangler W and Culbertson M (1991) Salivary gland disease in dogs and cats: 245 cases (1985–1988) *Journal of the American Veterinary Medical Association* **198**(3), 465–469

Stavropoulos A, Kostopoulos L, Randel Nyengaard J and Karring T (2003) Deproteinized bovine bone (Bio-Oss®) and bioactive glass (Biogran®) arrest bone formation when used as an adjunct to guided tissue regeneration (GTR). An experimental study in the rat. *Journal of Clinical Periodontology* **30**(7), 636–644

Tan B, Mordan NJ, Embleton J, Pratten J and Calgut P (2004) Study of bacterial viability within human supragingival dental calculus. *Journal of Periodontology* **75**(1), 23–29

University of Minnesota, Center for Companion Animal Health (1996) Preliminary data: National Companion Animal Study. *Journal of Veterinary Dentistry* **13**(2), 56

Walker K, Karpinia K and Baehni P (2004) Chemotherapeutics: antibiotics and other antimicrobials. *Periodontology 2000* **36**(1), 146–165

Wang H and Greenwell H (2001) Surgical periodontal therapy. *Periodontology 2000* **25**, 89–99

8

Feline inflammatory, infectious and other oral conditions

Dea Bonello

Periodontal disease, including periodontitis and gingivitis, is the most common inflammatory disorder affecting the oral cavity of cats and is caused by the accumulation of plaque on the teeth, gingiva and in the gingival sulcus.

A range of inflammatory oral conditions (e.g. stomatitis, eosinophilic granuloma complex, inflammation associated with carcinoma) caused by agents other than plaque also occur in the feline oral cavity (Figure 8.1). These generally affect the oral mucosa (oral mucositis) but may also involve the periodontium.

These inflammatory oral conditions may appear similar at various stages of their pathogenesis, resulting in difficulty distinguishing between them and in the formulation of an accurate diagnosis. This may be because they display common pathogenic behaviour at some stage of the inflammatory response. This response is usually similar regardless of the cause, and it occurs in response to antigenic stimulation but does not differentiate the origin of that stimulation. In fact, the cat responds to various noxious stimuli by the same mechanisms that trigger inflammatory hyper-reactivity of the oral mucosa. In addition to the imbalance between the local defensive response and the severity of the noxious stimuli (e.g. plaque, toxic, viral and unknown), there are mechanisms resulting in excessive degranulation of mucosal mast cells normally found in the oral cavity of dogs and cats. When disease is present, these cells are activated by numerous agonistic immune stimuli (e.g. IgE and IgA), neurogenic stimuli (e.g. substance P and nerve growth factor) and bacterial stimuli (e.g. plaque enzymes and toxins). Consequently, this results in the release of massive, uncontrolled amounts of numerous mediators, which may be preformed (e.g. cytokines, vasoactive amines, proteolytic enzymes, chemotactic and neurotropic factors) or synthesized *ex novo* (e.g. arachidonic acid derivatives). Once released into the extracellular environment, these mediators:

Aetiology	Condition
Immune system associated depression or dysfunction	Acute necrotizing ulcerative gingivitis (ANUG)
Autoimmune disorders	Systemic lupus erythematosus (SLE) Pemphigus vulgaris Idiopathic vasculitis Toxic epidermal necrolysis
Hypersensitivity	Drug eruptions Insect stings
Viral infection	Feline leukaemia virus (FeLV) Feline immunodeficiency virus (FIV) Calicivirus Feline herpesvirus type-1 Feline coronavirus (FCoV) (causes feline infectious peritonitis, FIP) Poxvirus
Bacterial infections	Dermatophylosis Actinomycosis Nocardiosis Mycobacteriosis
Mycotic infections	Candidiasis Cryptococcosis
Miscellaneous conditions	Feline eosinophilic granuloma complex (EG) Feline indolent ulcer Feline chronic gingivostomatitis (FCGS)

8.1 Feline inflammatory and infectious oral conditions.

- Trigger a series of vascular, epithelial and neurological responses that underlie the signs and symptoms of the early stages of oral inflammation
- Extend the duration of oral inflammation and pain due to their influence on the local lymph node response and functionality of the nerve fibres
- Cause or aggravate the destructive phenomena affecting the tissues of the oral cavity, which characterize the more advanced stages of periodontal disease and other inflammatory conditions.

Because oral tissues have a limited range of responses, pathological lesions with different aetiology frequently appear similar. Therefore, the diagnosis of an oral lesion is often a complex process involving a wide range of examinations and diagnostic tests. It is often advisable to obtain a biopsy sample from the lesion and submit this to the laboratory for histopathological evaluation.

Cytological examination of smears obtained from tissue fluids, needle aspirates or impression smears (of the cut tissue surface) can be quick and useful screening techniques. They may be performed in-house with little experience and training, or samples can be submitted to a pathologist experienced in cytology for a more accurate interpretation. Unfortunately cytology is often non-diagnostic, and even when it is, histology should be performed to confirm the diagnosis (Figures 8.2 and 8.3).

The management of inflammatory diseases of the oral cavity (e.g. gingivitis, periodontitis, stomatitis and stomatomucositis) is based on preventive and therapeutic medical and surgical measures. These measures include oral hygiene and dietary control, together with periodic removal of plaque and calculus (scaling and polishing). A maintenance programme of oral hygiene then helps to prevent the inflammatory response of the periodontal tissues from being triggered or, if already present, prevents the progression of existing lesions and the formation of new ones. Medical and surgical measures used to treat oral inflammation

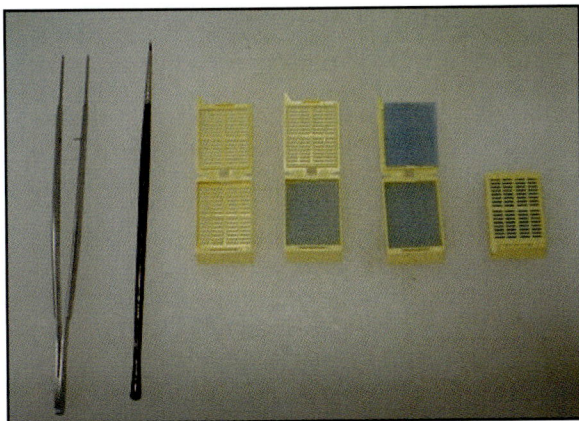

8.3 To obtain a correct diagnosis from a biopsy sample it is mandatory that the sample be of full-thickness and be correctly oriented.

depend on the aetiology of the inflammatory disease and mainly focus on the use of antibiotic and/or anti-microbial/antiseptic and/or anti-inflammatory treatments, possibly in association with specific conservative or surgical exodontic procedures. Treatment measures chosen depend on the degree of dental and periodontal tissue involvement, together with concurrent systemic factors (e.g. the animal's general state of health and age).

Periodontal disease

Periodontal disease is the most common inflammatory disease of the oral cavity of cats and is caused by plaque accumulation on the teeth, gingiva and in the gingival sulcus. It affects the majority (85–95%) of cats older than two years of age, particularly those that do not receive oral care, such as adequate dietary measures, daily oral hygiene or professional prophylactic treatment. Individual and breed susceptibility to periodontal disease is recognized particularly in pure-breed cats, with Persian, Maine Coon, Burmese and Siamese breeds being more prone to early or severe periodontal disease.

Some defence mechanisms that prevent plaque bacteria from accumulating and causing damage exist in healthy animals. The integrity of the oral cavity epithelium represents the first protective barrier. Saliva with its flushing action continuously removes a huge amount of bacteria, as do the movements of the tongue and lips, and the act of mastication. Saliva and crevicular fluid, produced in the gingival sulcus, contain substances that help to prevent bacteria from adhering to the surfaces of the oral mucosa and the teeth. They also contain substances with specific bacteriostatic and bactericidal properties. Normal intrinsic oral hygiene is also enhanced by normal occlusion and uniform occlusal force distribution, effective mastication, and a lightly abrasive and nutritionally balanced dry diet.

In predisposed, immunocompromised or geriatric patients, these mechanisms are not as effective and periodontal disease may occur. The end result of untreated periodontitis is destruction of the periodontal ligament and alveolar bone with eventual tooth loss.

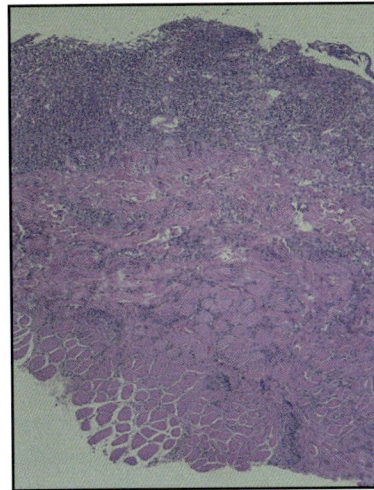

8.2 The normal technique of swabbing affected areas is prone to producing false results due to contaminants that often overgrow other species in the laboratory; this is especially true of ulcerated lesions. In these cases it is better to obtain a tissue sample and submit this to the laboratory.

There is also evidence in humans and dogs that infection in the oral cavity may cause systemic disease. The same may be true in cats affected by periodontal disease. For these reasons the veterinary surgeon's intervention is necessary to:

- Diagnose and treat periodontal disease (see Chapter 7)
- Identify the predisposing factors
- Prevent progression of the disease.

If possible the predisposing factors should be eliminated, to facilitate restoration of periodontal health. Professional intervention alone is not sufficient to arrest the progression of periodontal disease. The mainstay of treatment is meticulous daily plaque removal. The use of special diets or dietary adjuncts, although not eliminating the need for daily plaque removal and regular professional therapy, may serve to help improve gingival health during the interval between professional oral health assessments and treatment. Research results indicate that daily addition of dental chews to a dry diet is effective in reducing plaque and calculus accumulation on tooth surfaces in cats, as well as reducing the severity of gingivitis (Ingham *et al.*, 2002).

Aetiology

Periodontal disease is the collective term for a number of plaque-induced inflammatory conditions of the periodontium. Bacteria are normal inhabitants of the oral cavity but under some conditions they accumulate on the tooth surfaces and in the gingival sulcus, forming

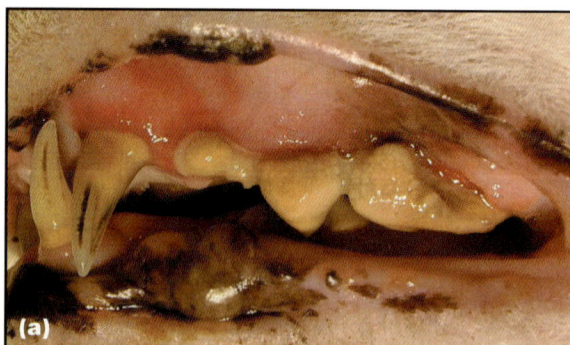

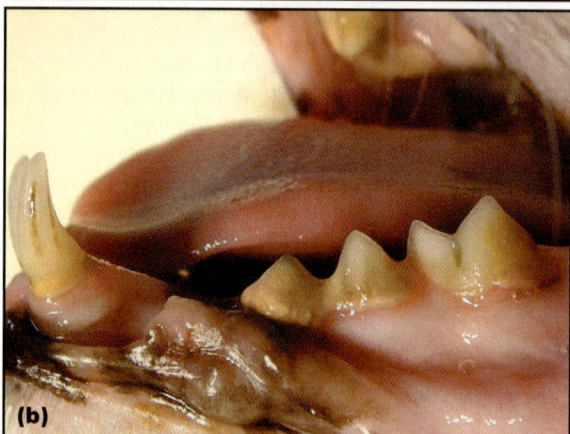

8.4 **(a)** Severe gingivitis, periodontitis and extensive build-up of calculus on the maxillary teeth. **(b)** Moderate periodontal disease and mild gingivitis on the mandibular teeth of the same cat.

Bacteria	Gram-positive: Aerobes/facultative anaerobes: • Streptococcus • Micrococcus • Actinomyces • Nocardia • Lactobacillus Anaerobes: • Peptostreptococcus • Actinomyces • Propionilbacterium • Bifidobacterium • Clostridium • Porphyromonas Gram-negative: Aerobes/facultative anaerobes: • Neisseria • Branhamella • Actinobacillus • Capnocytophaga • Campylobacter • Eikenella • Haemophilus • Coliforms Anaerobes: • Veillonella • Fusobacterium • Wolinella • Prevotella • Bacteroides • Campylobacter • Spirochaetes
Protozoa	Entamoeba Trichomonas
Yeast	Candida

8.5 Composition of oral flora.

dental plaque. The animal's response to the pathological presence of bacteria is expressed as an inflammatory reaction. If the inflammation only involves the gingiva, then the inflammation is termed gingivitis. Periodontitis is inflammation affecting all the tooth-supporting structures (i.e. gingiva, periodontal ligament, cementum and alveolar bone) (Figure 8.4).

The anaerobic plaque bacteria (spirochaetes, *Porphyromonas* and *Prevotella* species) are present in large numbers in periodontal pockets and are considered to play a major role as pathogenic agents in the aetiology of periodontal disease. Some unique *Porphyromonas* species have been identified in the cat (Figure 8.5). As mentioned previously, many different predisposing factors (functional or organic alterations) also play a fundamental role in that they affect the susceptibility of the animal to periodontal disease. Systemic factors predispose the periodontium to the initiation of the disease but the real causal agents are the bacteria within the plaque.

Plaque development

Teeth are coated by a thin film, the pellicle, derived from salivary and crevicular glycoproteins. The pellicle is firmly attached to the tooth surface and forms within minutes of brushing or scaling of the tooth. The bacteria present in the oral cavity adhere to this film and continue to accumulate. Early colonizers are mainly Gram-positive microorganisms, which produce a glycopolysaccharide that enables them to adhere to the pellicle and to each other. This binding allows the bacteria to produce colonies that protect and nourish the bacteria. Within 24 hours the entire tooth surface is covered by a layer of microorganisms incorporated into an organic matrix, the plaque. The main bacteria in supragingival plaque in cats are aerobes and facultative anaerobes (*Actinomyces* and *Streptococcus*). When the plaque matures and extends subgingivally, the environment becomes suitable for growth of anaerobic bacteria and spirochaetes due to the low redox potential. The subgingival plaque flora associated with periodontitis in cats consists of *Porphyromonas*, *Prevotella*, *Peptostreptococcus*, *Fusobacterium* and spirochaetes.

The structure of plaque is immensely complicated and what has been called the 'climax community' of mature plaque represents a balanced equilibrium of organisms or microbial ecosystem on the tooth surface. Plaque can often be seen as a soft, non-calcified layer present on the tooth surface. In thin layers it is scarcely visible but its presence is confirmed by scraping the tooth surface with a periodontal probe or by the use of plaque-disclosing agents. Plaque forms most readily in sheltered regions of the mouth, for example the gingival crevice. It is unusual to find it on the masticatory surface of the tooth unless that tooth is out of function. The plaque must be removed mechanically by brushing every day. When tooth brushing is not possible it is helpful to use products containing substances able to slow down the rate of plaque deposition (e.g. chlorhexidine gluconate). In addition, the daily incorporation of dental chews to a dry diet is effective in reducing plaque and calculus accumulation on tooth surfaces in cats, as well as reducing the severity of gingivitis.

Calculus formation
With time, undisturbed supragingival and subgingival plaque can undergo mineralization as a result of the formation of calcium and phosphate crystals. Mineralized bacterial plaque is called calculus. Precipitation of mineral salts within plaque can be seen only hours after plaque deposition, but is more commonly seen from 2–14 days after plaque is formed. The minerals in supragingival calculus are derived from saliva, while those in subgingival calculus are derived from the crevicular fluid. Plaque mineralization mechanisms have not been definitively clarified yet, but it is generally believed that an element in plaque acts as a seeding site or nidus where crystallization can start.

There is large individual variability in the capacity to form calculus. Calculus accumulation reaches a maximum within a period of 10–24 weeks, after which the deposition rate progressively diminishes as a result of reduced space and mechanical abrasion. In cats, calculus deposition takes place mostly on the maxillary fourth premolar teeth (the ducts of the parotid and

zygomatic salivary glands open near these teeth) and on the mandibular first molars. Feline canine teeth are less affected when compared with the same teeth in dogs. Calculus plays a less important role than plaque in the pathogenesis of periodontal disease. However, its rough surface supports a continuous accumulation of organic substances and bacteria, and contributes to keeping the plaque in close contact with the periodontal tissues. The resulting effect is that the inflammatory response continues.

Pathogenesis

Gingivitis
Plaque bacteria and their byproducts (e.g. endotoxins) penetrate the sulcular and junctional epithelium, and gain access to the underlying connective tissue. This results in an acute exudative inflammatory reaction that is initially confined to the area of the gingival sulcus (sulcus epithelium, junctional epithelium, perivascular connective tissue). This process is characterized by the extravascular migration of polymorphonuclear (PMN) leucocytes and lymphocytes. Host-derived tissue destruction results in alterations to fibroblasts, collagen loss and junctional epithelial cell proliferation. The resulting lesion is termed gingivitis and is comparable to a type IV immunopathological reaction (delayed or cellular hypersensitivity). Progression of the lesion occurs as the inflammatory cells (B lymphocytes and plasma cells) invade further down the connective tissue and the vessels of the vascular plexus increase in number and volume. Additional accumulation and development of subgingival plaque also occurs.

The junctional epithelium detaches from the enamel and, together with the sulcular epithelium, forms the pocket epithelium. If the pocket epithelium is thin and ulcerated it bleeds easily. In other areas it may become thickened.

Stages:

- Acute gingivitis – the gums appear red and swollen and bleed easily. Bacterial plaque is not always visible to the naked eye.
- Chronic gingivitis – the presence of calculus and plaque causes chronic inflammation of the gingiva. Halitosis is the main presenting sign. Chronic gingivitis can persist indefinitely or progress to periodontitis (Figure 8.6).

Gingivitis is a reversible inflammation of the gingiva, except in cases where the chronic inflammatory stimulus results in gingival hypertrophy. In some cat breeds (Persians, Abyssinians and Domestic Shorthair kittens) gingivitis can have proliferative characteristics. In some animals the inflammatory stimulus causes the formation of gingival masses, called epulides (Figure 8.7; see Chapter 10 regarding controversy over the use of this term). These masses can enlarge with time, and may interfere with mastication and prevent the maintenance of efficient oral hygiene. These lesions must be removed surgically (gingivectomy) and should always be submitted for histopathological examination.

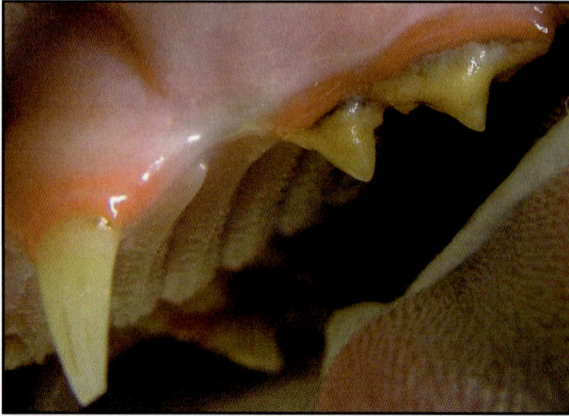

8.6   Chronic gingivitis with heavy plaque and calculus deposits.

Aetiology	Condition
Reactive lesions (not neoplastic)	Pyogenic granuloma Focal fibrous hyperplasia
Benign neoplasia (odontogenic)	Peripheral odontogenic fibroma
Epithelial neoplasia (infiltrating)	Peripheral acanthomatous ameloblastoma
Malignant neoplasia (not odontogenic)	Squamous cell carcinoma Fibrosarcoma

8.7   Differential diagnosis of gingival overgrowth in cats.

Periodontitis

Untreated gingivitis can progress to periodontitis. In the deeper tissues affected by the inflammatory reaction the oxygen gradient is reduced and Gram-negative anaerobic motile bacteria increase to approximately 90% of the total number. These bacteria are responsible for the progression of the disease, the breakdown of the epithelial attachment, migration of the cellular infiltrate (acute inflammation) in an apical and lateral direction, and destruction of the periodontal ligament and alveolar bone. Disease progression is often episodic in nature rather than a continuous process.

Tissue destruction, characterized by apical migration of the epithelial attachment and alveolar bone loss, is the result of injury caused by plaque bacteria, both directly and indirectly via activation and maintenance of the host inflammatory response. Periodontitis is an irreversible condition, but its progression can be arrested and periodontal health stabilized with appropriate treatment. Despite the presence of bacteria-induced inflammation, antibiotic therapy is not commonly indicated in the treatment of gingivitis and periodontitis. In some instances it may even be contraindicated.

Stages:

- Periodontitis – characterized by the deposition of calculus and plaque, with gingival recession, periodontal pocket formation, alveolar bone loss and furcation exposure. The symptoms of periodontitis are halitosis, bleeding gums and difficulty eating. The pulp is often significantly

affected in periodontal disease as a result of accessory pulp canals being exposed following alveolar bone loss. A light and transmission electron microscopic study (Ghoddusi, 2003) conducted on dental pulps of cats suffering from periodontal disease, revealed that all sections of the pulp examined displayed a generalized infiltration of chronic inflammatory cells. Some capillaries located within the odontoblastic layer had several fenestrations, and odontoblasts showed many mitochondria and secretary vesicles. Fibroblasts displayed lytic changes in some areas. These findings indicate that special care should be taken when planning treatment for teeth with moderate bone loss and especially for those with furcation involvement.

- Advanced periodontitis – can compromise tooth vitality. When the periodontium is affected such that the periapical tissues are involved, the infection can spread to the dental pulp. This is known as a combined periodontic–endodontic lesion. As a general rule, these teeth should be extracted (Figures 8.8 and 8.9).

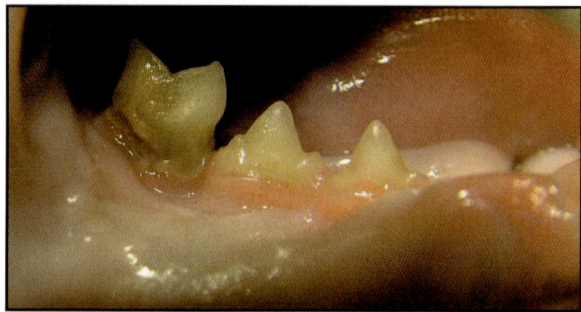

8.8   Periodontitis may be a localized 'focal' disease. This tooth should be extracted.

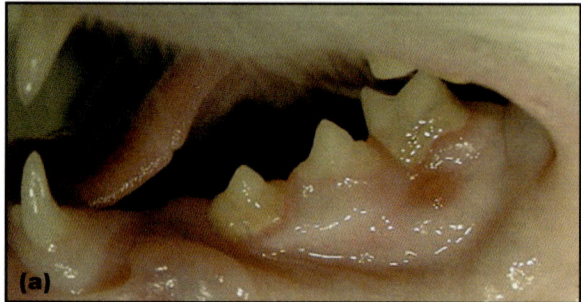

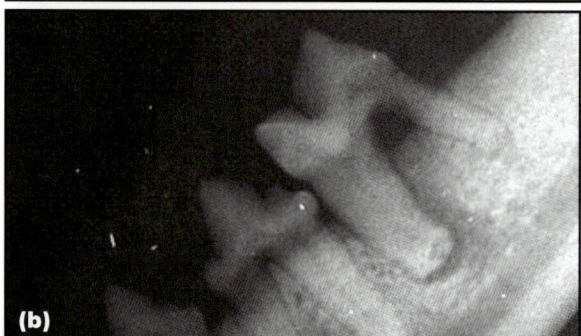

8.9   **(a)** Severe periodontitis and periodontal abscessation of the mandibular first molar. **(b)** Radiograph of the same tooth, illustrating the periodontic–endodontic nature of this lesion.

Periodontitis is a cyclical disease (Goodson *et al.*, 1982; Socransky *et al.*, 1984). It is a chronic illness, characterized by periods of intense destructive activity and periods of quiescence. The resulting tissue damage is irreversible. This alternation is probably related to the features of the causative bacterial flora. Gramnegative, anaerobic, motile bacteria cause an acute inflammatory response, which leads to periodontal tissue destruction. During periods of quiescence, Grampositive aerobic bacteria prevail, adhering to the tooth surface and forming the plaque that in due course can mineralize to form calculus.

During the acute phase of the disease the nature of the inflammatory response changes, with increased prevalence of neutrophils and the formation of a purulent exudate. If the host's immune response is not compromised, the chronic phase follows the acute phase and is characterized by the presence of lymphocytes and plasma cells. The mechanism of alternation leads to progressive tissue destruction (gingival epithelium, connective tissue, bone and periodontal ligament) with a consequent increase in the severity of the lesion. Lesions may appear to remain clinically stable for a long time but damage is often being caused to the alveolar bone, which is not visible on oral examination.

The final outcome of periodontitis is loss of the tooth, which leads to resolution of the pathology, i.e. when the periodontium is severely compromised the tooth is lost from the alveolus and the gingiva heals. However, tooth loss is not an acceptable outcome for periodontitis! The persistence of a chronic bacterial infection in the oral cavity exposes the animal to the risk of bacteraemia and colonization of other distant organs (e.g. heart, kidneys). In the healthy animal these transient bacteraemias together with their associated inflammatory mediators and bacterial toxins are quickly cleared. However, severe consequences may be experienced by immunocompromised animals or those with organs affected by a bacteraemia. Other systemic complications associated with periodontal disease may occur and are the subject of much research in humans. However, a link is difficult to prove.

Clinical features of specific types of periodontal disease

Juvenile hyperplastic gingivitis: This condition is seen in some young pure breeds (Abyssinians and Persians) and also in other kittens. Proliferative tissue of gingival origin begins to cover the teeth at the time of permanent teeth eruption (6–8 months), seriously impairing mastication and maintenance of oral hygiene. The treatment of choice is gingivectomy to remove the hyperplastic tissue, together with scaling and polishing (Figure 8.10). Patients should be re-examined at regular intervals at least in the first year, as the condition may recur. Good dental home care is necessary.

Juvenile early-onset gingivitis: This is a non-proliferative gingivitis seen in the deciduous and permanent dentitions of young Persian kittens. The gingiva appears as an erythematous strip extending from the

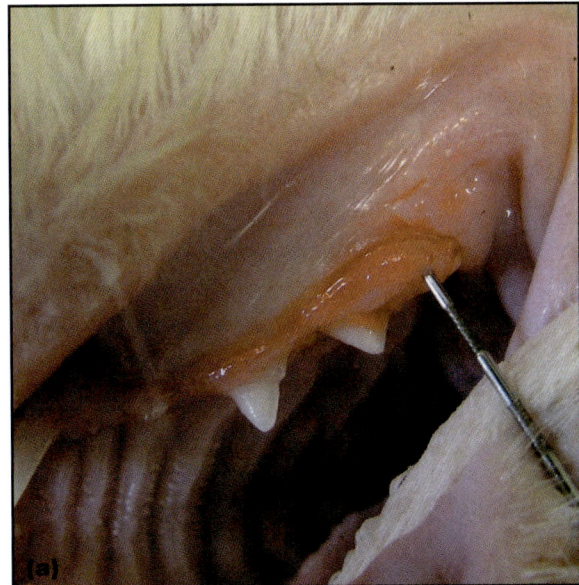

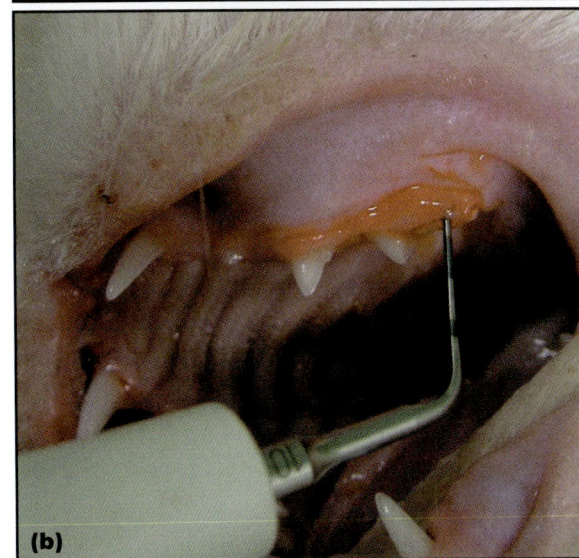

8.10 Juvenile hyperplastic gingivitis in a Persian cat. **(a)** False gingival pocket made of hyperplastic tissue. **(b)** Subgingival scaling, with a subgingival perio tip mounted on an ultrasonic scaler. Subsequent removal of the hyperplastic tissue was carried out by means of a gingivectomy/gingivoplasty.

incisors to the molars. Treatment consists of meticulous home care, together with periodic professional scaling and polishing. Appropriate treatment of juvenile early-onset gingivitis will prevent progression to early periodontitis.

Juvenile onset gingivitis–periodontitis: This occurs in pure-breed kittens, particularly Maine Coon and Siamese, as well as in Domestic Shorthair kittens. Thick deposits of plaque and calculus accumulate, resulting in gingiva that appear red and swollen. The gingivitis rapidly progresses to severe periodontitis with loss of gingival attachment, deep periodontal pockets and/or gingival recession and extensive bone resorption. Often this condition progresses without evidence of clinical signs, but detailed examination will reveal gingival bleeding and difficulty with mastication.

Frequent professional scaling and polishing is required and efficient dental home care must be instituted. However, many of these patients do not respond favourably to treatment and may loose many teeth at a young age (Figure 8.11).

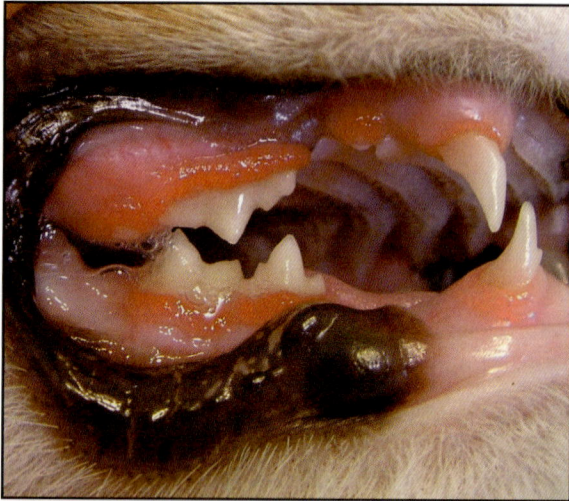

8.11   Juvenile onset gingivitis–periodontitis in a Maine Coon kitten.

Diagnosis

Symptoms of periodontal disease (but also of other oral cavity diseases) include but are not limited to:

- Halitosis
- Difficulties in mastication and/or deglutition
- Inappetence
- Weight loss
- Chattering of teeth (jaw-opening reflex)
- Poor grooming
- Pawing at the mouth
- Nasal discharge (often unilateral) and sneezing
- Spontaneous gingival bleeding or bleeding on chewing.

The cat affected with periodontal disease must be submitted to a careful general clinical examination, followed by evaluation of the oral cavity and the surrounding structures. Examination under general anaesthesia enables more detailed evaluation of the oral cavity, the teeth and periodontium, but may also mask the severity (redness) of some inflammatory conditions.

Clinical examination

Many generic symptoms are associated with the presence of periodontal disease in cats, but they often go unobserved because of the brevity of their duration or their poor intensity. With the exception of halitosis and difficulties in mastication, owners may not notice the symptoms of periodontal disease or only notice them when the disease process is advanced. The veterinary surgeon can not and must not rely upon owner's ability to detect early symptoms of the disease. Similarly in evaluating the case history, the veterinary surgeon should not only focus on the diet or home oral hygiene regimen but also gather all the information on the

environment in which the animal lives, on its interaction with the environment, its family history and past and/or present health problems.

Periodontal examination

The periodontal examination is performed with the aid of a periodontal probe. The periodontal probe should be gently run under the gingival margin of each tooth. Many cats react to this manoeuvre by 'chattering' their jaws. Initially, this reaction was assumed to be caused by oral pain (periodontal disease or feline odontoclastic resorptive lesions, FORLs) causing a local reflex arc. However, in cats followed up serially, there was poor correlation between chattering, the extent of gingivitis and the presence of a FORL located at the gingival margin. Regardless of oral disease status, some cats do 'chatter' under general anaesthesia and others do not.

The periodontal examination enables evaluation of the:

- Amount of plaque and calculus present on the tooth surface
- Degree of gingivitis
- Presence of gingival hyperplasia or recession
- Degree of attachment loss
- Bony resorption at the furcation
- Mobility of individual teeth.

Periodontitis indices numerically express the existence and/or severity of pathological conditions in the patient and indicate the necessity for treatment. Each value should be recorded on the patient's dental chart (see Chapters 2 and 5 for more information on charting). Some of these evaluations require integration with other information, e.g. that provided by radiographs. The scores for each tooth (or in the case of some indices, e.g. gingivitis index (GI) and periodontal disease index (PDI), the total score of the various measurements taken for the tooth) are added and then divided by the number of evaluated teeth (Figures 8.12 and 8.13). This 'total index' is useful when comparing evaluations performed at different times on the same cat, and facilitates objective comparison of improvement, stabilization or dis-

Original terminology	Abbreviated terminology	Index range
Plaque index	PI	0—3
Calculus index	CI	0—3
Gingivitis index	GI	0—3
Gingival hyperplasia	GH	mm
Pocket depth	PD	mm
Periodontal disease	PDI	0—4
Attachment loss	AL	mm
Furcation	F	0—3
Mobility	M	0—3

8.12   Original and modified indices for use in veterinary medicine.

PDI grade	Periodontal disease	AL (%)	Pocket depth (mm)
0	Healthy	0	<0.5
1	Gingivitis	0	<0.5
2	Initial	<25	<1.0
3	Moderate	>25; <50	<2.0
4	Severe	>50	>2.0

8.13 Periodontal disease index used in veterinary medicine.

ease progression in the patient. Charting is indispensable for the correct formulation of a diagnosis of periodontal disease, for appropriate treatment planning and to evaluate the changes in the disease condition over time. Standard dental charts can be modified to suit personal preferences.

Periodontal probing: The periodontal probe is inserted, using gentle pressure, between the tooth and the soft tissues until resistance is felt. Except for the canine teeth, in the majority of healthy cats, gingival height is only 1–2 mm, making it sometimes difficult to insert the probe. Probing depths are affected not only by the force that the examiner exerts on the probe but also by the degree of tissue inflammation. A very light force of about 25 grams is necessary during gentle probing. Special attention must be paid to the insertion of the probe. It may be necessary to angle the probe to insert it, especially in the interproximal spaces. Once in the pocket the probe should be oriented parallel to the tooth surface. At times, the presence of thick calculus will prevent the introduction of the probe into the gingival sulcus; in these cases it is necessary to remove the gross calculus prior to periodontal examination.

Radiographic examination

The diagnosis of periodontal disease cannot be based on visual inspection of the oral cavity alone. To diagnose periodontal disease it is mandatory to perform a detailed oral examination, including periodontal probing of each tooth and a full-mouth intraoral radiographic examination of the teeth under general anaesthesia. Radiology enables the clinician to perform a more complete evaluation of the periodontal status than clinical examination alone.

Pathology affecting the tooth root within the alveolar bone can only be evaluated using radiography. It is very important to determine the amount and quality of bone that surrounds the tooth roots. The importance of radiographic findings in therapeutic decision-making was assessed in a study of 115 cats, and whilst the main clinical findings were confirmed radiographically in all cats, radiographs of teeth without clinical lesions yielded clinically important findings in 41.7% of cats. Radiographs of teeth with clinical disease yielded additional or clinically essential information in 53.9% and 32.2% of cases, respectively (Verstraete *et al.*, 1998). The severity of periodontal pathology is not always directly correlated to the amount of plaque and calculus present on

the tooth surface, or to the mobility of a single tooth. If correct diagnostic procedures are not followed severe and extensive lesions may not be detected.

Radiographic signs of periodontal disease: The radiographic signs of periodontal disease (Figures 8.14 and 8.15) include:

- Rounding of the alveolar margin at the cementoenamel junction
- Periodontal space widening
- Disruption of the lamina dura
- Lysis of perialveolar bone
- Canine perialveolar bone reaction with moth-eaten appearance
- Erosion of the alveolar margin.

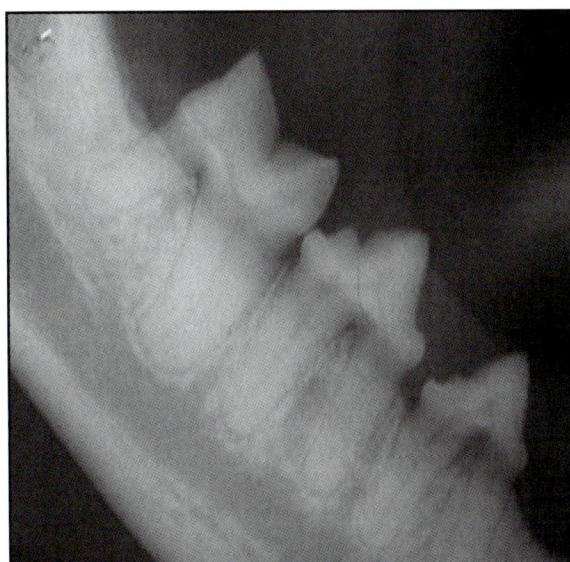

8.14 Horizontal bone loss. Recession of the alveolar margin parallel to the cementoenamel junction.

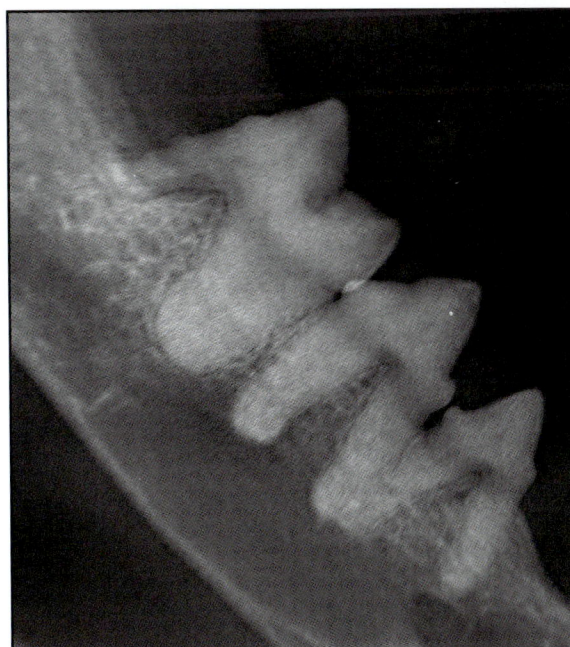

8.15 Vertical bone loss. Alveolar bone loss in an apical direction, localized to one or more roots.

Treatment

Gingivitis

The treatment plan for gingivitis involves:

- Describing the disease process to the pet owner
- Educating the owner in daily dental home care
- Professional periodontal therapy: supra- and subgingival scaling and polishing
- Regular follow-up examinations.

Periodontitis

The treatment plan for periodontitis involves:

- Describing the disease process to the pet owner
- Educating the owner in daily dental home care
- Professional periodontal therapy: supra- and subgingival scaling and polishing, root surface debridement, extraction of teeth with advanced periodontitis
- Regular follow-up examinations
- Periodontal surgery may be indicated. In cats gingival height is only 1–2 mm, which rules out most surgical periodontal procedures. Guided tissue regeneration is a possible surgical option in cats (Takahashi *et al.*, 2005) but should be performed by a suitably experienced colleague in a referral practice.

See also Chapters 7 and 11.

Home care

Tooth brushing is not easily applied to the cat, but with patience many cats can be trained to have their teeth brushed daily.

Feline odontoclastic resorptive lesions

The clinical and radiographic examination of cats with periodontal disease may reveal the presence of resorptive lesions of cementum and/or dentine and enamel. These defects are often covered by inflammatory gingival tissue or by granulation tissue of pulpal or gingival origin. These lesions are termed feline odontoclastic resorptive lesions (FORLs or neck lesions).

FORLs are one of the most common dental conditions seen in feline practice, affecting from 25% to 75% of cats. There are no sex or breed predispositions. However, FORL prevalence increases with increasing age. FORLs are distinct from caries. Caries is the result of demineralization of the inorganic portion of teeth and consequent destruction of the organic portion, as a result of acid production by plaque bacteria via sugar fermentation. FORLs are also distinct from other conditions causing tooth substance loss, e.g. attrition, abrasion and erosion.

Aetiology and pathogenesis

FORLs were initially classified as periodontal disease (Schneck, 1976) as it was assumed that these lesions resulted from periodontal disease. One hypothesis for the aetiology of FORLs is that plaque and its bacterial byproducts (extrinsic factors) and inflammation-induced cytokines (mediators) appear to activate the odontoclasts and osteoclasts (present in the periodontal space and around the blood vessels), which progressively destroy the dental tissues via a mechanism similar to the destruction of the alveolar bone in periodontitis (Figure 8.16).

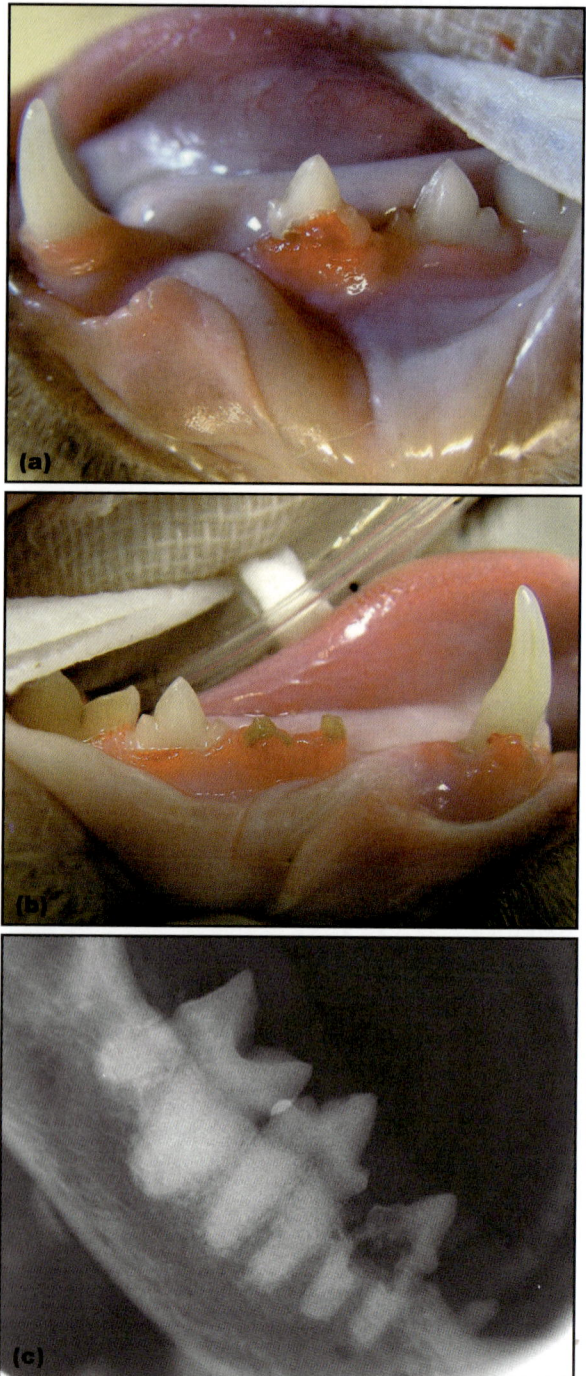

8.16   **(a)** Clinical presentation of a FORL with concurrent gingivitis. **(b)** FORLs are often bilateral and covered by inflamed gingiva or granulation tissue. The tooth affected most often is the mandibular third premolar. **(c)** Radiograph showing large defects in the gingival third of the crown and roots of the mandibular third premolar as a result of FORLs.

Recent studies have questioned the relationship between periodontal disease and FORLs and have been unable to demonstrate a good correlation between the severity of gingivitis and development of resorptive lesions. This was demonstrated on teeth in a group of cats that had serial dental examinations over a five-year period. Cat teeth with resorptive lesions and periodontitis may have a distinctly different clinical and radiographic appearance compared with teeth that have focal, lesion-associated gingivitis. Other hypotheses for the aetiology of FORLs include:

- Dietary texture
- Abnormal calcium regulation
- Hypervitaminosis A
- Mechanical stress
- Anatomical abnormalities of teeth
- Viral infection.

At present the increased vitamin D activity hypothesis (Reiter and Mendoza, 2002) on FORL aetiopathogenesis has received further consideration. Excess of vitamin D and vitamin D metabolites administered to experimental animals may cause dental and periodontal changes similar to the clinical, radiographic and histopathological features of FORLs.

Diagnosis

FORLs are often covered with plaque, calculus, hyperplastic gingiva or proliferative tissue of pulpal origin. They are most often located at the cementoenamel junction and at the furcation area of multi-rooted teeth. Clinically, FORLs appear as defects of the crown and root surfaces, and are extremely variable in size and depth. Some defects may appear small but extend into the tooth structure, resulting in teeth that are prone to fracture easily. Root replacement resorption and ankylosis may also be present in more advanced stages. Full-mouth radiographs are necessary to determine the distribution of the lesions, the extent of each lesion and to identify the presence of any root abnormalities that might complicate treatment of the lesions (Figure 8.17).

When confined below the gingival margin, and not affecting the dental pulp, FORLs are usually not painful. This initial lesion may be asymptomatic for a long time with halitosis being the only clinical sign. In the more advanced stages of the disease difficulty in mastication or rarely anorexia and weight loss are the most frequent symptoms. The most commonly affected teeth are the mandibular third premolars, the maxillary fourth premolars and the mandibular molars.

Radiographic signs of FORLs
The radiographic signs of FORLs (Figure 8.18) include:

- Erosion of the alveolar margin at the cementoenamel junction
- Resorption of dental tissues of the crown
- Disruption of the lamina dura
- Root resorption (diffuse or focal)
- Root ankylosis and periodontal space loss.

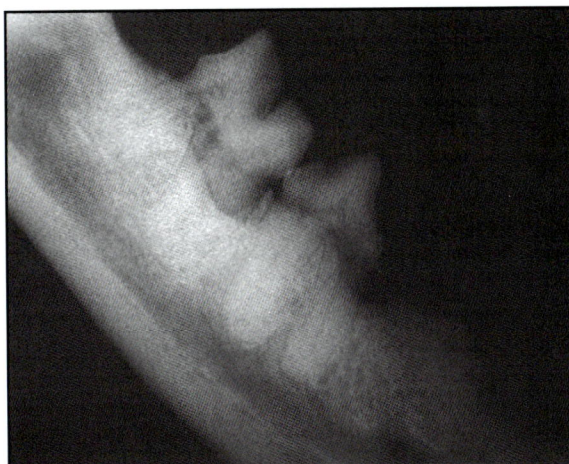

8.18 Small defects are present on the distal part of the mesial root of the mandibular first molar. Remnants of the third premolar appear as 'ghost roots'.

Stage	Clinical appearance	Radiographic appearance
1	Lesions extend into the cementum only, do not enter the dentine and are not sensitive. May be difficult to detect	Minute radiolucent defects. May be difficult to see radiographically
2	Lesions progress into crown or root dentine and are painful. Hyperplastic gingiva and inflammatory granulation tissue often overlies defects	Notched radiolucent areas with sharp or scalloped margins, often found at the cementoenamel junction
3	Lesions extend into the pulp chamber and root canal and are painful. Bleeding of pulp tissue and gingival or pulpal granulation tissue is evident on probing. The tooth crown may fracture spontaneously	The tooth shows extensive radiolucent areas, and may have a moth-eaten or striated appearance. Replacement resorption may be present, with root dentine being replaced by bone
4	Extensive structural damage, and dentoalveolar ankylosis of roots with alveolar bone may occur. These teeth are fragile and prone to fracture	When dentoalveolar ankylosis is present the cementum and the bone are fused, and the lamina dura is disrupted or absent
5a	Teeth with no crown, only root remnants remain. May appear as a bulge covered by healthy intact gingiva or inflamed gingiva	Roots or roots fragments visible in the alveolar bone, and may be resorbed or become sequestrated or cause osteomyelitis
5b	The crown is intact, the root structure is lost because of extensive root replacement resorption	The tooth root structure is replaced by bone, the root contour becomes irregular and gradually disappears (ghost roots)

8.17 Classification of FORLs. (Modified after Reiter and Mendoza, 2002)

Stage	Treatment	Result
1–2	Scaling and polishing Adequate cavity preparation Fluoride treatment Dentinal bonding and use of a pit and fissure sealant	Preventive treatment? Controversial
2	Scaling and polishing Adequate cavity preparation Restoration (glass ionomer, compomer or composite)	Controversial Poor long-term success rate
2–3	Extraction Crown amputation and intentional root retention (selected patients)	Good
4	Extraction Crown amputation and intentional root retention (selected patients)	Good
5a	Extraction Intentional root retention (selected patients)	Good
5b	Crown amputation (selected patients)	Good

8.19 Treatment of FORLs.

In a recent study of full-mouth survey radiographs to determine patterns of alveolar bone loss (periodontitis) and other lesions in almost 150 cats, it was evident that horizontal bone loss is the most common radiographic pattern of alveolar bone loss. Pure-breed cats were not more likely than mixed-breed cats to have periodontitis, but when they did have periodontitis it was more likely to be moderate to severe. Severe focal vertical bone loss was more frequent in cats with periodontitis and FORLs than in cats without FORLs (DuPont *et al.*, 2002). The prevalence of root replacement resorption in teeth with FORLs was significantly lower in cats suffering from concurrent periodontitis.

Treatment

Many treatments to arrest the progression of a FORL have been attempted, unfortunately, without satisfactory results. Currently, the treatment of choice for any tooth affected by a FORL is extraction. Extracting teeth with extensive FORLs may be difficult because they are brittle and liable to fracture. Furthermore, these teeth are often affected by root ankylosis and replacement resorption, making extraction even more difficult. 'Pulverization' or 'atomization' of retained roots is contraindicated as this process is associated with numerous complications. 'Crown amputation' with root retention has been suggested as a possible treatment option, after *in vivo* observation that retained root fragments of teeth affected by FORLs undergo complete resorption, without causing pain or apparent discomfort. Many different studies suggest that crown amputation with intentional root retention may be a valid alternative to extractions in selected cats with FORLs.

Selection of cases is the most important part of treatment planning. Teeth affected by periodontal or endodontic disease should be completely extracted. Cats affected by chronic stomatitis, and feline immunodeciency virus (FIV) or feline leukaemia virus (FeLV) positive cats should also have their teeth extracted.

To perform a crown amputation, an envelope flap is elevated to expose the alveolar bone and the roots. Using a round bur mounted on a high-speed handpiece and with water cooling, the crown substance should be removed to slightly below the alveolar bone level. The gingiva is then sutured back in position. Patients undergoing this treatment should be closely monitored for at least 12 months with periodic radiographic examinations to ensure that complete resorption of the retained root occurs.

Other possible suggested treatment options are fluoride application to stage 1 lesions and restoration of stage 2 lesions, using glass ionomer fillings. The results of these treatments are controversial, as reported in many studies, probably because of the progressive nature of the disease and its unknown aetiology (Figure 8.19).

Reactive supereruption of the canine teeth

The canine teeth of cats are a common site of periodontal disease and resorptive lesions. Maxillary canines, and less frequently mandibular canines, are affected by a perialveolar bone reaction, enlarging the bony juga and resulting in extrusion of the tooth out of the alveolus. This reactive supereruption is easily detect-

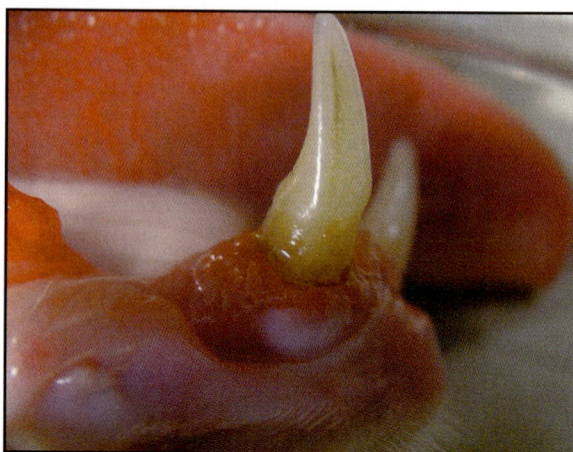

8.20 Reactive supereruption of the mandibular canine.

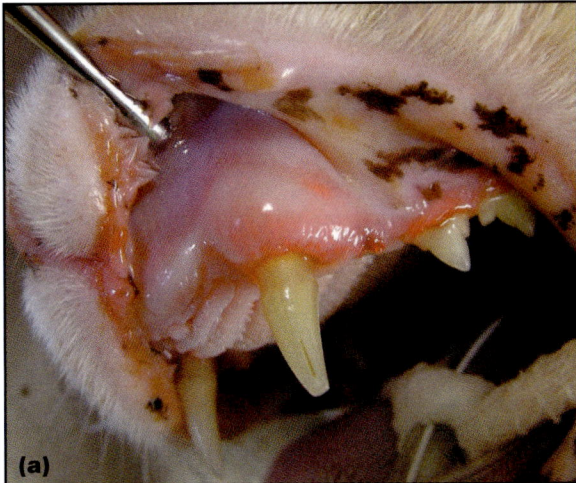

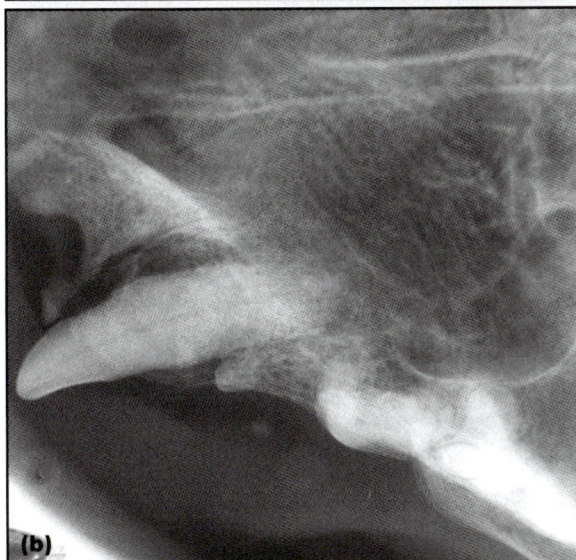

8.21 **(a)** Reactive supereruption and alveolar bone reaction of the maxillary canine. **(b)** Radiograph of the same tooth. Note the characteristic moth-eaten appearance of the alveolar bone.

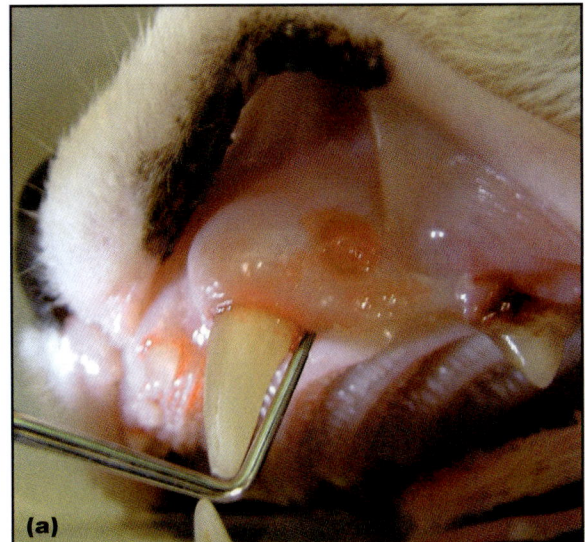

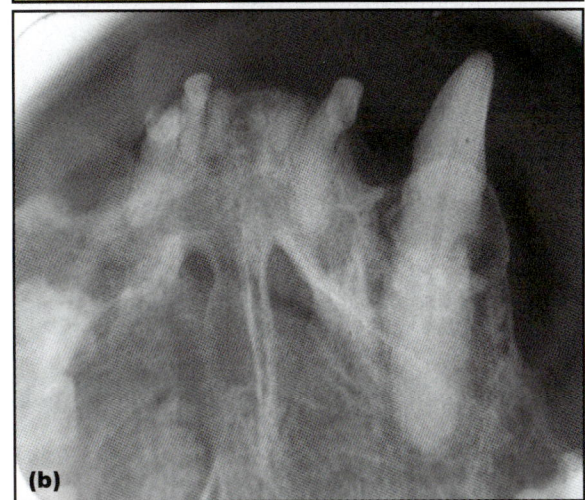

8.22 **(a)** Deep periodontal pocket of a supererupted maxillary canine with abscessation and a draining sinus tract. **(b)** Radiograph of the same tooth.

able on clinical examination of the oral cavity. The cementoenamel junction of the canines is easily distinguishable and positioned away from the gingival margin. Radiographic examination of supererupted teeth shows a reactive process of the perialveolar bone, which displays a moth-eaten appearance. These teeth can be firmly attached but deep periodontal pockets are often present, sometimes with abscessation or tract drainage (Figures 8.20, 8.21 and 8.22). In these cases extraction is the treatment of choice. Special care should be paid to the closure of the extraction site.

Feline chronic gingivostomatitis

Aetiology and pathogenesis

Feline chronic gingivostomatitis (FCGS) is a common, yet poorly understood, syndrome. Erosive/ulcerative feline stomatitis commonly manifests as one of two histological presentations: the first is characterized by a dense band-like submucosal lymphocytic–

plasmacytic infiltrate (Figure 8.23); the other by a chronic active inflammation of the mucosa and submucosa, which histologically also includes a neutrophilic infiltrate (Figure 8.24). The number of inflammatory cells increases with the severity of the disease.

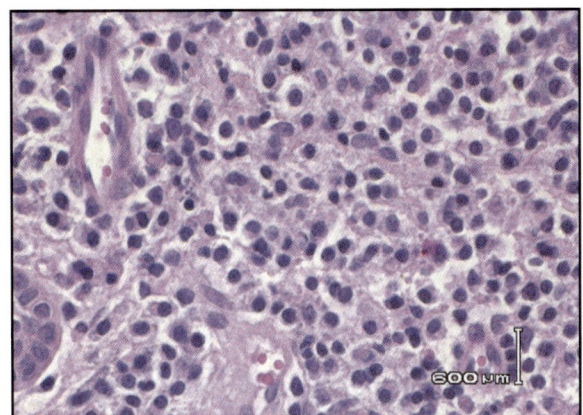

8.23 Dense band-like submucosal lymphocytic–plasmacytic infiltrate.

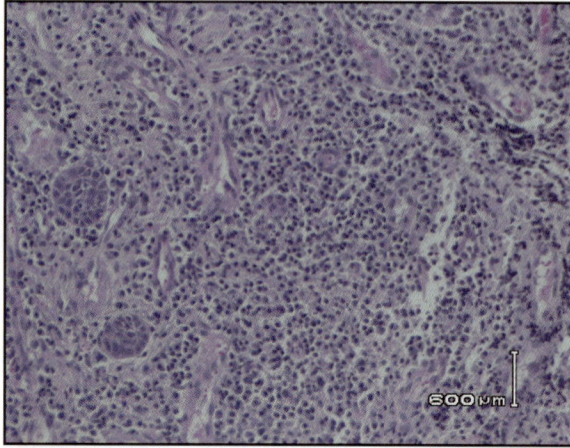

8.24   Chronic active inflammation (neutrophils) of the mucosa and submucosa.

Bacteria (particularly in dental plaque), viruses (feline calicivirus (FCV), feline herpesvirus (FHV), FIV, FeLV, feline coronavirus (FCoV)) and excessive or abnormal immune reactions have been considered as possible aetiologies. Calicivirus has been isolated from the oral cavity of FCGS-affected cats, although no direct aetiological link has been shown and only transient caudal oral inflammation is caused by experimental FCV infection. Nevertheless, cats with FCGS are significantly more likely to concurrently shed both FCV and FHV type-1 than are cats with classic periodontal disease (Figure 8.25). It is possible that the virus shedding seen in many cases is related to the stress caused by FCGS suppressing the local immune response, permitting viral replication. Cats with established FIV infection also have an increased risk of developing FCGS. However, there is no evidence of a direct correlation between FCGS and this virus.

Co-infection of *Haemobartonella henselae* has been reported in FIV positive cats, some of which were affected by FCGS, but no obvious correlation has been found between the presence of the parasite and the severity of clinical lesions (Ueno *et al.*, 1996).

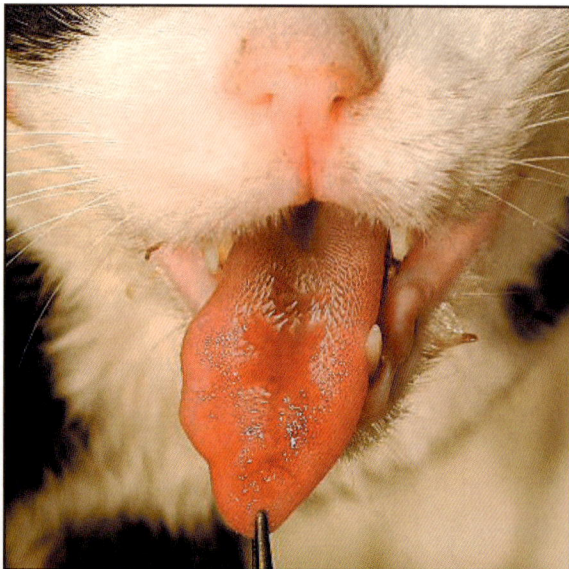

8.25   Ulcers on the tongue are suggestive of FHV and FCV infection.

The specific pathogenesis of feline stomatitis is unknown. It is thought that the inflammation is a result of plaque intolerance, and that it occurs due to an alteration in the immune response with either, or both, immunosuppression and type III hypersensitivity reactions playing a part (Figure 8.26). The characteristics of the inflammatory infiltrate and the presence or absence of a polyclonal gammopathy may indicate persistence of intracellular or extracellular antigenic stimulation, and a cell-mediated or humoral immune response. Cats with FCGS have typically higher salivary concentrations of IgG and IgM, but a lower concentration of IgA compared with unaffected cats. A reduction in IgA levels impairs local defence mechanisms against oral bacteria, viruses and soluble antigens and therefore may contribute to the development or persistence of pathology.

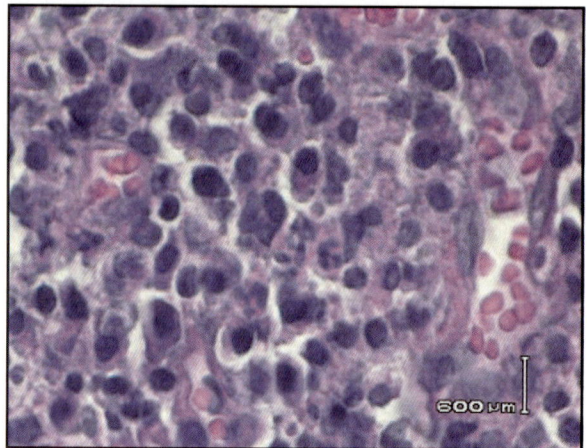

8.26   Lymphoplasmacellular stomatitis with eosinophils.

In type III hypersensitivity reactions antigen–antibody (IgG, IgM) complexes form within the tissues with the release of complement, causing increased inflammation. Continuous exposure to antigens, such as those in dental plaque, results in persistent reactions, which may explain the severity of damage that can occur to the oral tissues and bone (Figure 8.27). Furthermore, the location of the lesions can be ex-

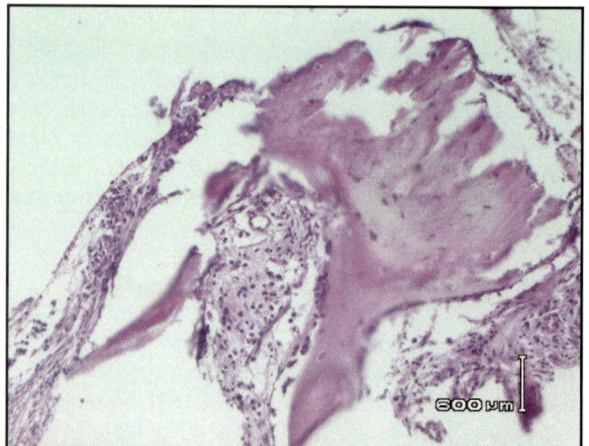

8.27   Bone involvement, characterized by mixed cellular inflammatory infiltration and osseous lytic changes, may complicate the clinical outcome of FCGS.

plained by the concentration of antibody and antigenic factors; lesions appear where antigens and antibodies occur in the necessary volume for precipitation of complexes to occur. The extension of disease into the pharynx can also be explained by the normally high levels of lymphoid tissue here, and the presence of bacterial plaque on the base of the tongue as well as on the teeth.

A significant increase in inflammatory cytokine levels, including interleukin-2 (IL-2), IL-4, IL-5, IL-6, IL-10, IL-12 and gamma interferon (IFN-gamma), is seen in tissue samples taken from the oral cavity of cats affected by FCGS. However, no correlation has been found between these values and the severity of clinical lesions. Other significant findings include the prevalence of CD8+ cells at all stages of the disease and a mixed T helper cell type 1/type 2 profile. When studied, serum melatonin levels were found to be lower in cats with FCGS than in a control group, but the rationale for this is uncertain. An algorithm of the aetiology of FCGS is given in Figure 8.28.

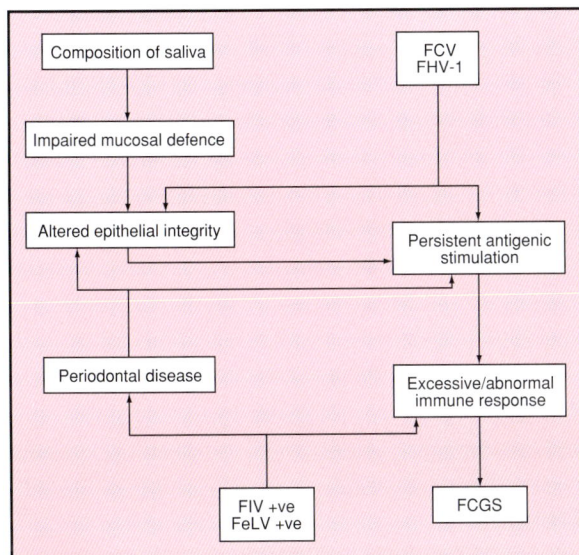

8.28 Algorithm showing the aetiology of FCGS.

Diagnosis

Clinical presentation

FCGS is a condition seen in cats and has no sex, age or breed predilection. However, a few studies indicate that pure-breed cats (e.g. Siamese, Abyssinian, Persian, Himalayan and Burmese) seem to develop more severe disease, possibly due to a genetic tendency in these breeds. The median age of affected cats is 7 years (range 4 months to 17 years).

The most obvious clinical lesions are bilateral erythematous, ulcerative and/or proliferative lesions of the gingiva (Figure 8.29), buccal mucosa, lips, palatoglossal folds (often incorrectly termed faucitis) and the lateral pharyngeal walls (the fauces) (Figures 8.30 and 8.31). Lesions can also be found on the lateral aspect of the tongue, from contact with the lingual surface of mandibular molars and premolars. The palatal mucosa

adjacent to the upper molars and premolars may be inflamed too, appearing flattened, ulcerated or depigmented. Regional lymphadenopathy may also be present. Prolifero-ulcerative pharyngitis may be seen as a caudal extension of gingivostomatitis. The latter is considered to be a separate pathological entity by some authors who believe it to be related to FCV infection.

Various degrees of dental and periodontal disease may be present, with or without large accumulations of plaque and calculus. The clinical symptoms and signs of FCGS (Figure 8.32) include halitosis, difficulty in prehending or chewing food, dysphagia, pain on opening the mouth, ptyalism and weight loss. Behavioural changes may also be noticed, the affected cats becoming less active and reluctant to groom themselves, or more aggressive towards the owners or other pets.

Diagnosis of FCGS can easily be made on the basis of clinical appearance. Lesions and symptoms, together with the lack of response to professional tooth cleaning and home oral hygiene measures, are typically suggestive of this disease. History of failure to cure the condition using different medical treatments can also be suggestive of FCGS. Biopsy is rarely necessary, but is helpful in excluding neoplastic conditions and confirming the diagnosis. Biopsy samples

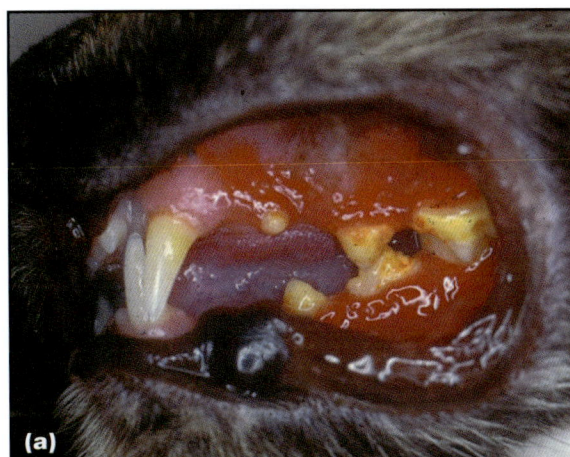

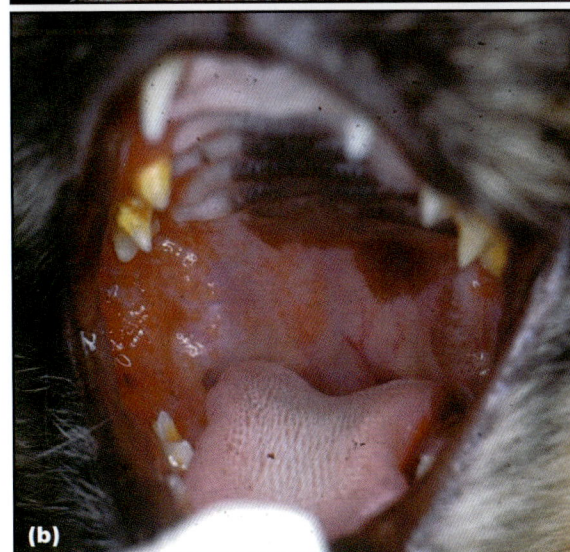

8.29 **(a)** Ulcerative gingivostomatitis involving the gingiva and **(b)** the vestibular mucosa.

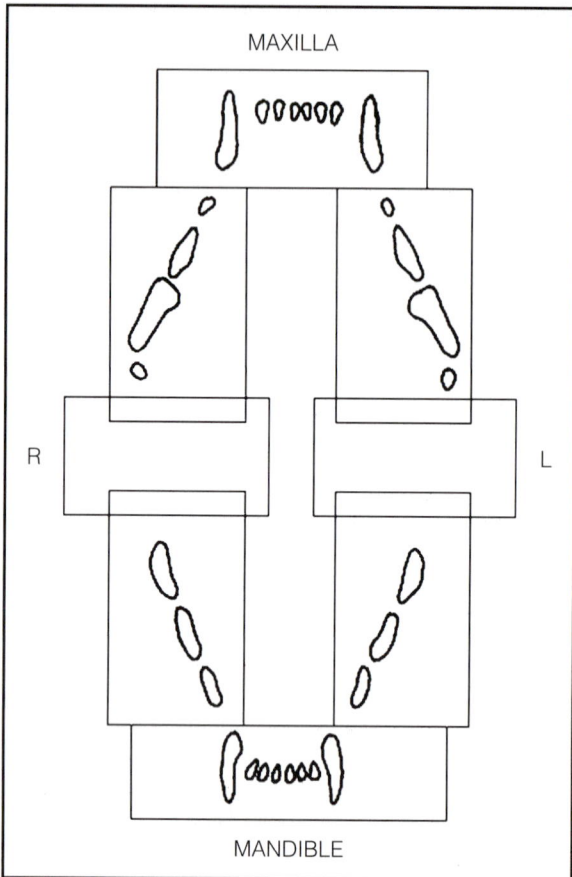

MAXILLA

R

L

MANDIBLE

8.30 An example of a dental chart, showing all the possible localizations of FCGS lesions.

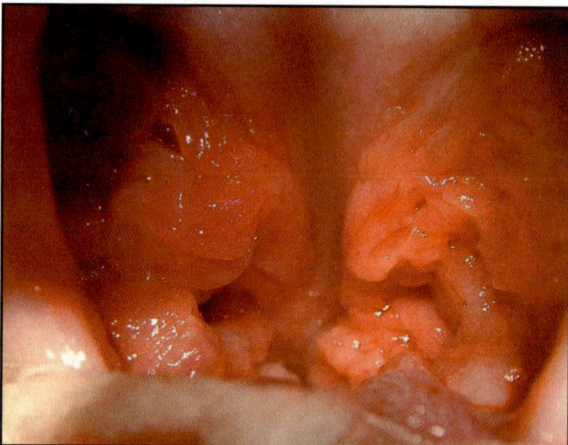

8.31 Severe proliferative faucitis; the term 'faucitis' is commonly but incorrectly used to indicate lesions confined to the palatoglossal folds and regions lateral to the folds.

can also provide useful information on the extent and nature of the inflammatory process involving the tissues. In some cases the alveolar bone can be affected, and this should be taken into consideration when planning the medical therapy. Routine laboratory examinations (Figure 8.33) are mandatory to reveal the patient's general medical condition, and as part of the preoperative diagnostic work-up. However, they often do not provide additional relevant information.

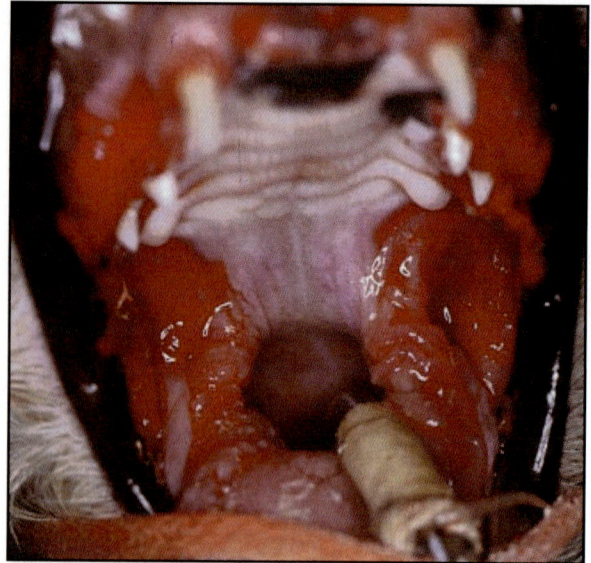

8.32 FCGS in a coronavirus carrier Maine Coon; spontaneous bleeding occurred when opening the mouth.

Complete blood count (CBC)
Blood biochemical profile (including urea, creatinine and glucose)
Protein electrophoresis
Serological assays (e.g. FIV; FeLV; feline infectious peritonitis, FIP)
Fungal cultures (e.g. *Candida* spp.)
Viral isolation (e.g. FCV; FHV-1)
Cytology
Histology

8.33 Suggested laboratory examinations for cats with FCGS.

Treatment

Reported treatments include administration of antibiotics, corticosteroids, megestrol acetate, sodium salicylate, gold salts, lactoferrin, interferon, use of chlorhexidine containing mouth rinses, professional tooth cleaning, dental home care and extraction of multiple or all of the teeth (full-mouth extraction) (Figure 8.34).

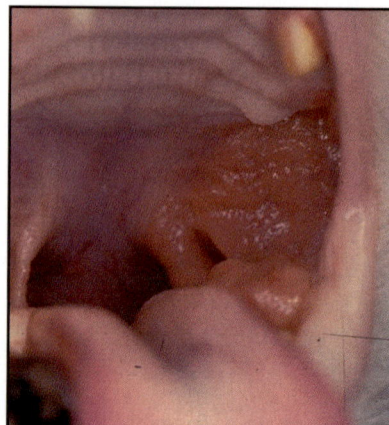

8.34 Unilateral lesion, localized on the side of the mouth where the teeth are still in place.

Medical

Medical treatment (Figure 8.35) of feline stomatitis using corticosteroids is very common; however, full remission of signs is rare and treatment must be repeated to maintain control of the oral symptoms and signs. Corticosteroid efficacy often decreases with repeated use, so that higher doses or more frequent administration is required. As steroids have numerous side effects this form of treatment is less than ideal, but it is effective in the initial management of inflammation, reducing pain and stimulating appetite. Megestrol acetate has been widely used in the past, but its well known side effects suggest that its use should be avoided. Several immuno-modulating drugs that are not licensed for feline use have been used to treat affected cats. These include: levamisole (supposedly restoring suppressed immunity), ciclosporins (suppressing cell mediated responses) and thalidomide (an anti-neovascular agent and tranquillizer), but evidence of efficacy is lacking. Clinical use of such untested agents can not be recommended. Interferon and immunostimulatory drugs have also been used in cats with stomatitis, with poor results. Antiviral agents, such as azidotimidine (AZT) and 9-(2-phosphonyl-methoxy-ethyl) adenine (PMEA), have been tried in FIV positive cats with remission of clinical signs reported in some cases.

Antibiotic therapy using drugs effective against both Gram-positive aerobic and Gram-negative anaerobic bacteria, and able to concentrate adequately in the oral soft tissues and bone, is generally suggested (Figure 8.36). Long-term antibiotic therapy becomes almost ineffective in controlling the disease within weeks to months, and may select for resistance or permit mycotic super-infections. Oral rinses or gels containing chlorhexidine gluconate are useful in maintaining oral hygiene or as a postoperative adjunctive therapy, and due to their mode of action do not induce resistance. Long-term oral rinse application is often not tolerated by cats and, furthermore, chlorhexidine may have harmful effects on the gingival tissues when administered over a long period of time (Mariotti and Rumpf, 1999). None of the suggested medical treatments (e.g. megestrol acetate, gold salts and chlorhexidine) or soft laser application are curative or able to guarantee clinical remission of signs and symptoms in the long term. The lack of efficacy is not surprising when one considers that there is no medical therapy effective in controlling dental plaque, which is a major factor in the aetiology of the inflammation seen in FCGS (Figures 8.37 and 8.38).

Surgical

General anaesthesia is necessary to perform a complete oral examination and obtain full-mouth dental radiographs for accurate diagnosis and treatment planning. The primary aim of surgical treatment is to remove plaque bacteria and cure any pathological condition of the teeth in order to decrease the inflammatory response. Therefore, every diseased tooth (periodontal disease, FORL, pulp necrosis, fractures) should be extracted (see Chapter 11). Professional

Patient	Treatment			
First opinion case: A + B ± C	**A**	**B**	**C**	**D**
Referred case unresponsive to medical treatment: A + C ± D	Clinical examination Blood work Full-mouth radiographs Biopsy Medical treatment	Dental prophylaxis Extraction of diseased teeth Medical treatment Home oral hygiene	Dental prophylaxis Extraction of premolar and molar teeth ± Medical treatment Home oral hygiene	Dental prophylaxis Extraction of canine and incisor teeth Biopsy ± Medical treatment
Referred case unresponsive to surgical treatment: A + D				
If the previous fail, start again: A + others (PCR for FCV, FHV-1)				

8.35 Treatment protocols for FCGS. Note that treatment does not result in a cure in all cases.

Drug	Route of administration	Dosage
Amoxicillin/clavulanate	Orally; s.c.; i.m.	12.5 mg/kg q12h
Clindamycin	Orally; i.m.	5.5–11 mg/kg q12h
Doxycycline	Orally	10 mg/kg q24h
Metronidazole/spiramycin	Orally	(12.5 mg M + 75.000 UI S)/kg q24h
Metronidazole	Orally; i.v.	10–25 mg/kg q8–12h

8.36 Commonly used antimicrobial drugs for the treatment of FCGS.

Drug	Route of administration	Dosage
Tolfenamic acid	Orally; s.c.; i.m.	2–4 mg/kg q24h
Meloxicam	i.v.; s.c.	0.2 mg/kg q24h
Carprofen	i.v.; s.c.	2–4 mg/kg q24h
Methylprednisolone	Orally; s.c.; i.m.	1–2 mg/kg q24h

8.37   Commonly used anti-inflammatory drugs for the treatment of FCGS.

Drug	Route of administration	Dosage
Fentanyl patch	Transdermal	
Butorphanol tartrate	i.v.; s.c.; i.m.	0.11—0.22 mg/kg q4h
Buprenorphine	s.c.; i.m.; sublingual	0.01 mg/kg q8—12h

8.38   Commonly used analgesic drugs for the treatment of FCGS.

tooth cleaning removes plaque and leads to a reduction in the associated inflammation, but without thorough dental home care (tooth brushing) bacterial deposits will rapidly reform, stimulating further inflammation. It is mandatory to carefully explain this to the owners so that they understand the need for exemplary plaque control. If an owner is willing and able to perform meticulous home care, then it should immediately follow professional tooth cleaning. Initially in the postoperative period an oral gel containing chlorhexidine and short-term antibiotic therapy are advantageous. Once the condition has improved (oral soft tissues have healed following surgery), daily tooth brushing should be the primary method of choice to control plaque accumulation.

However, few cat owners are able or willing to perform dental home care to a sufficient level to avoid plaque accumulation and consequently reduce the inflammatory reaction. Therefore, it is often necessary to adopt a more aggressive treatment approach. This involves removing the primary solid surfaces on which plaque forms, i.e. the teeth. It is not possible to prevent plaque accumulation on the tongue base, so total plaque control is not achieved even if all the teeth are extracted. Extraction seems to be the best long-term option in most cases (93% of cats will recover within about 2 years following 'full-mouth' extraction) (Figure 8.39). Subtotal or whole mouth extraction is effective in inducing clinical remission of symptoms in many cases, and is curative in others. Owners may be reluctant to accept extraction of healthy teeth but in time the evidence of the ineffectiveness of medical treatments, their associated side effects and the difficulty in maintaining satisfactory oral hygiene, usually convinces them of the benefits of the treatment plan.

When extracting the teeth it is necessary to take both pre- and postoperative radiographs to establish root morphology, identify associated pathology and to confirm that all root remnants have been extracted. It is mandatory to identify and extract any residual root fragments as they are likely to act as foci of bacterial infection, leading to persistence of the inflammatory

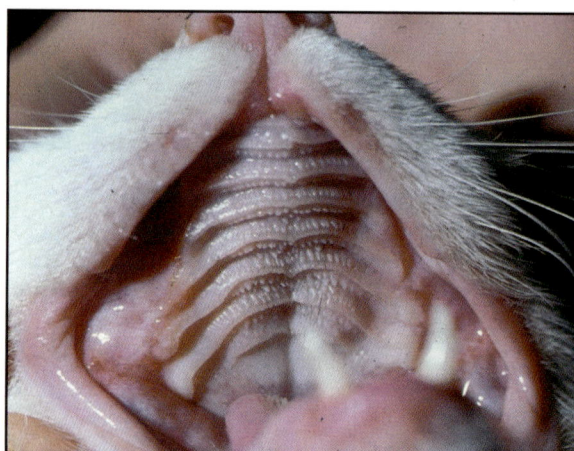

8.39   Outcome of a full-mouth extraction procedure; complete resolution of the disease.

response (Figure 8.40). Dental extraction is a surgical procedure requiring aseptic technique for optimum results. An essential initial step is to perform a thorough dental scaling and polishing, following flushing of the oral cavity with an effective oral antiseptic. The extraction sites should be carefully sutured using a rapidly absorbable monofilament synthetic material, even if the mucoperiosteal flaps are not elevated (Figures 8.41, 8.42 and 8.43). If there is any doubt about undertaking the surgery oneself, referral of the case to a specialist is indicated. FeLV and FIV positive status does not alter the treatment recommendations. Cats with these infections usually respond to whole mouth extraction providing their general medical condition is satisfactory. For details of radiographic and extraction techniques see Chapters 2 and 11.

Whole mouth extraction can be a major procedure and it is often advisable to stage the surgery. All diseased teeth and any remaining healthy premolars and molars should be extracted during the first procedure; canine and incisor extraction should be scheduled later unless it proves necessary to extract them at the initial procedure. Usually, the majority of the inflammation is associated with the molar and premolar teeth and the

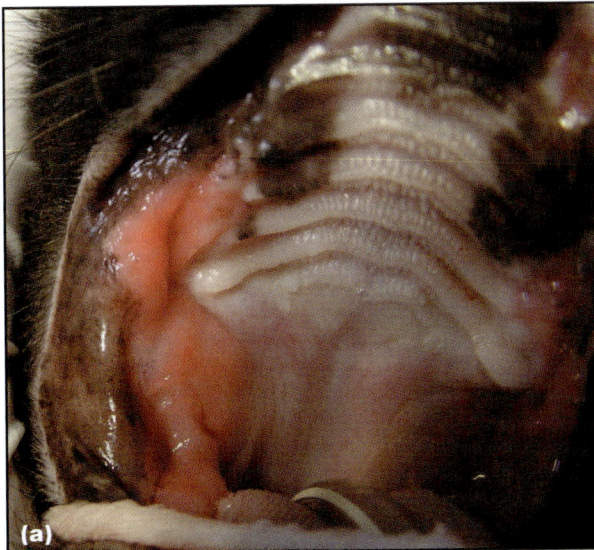

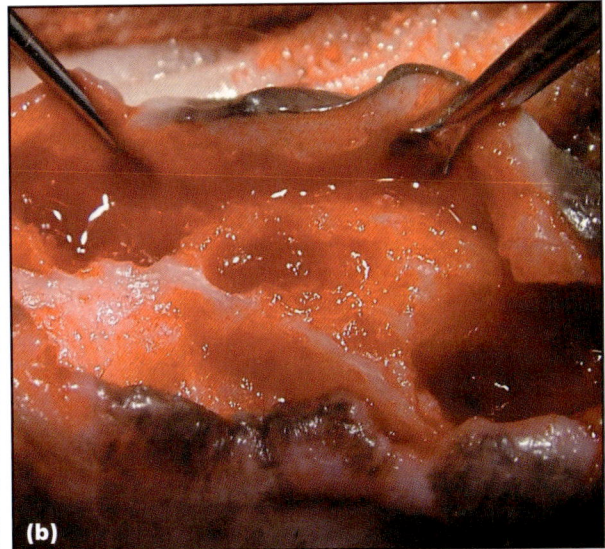

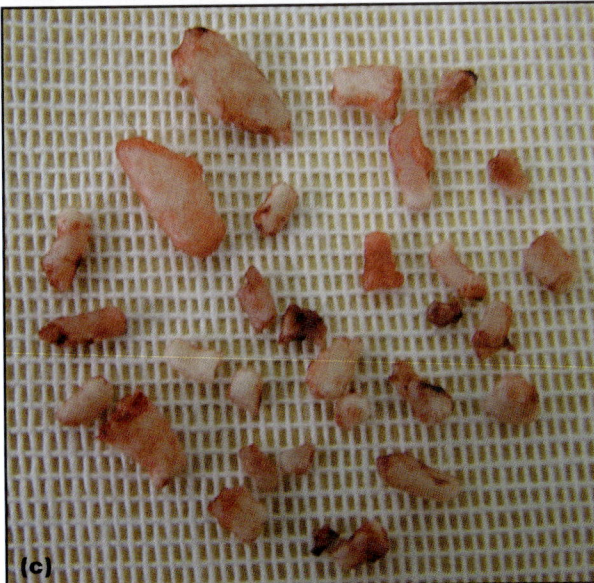

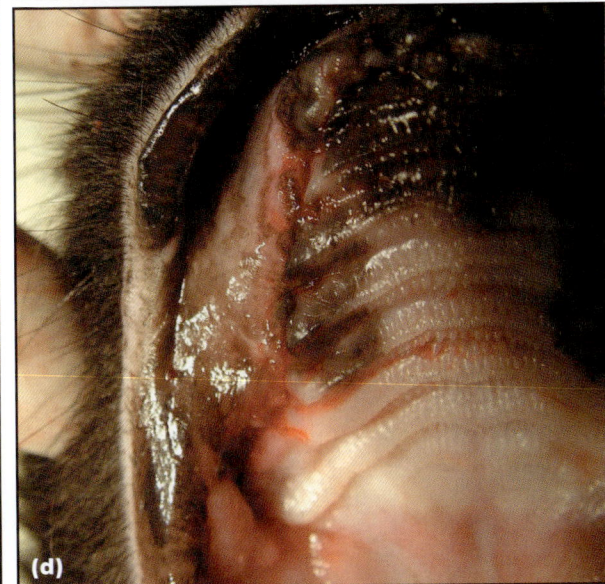

8.40 **(a)** Persistence of tissue inflammation after removal of the molar and premolar teeth, due to a poor extraction technique. **(b)** It is necessary to elevate full-thickness flaps to localize all the root fragments that are embedded in the alveolar bone. **(c)** All the root fragments must be completely removed and **(d)** the gingival tissue sutured back in place.

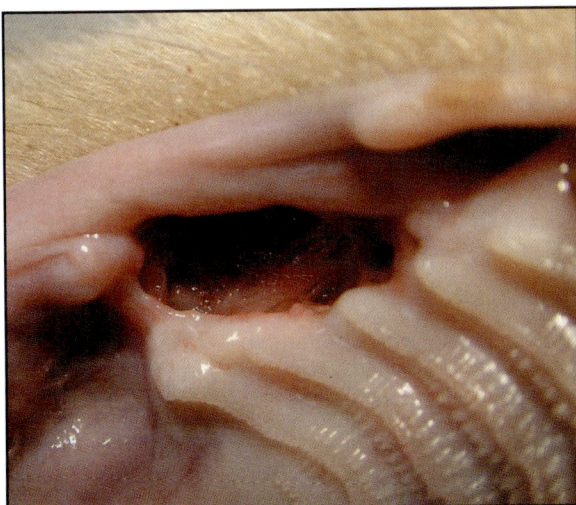

8.41 A large oronasal communication. An unusual postoperative complication following full-mouth extraction.

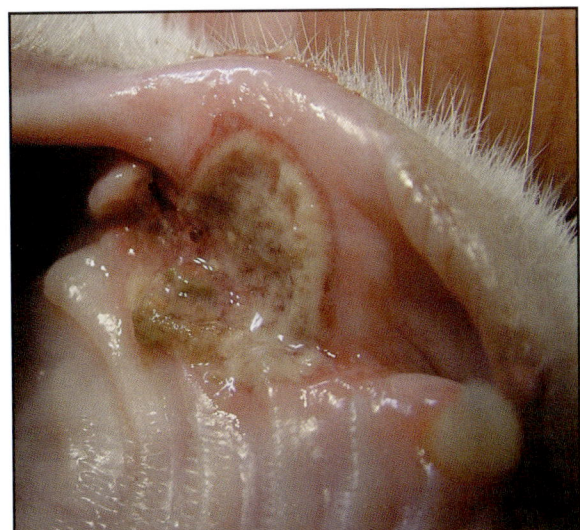

8.42 Extensive tissue necrosis. A postoperative complication following full-mouth extraction.

canines and incisors can be maintained (Figure 8.44).

Some cats have proliferative gingival lesions that should be excised if they cause difficulty in prehension, mastication or swallowing of food. Gingivectomy (or gingival reduction) can be performed with cold steel (blade and scissors), electrosurgery, cryotherapy or laser ablation surgery. Electrosurgery, cryosurgery and laser surgery are more effective in controlling haemorrhage, but it is easy to inadvertently damage the dental tissues, periodontal ligament and alveolar bone. Proper technique and prior experience of these modalities are mandatory. The cold steel technique is safer for adjacent tissues, but haemorrhage is more difficult to control.

Whilst neoplastic lesions are less common than FCGS, it is important to recognize them so that an appropriate prognosis can be given. Any atypical lesions should be biopsied and samples submitted to an oral pathologist who has experience in the evaluation of FCGS lesions. Oral lymphoma is rare but may appear as bilateral inflammation similar to FCGS. Squamous cell carcinoma is typically unilateral but again usually presents as an area of visible inflammation.

Postoperative care and assessment

Preoperative, intraoperative and postoperative pain control (opioids, regional or local nerve blocks, non-steroidal anti-inflammatory drugs (NSAIDs) plus a transdermal fentanyl patch or intravenous buprenorphine) is essential to help get the cats eating unaided as soon as possible. In some cases it may be necessary to provide postoperative alimentary support via an oesophagostomy tube. These patients should be nursed in a hospital setting until the cat is eating unaided. Some cats may eat dry food within a few days; most will eat moist food, but homemade food may be offered. It is best to avoid sticky or excessively sloppy foods to prevent accumulation of food debris in the oral cavity (i.e. adjacent to the suture material). Antibiotics are often advocated for one to three weeks post-surgery, depending on the drug prescribed. However, many cats do well without antibiotics. It is mandatory to review the patient frequently after surgery, ideally once a week for at least a month, and subsequently every two or three weeks as indicated, in order to adjust any therapy if necessary.

Prognosis

FCGS is a frustrating condition to treat. Even following full-mouth extraction some patients, especially those who have already been subjected to prolonged medical treatment, fail to respond appropriately. In some cases the oral bacteria (ever present in the mouth), particularly on the tongue base are sufficient to maintain inflammation. It is likely that there are also other factors at work in these cases. The longer ineffective medical therapy is prolonged, the more refractory FCGS seems to become. The response to caudal (premolars and molars) and whole mouth extraction varies: complete resolution occurs within several weeks in about 60% of cases, a further 20% have minimal residual inflammation and no oral pain, 13% have partial improvement but require continued medical therapy, and approximately 7% show no improvement. In some cases the response to extraction takes a long time (up to two years). Pain control together with prolonged aggressive antibiotic therapy (clindamycin 11 mg/kg orally q12h) and avoidance of the use of steroids is important in poorly responding cases. Interferon and other immune-modulators are possibly indicated in these cases.

8.43   Osteitis and osteomyelitis. Postoperative complications following a full-mouth extraction.

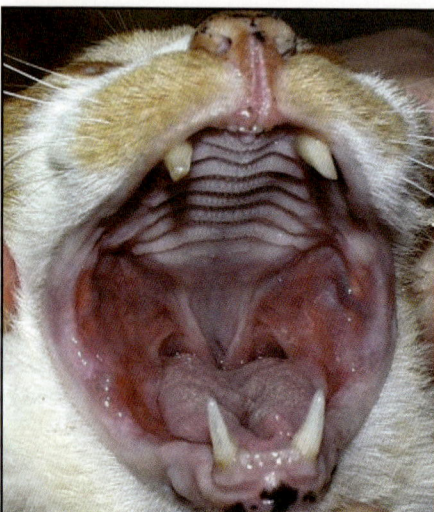

8.44   Incisors and canine teeth may be removed later if necessary. In some cases resolution is only achieved after all teeth have been extracted.

Eosinophilic granuloma complex

Eosinophilic granuloma complex in the cat consists of three clinical entities:

- Eosinophilic granuloma
- Eosinophilic ulcer
- Eosinophilic plaque.

These lesions can occur simultaneously in the same animal and have many common aspects, for

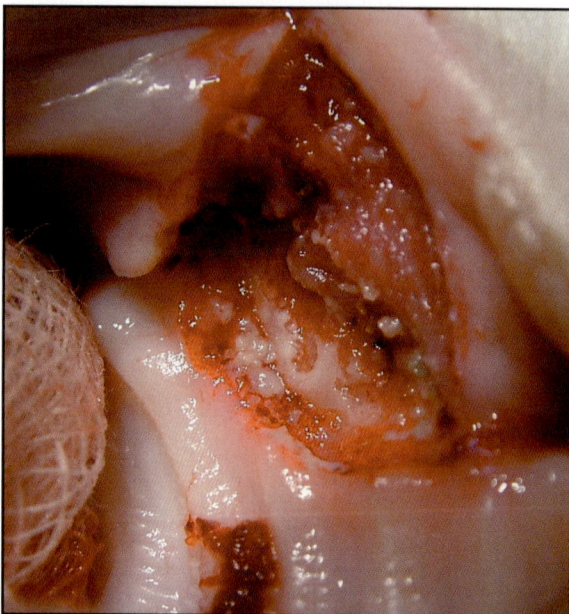

example an occasional peripheral blood eosinophilia and an eosinophilic tissue infiltrate. They can also occur in association with various allergies.

Eosinophilic granuloma

Aetiology and pathogenesis
Eosinophilic granuloma may be an isolated lesion or manifest as part of the eosinophilic granuloma complex, associated with eosinophilic plaques or deep ulceration (so-called *rodent ulcers*). Eosinophilic granulomas may be seen in the oral cavity as raised linear lesions, yellowish-pink in colour. Oral lesions can involve the oral mucosa, hard palate mucosa, the soft palate (Figure 8.45) or the base of the tongue, and cause dysphagia or ptyalism.

Eosinophilic granuloma is more commonly found in young animals (2–6 years), with twice the prevalence in females than males. It has been associated with insect bite allergies (e.g. flea and mosquito salivary antigens), food allergy, atopy, immunosuppression, bacterial and viral (calicivirus) infections. The aetiology of oral eosinophilic granulomas is rarely determined and for this reason they are still often considered idiopathic.

The histology of eosinophilic granulomas resembles a foreign body reaction. These lesions may resolve spontaneously or persist for a prolonged period.

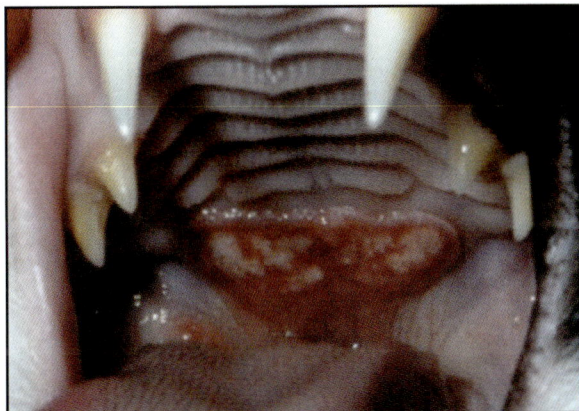

8.45 Eosinophilic granuloma complex: ulcerative lesion located on the soft palate. (Courtesy of Dr Chiara Noli.)

Eosinophilic ulcer

Aetiology and pathogenesis
An eosinophilic ulcer may present as part of the eosinophilic granuloma complex, or occur as a single lesion. It is typically a well circumscribed lesion, most frequently located on the upper lip (Figure 8.46), with raised edges and necrosis of the superficial layers. The lesions vary in size and are usually not painful. The eosinophilic ulcer has a higher prevalence in middle-aged and female cats. The aetiology of eosinophilic ulcers may be traumatic, as seen in cases where the lower canines contact the upper lip resulting in a secondary bacterial infection and fibrosis.

The histological features of eosinophilic ulcers are often non-specific. The transformation of a chronic

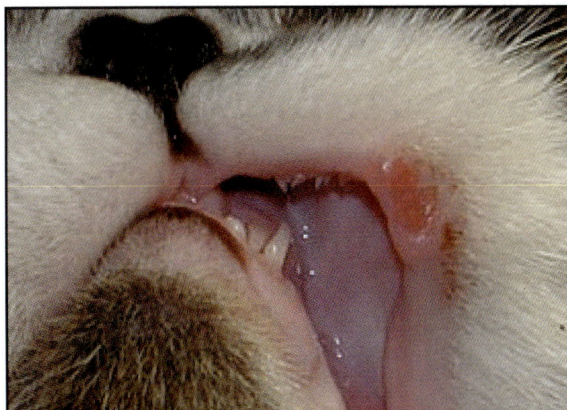

8.46 Indolent ulcer on the upper lip, probably caused by the deviated mandibular canine traumatizing the upper lip.

eosinophilic ulcer into a squamous cell carcinoma has been reported, although this is a rare occurrence. Biopsy is useful to exclude the possibility of neoplasia.

Treatment

Medical
Thorough control of ectoparasites is essential. To rule out food allergy and atopy, a restricted-ingredient diet can be used and skin testing performed. If there is no response to dietary change, or if there is evidence of secondary infection, antibiotic treatment (amoxicillin/clavulanate at 20 mg/kg or cefalexin at 20–30 mg/kg q12h) is often required for prolonged periods (4–6 weeks).

For patients refractory to these measures, corticosteroid treatment is indicated. Prednisolone (1–2 mg/kg q12h, gradually reducing the dosage and progressing to alternate day treatment when a response is seen) is usually effective. Therapy should be continued until the lesion or at least the signs completely disappear. It is best to start with the minimum effective dose and avoid unnecessarily prolonged or repeated treatment. Other therapeutic options that have been suggested include ascorbic acid, gold salts, megestrol acetate, interferon, chlorambucil, ciclosporin and essential fatty acids, as well as intralesional administration of corticosteroids.

Surgical
Conventional surgical excision is indicated for excessively proliferative lesions that interfere with breathing or swallowing. Electrosurgery can also be used, with the aim to minimize haemorrhage, but caution is needed to avoid thermal injuries to the adjacent tissues. Before performing any kind of surgery it is recommended to biopsy the lesion to confirm the diagnosis of an eosinophilic lesion. Other reported treatments are CO_2 laser tissue ablation and cryotherapy.

Postoperative pain control is essential to help get cats eating as soon as possible. Cases should be followed up long term to monitor for recurrence, particularly when the aetiology has not been determined. Idiopathic eosinophilic lesions tend to recur and require ongoing, sometimes lifelong treatment.

Chapter 8 Feline inflammatory, infectious and other oral conditions

References and further reading

Bollmer BW, Sturzenberger OP, Lehnhoff RW, Bosma ML, Lang NP, Mallatt ME and Meckel AH (1986) A comparison of 3 clinical indices for measuring gingivitis. *Journal of Clinical Periodontology* **13(5)**, 392–395

Clarke DE (2001) Clinical and microbiological effects of oral zinc ascorbate gel in cats. *Journal of Veterinary Dentistry* **18(4)**, 177–183

Clarke DE and Cameron A (1998) Relationship between diet, dental calculus and periodontal disease in domestic and feral cats in Australia. *Australian Veterinary Journal* **76(10)**, 690–693

Colgin LMA, Schulman FY and Dubielzig RR (2001) Multiple epulides in 13 cats. *Veterinary Pathology* **38**, 227–229

Crossley DA and Penman S (1995) *BSAVA Manual of Small Animal Dentistry, 2nd edition*. BSAVA Publications, Cheltenham

DeBowes LJ, Mosier D and Logan E (1996) Association of periodontal disease and histological lesions in multiple organs from 45 dogs. *Journal of Veterinary Dentistry* **13(2)**, 57–60

DuPont GA and DeBowes LJ (2002) Comparison of periodontitis and root replacement in cat teeth with resorptive lesions. *Journal of Veterinary Dentistry* **19(2)**, 71–75

Fleiss JL, Park MH, Bollmer BW, Lehnhoff RW and Chilton NW (1985) Statistical transformations of indices of gingivitis measured non invasively. *Journal of Clinical Periodontology* **12(9)**, 750–755

Gelberg HB, Lewis RM, Felsburg PJ and Smith CA (1985) Antiepithelial autoantibodies associated with the feline eosinophilic granuloma complex. *American Journal of Veterinary Research* **46(1)**, 263–265

Ghoddusi J (2003) Ultrastructural changes in feline dental pulp with periodontal disease. *Microscopy Research and Technique* **61(5)**, 423–427

Goodson JM, Tanner AC, Haffajee AD, Sornberger GC and Socransky SS (1982) Patterns of progression and regression of advances destructive periodontal disease. *Journal of Clinical Periodontology* **9(6)**, 472–481

Gorrel C, Inskeep G and Inskeep T (1998) Benefits of a 'dental hygiene chew' on the periodontal health of cats. *Journal of Veterinary Dentistry* **15(3)**, 135–138

Gross TL, Ihrke PJ and Walder E (1992) *Veterinary Dermatopathology*. Mosby, St. Louis

Harbour DA, Howard PE and Gaskell RM (1991) Isolation of FCV and FHV from domestic cats 1980 to 1989. *Veterinary Record* **128(4)**, 77–80

Hargis AM and Ginn PE (1999) Feline herpesvirus 1-associated facial and nasal dermatitis and stomatitis in domestic cats. *Veterinary Clinics of North America: Small Animal Practice* **29(6)**, 1281–1290

Harley R, Gruffydd-Jones TJ and Day MJ (2003) Characterization of immune cell populations in oral mucosal tissues of healthy adult cats. *Journal of Comparative Pathology* **128**, 146–155

Harley R, Helps CR, Harbour DA, Gruffydd-Jones TJ and Day MJ (1999) Cytokine mRNA expression in lesions in cats with chronic gingivostomatitis. *Clinical and diagnostic laboratory immunology* **6(4)**, 471–478

Harvey CE and Emily PP (1993) *Small Animal Dentistry*. Mosby, St. Louis

Harvey CE, Thornsberry C and Miller BR (1995) Subgingival bacteria – comparison of culture results in dogs and cats with gingivitis. *Journal of Veterinary Dentistry* **12(4)**, 147–150

Harvey CE, Thornsberry C, Miller BR and Shofer FS (1995) Antimicrobial susceptibility of subgingival bacterial flora in cats with gingivitis. *Journal of Veterinary Dentistry* **12(4)**, 157–160

Harvey HJ (1980) Cryosurgery of oral tumours in dogs and cats. *Veterinary Clinics of North America* **10**, 821–830

Hennet P (1995) Trattamento delle stomatiti croniche del gatto. *Summa* **6**, 63–69

Ingham KE, Gorrel C and Bierer TL (2002) Effect of a dental chew on dental substrates and gingivitis in cats. *Journal of Veterinary Dentistry* **19(4)**, 201–204

Juliff WF and Helman RG (1984) Linear granuloma involving the tongue of a cat. *Feline Practice* **14(1)**, 39–42

Kalaitzakis CJ, Tynelius-Bratthall G and Attstrom R (1993) Clinical and microbiological effects of subgingival application of a chlorexidine gel in chronic periodontitis: a pilot study. *Swedish Dental Journal* **17(4)**, 129–137

Knowles JO, Gaskell RM, Gaskell CJ, Harvey CE and Lutz H (1989) The prevalence of feline calicivirus, feline leukemia virus and antibodies to FIV in cats with chronic stomatitis. *Veterinary Record* **124**, 336–338

Kozakiewicz M and Godlewski A (2003) Modulation of the mitotic activity and population of the mast cells in the oral mucosa by substance P. *Cellular & Molecular Biology Letters* **8**, 727–734

Legendre LFJ (1993) Management and long term effects of electrocution in a cat's mouth. *Journal of Veterinary Dentistry* **10(3)**, 6–8

Loe H (1967) The gingival index, the plaque index and the retention index systems. *Journal of Periodontology* **38**, 610–616

Lommer M and Verstraete FJ (2001) Radiographic patterns of periodontitis in cats: 147 cases (1998–1999). *Journal of the American Veterinary Medical Association* **218(2)**, 230–234

Lommer MJ and Verstraete FJM (2003) Concurrent oral shedding of feline calicivirus and feline herpesvirus 1 in cats with chronic gingivostomatitis. *Oral Microbiology and Immunology* **18**, 131–134

Lund EM, Armstrong PJ, Kirk CA, Kolar LM and Klausner JS (1999) Health status and population characteristics of dogs and cats examined at private veterinary practices in the United States. *Journal of the American Veterinary Medical Association* **214(9)**, 1336–1341

MacEwen EG and Hess PW (1987) Evaluation of effect of immunomodulation on the feline eosinophilic granuloma complex. *Journal of the American Animal Hospital Association* **23**, 519–526

Manning TO, Crane SW, Scheidt VJ and Osuna DJ (1987) Three cases of feline eosinophilic granuloma complex (eosinophilic ulcer) and observations on laser therapy. *Seminars in Veterinary Medicine and Surgery (Small Animal)* **2(3)**, 206–211

Mariotti AJ and Rumpf DAH (1999) Chlorhexidine-induced changes to human gingival fibroblast collagen and non-collagen protein production. *Journal of Periodontology* **70**, 1443–1448

Mason KV and Evans AG (1991) Mosquito bite-caused eosinophilic dermatitis in cats. *Journal of the American Veterinary Medical Association* **198(12)**, 2086–2088

Muller GH, Kirk RW and Scott DW (1989) *Small Animal Dermatology, 4th edition*. WB Saunders, Philadelphia

Norris JM and Love DN (1999) Associations amongst three feline *Porphyromonas* species from the gingival margin of cats during periodontal health and disease. *Veterinary Microbiology* **65(3)**, 195–207

Norris JM and Love DN (2000) *In vitro* antimicrobial susceptibilities of three *Porphyromonas* spp. and *in vivo* responses in the oral cavity of cats to selected antimicrobial agents. *Australian Veterinary Journal* **78(8)**, 533–537

Odom T and Anderson J (2000) Proliferative gingival lesion in a cat with disseminated cryptococcosis. *Veterinary Dentistry* **17(4)**, 177–181

Pedersen NC (1992) Inflammatory oral cavity diseases of the cat. *Veterinary Clinics of North America: Small Animal Practice* **22**, 1323–1345

Ramfjord SP (1967) The periodontal index. *Journal of Periodontology* **38(6)**, 602–610

Reiter AM and Mendoza KA (2002) Feline odontoclastic resorptive lesions. An unsolved enigma in veterinary dentistry. *Veterinary Clinics of North America: Small Animal Practice* **32**, 791–837

Roudebush P, Logan E and Hale F (2005) Evidence-based veterinary dentistry: a systematic review of homecare for prevention of periodontal disease in dogs and cats. *Journal of Veterinary Dentistry* **22(1)**, 6–15

Russel RG, Slattum MM and Abkowitz J (1988) Filamentous bacteria in oral eosinophilic granuloma of cat. *Veterinary Pathology* **25**, 249–250

Scarampella F, Abramo F and Noli C (2001) Clinical and histological evaluation of an analogue of palmitoylethanolamide, PLR 120 (comicronized Palmidrol INN) in cats with eosinophilic granuloma and eosinophilic plaque: a pilot study. *Veterinary Dermatology* **12(1)**, 29–39

Schneck GW and Osborn JW (1976) Neck lesions in the teeth of cats. *Veterinary Record* **99(6)**, 100

Scott DW (1975) Observations on the eosinophilic granuloma complex in cats. *Journal of the American Animal Hospital Association* **11**, 261–270

Sims TJ, Moncla BJ and Page RC (1990) Serum antibody response to antigens of oral Gram-negative bacteria in cats with plasma cell gingivitis-stomatitis. *Journal of Dental Research* **69**, 877–882

Socransky SS, Haffajee AD, Goodson JM and Lindhe J (1984) New concepts of destructive periodontal disease. *Journal of Clinical Periodontology* **11(1)**, 21–32

Takahashi D, Odajima T, Morita M, Kawanami M and Kato H (2005) Formation and resolution of ankylosis under application of recombinant human bone morphogenetic protein-2 (rhBMP-2) to class III furcation defects in cats. *Journal of Periodontal Research* **40(4)**, 299–305

Ueno H, Hohdatsu T, Muramatsu Y, Koyama H and Morita C (1996) Does co-infection of *Bartonella henselae* and FIV induce clinical disorders in cats? *Oral Microbiology and Immunology* **40**, 617–620

Valdez M, Haines R, Riviere KH, Riviere GR and Thomas DD (2000) Isolation of oral spirochetes from dogs and cats and provisional identification using polymerase chain reaction (PCR) analysis specific for human plaque *Treponema* spp. *Journal of Veterinary Dentistry* **17(1)**, 23–26

Verstraete F (1995) Biopsy. In: *BSAVA Manual of Small Animal*

Dentistry, 2nd edition, eds. D Crossley and S Penman. BSAVA Publications, Cheltenham

Verstraete FJ, Kass PH and Terpak CH (1998) Diagnostic value of full-mouth radiography in cats. *American Journal of Veterinary Research* **59(6)**, 692–695

Vogel G and Cattabriga M (1986) *Parodontologia*. USES, Firenze

Walsh LJ (2003) Mast cells and oral inflammation. *Critical Review in Oral Biology and Medicine* **14(3)**, 188–198

Walsh LJ, Davis MF, Xu LJ and Savage NW (1995) Relationship between mast cell degranulation and inflammation in the oral cavity. *Journal of Oral Pathology and Medicine* **24**, 266–272

White SD, Rosychuk RAW, Janik TA, Denerolle P and Schultheiss P (1992) Plasma cell stomatitis-pharyngitis in cats: 40 cases (1973–1991). *Journal of the American Veterinary Medical Association* **9**, 1377–1380

Wiggs RB and Lobprise HB (1997) *Veterinary Dentistry Principles and Practice*. Lippincott-Raven, Philadelphia

Willemse A and Lubberink AA (1978) Cryosurgery of eosinophilic ulcers in cats. *Tijdschr Diergeneeskd* **103(20)**, 1052–1056

Williams CA and Aller MS (1992) Gingivitis/stomatitis in cats. *Veterinary Clinics of North America: Small Animal Practice* **22(6)**, 1361–1383

Zetner K, Steurer I, Kampfer PH and Maier H (1998) Melatonin and chronic inflammatory disease in the feline oral cavity. *Praktischer Tierartzt* **79**, 410–416

9

Physical orodental conditions

Thomas Eriksen

Traumatic lesions of teeth and other structures of the oral cavity are common and are dependent on the animal breed, their environment, lifestyle and habits. Large, active or working dogs, and dogs and cats living in more densely populated areas with high traffic intensity, are prone to traumatic orodental lesions. Animals falling from great heights will often sustain multiple orodental and craniofacial lesions.

In some trauma patients oral lesions may be present, but can be overlooked if they do not exhibit obvious signs. Trauma patients may also present as emergencies with multiple life-threatening injuries. Oral lesions in these patients may also be overlooked due to the severity of the concurrent conditions. Once the animal is medically stable, attention should be given to the oral cavity and teeth, particularly in those patients showing reduced appetite, changes in eating habits or whose general condition is suboptimal. Most dental and oral problems in the trauma patient are not of initial concern, but if neglected the lesions can cause chronic problems, resulting in discomfort for the animal and in some cases may be very difficult to treat.

Dental pulp pathology

Aetiopathogenesis

Before further discussion of dental disorders, the pulpal consequences of physical trauma to the tooth need to be addressed. Inflammation is the single most important disease process affecting the dental pulp and accounts for virtually all pulpal disease of any clinical significance. Irritants to the pulp, which may lead to pulpitis, can be grouped under the following headings:

- *Bacterial.* Bacteria can reach the pulp as a result of tooth fractures, periodontal disease (bacteria may pass along the lateral canals from the exposed root surface to the pulp), abnormal wear (attrition and abrasion) exposing the pulp, caries or through marginal leakage of cavity restorations (Figure 9.1). Haematogenous infection is also possible. Animals suffering from dentinal or enamel dysplasia are prone to pulpitis
- *Thermal.* Frictional heat generated during scaling and polishing or cavity preparations, particularly in those teeth with appreciable cavity depths, is a significant pulpal irritant and may cause pulpitis. The importance of adequate cooling during these

operative procedures cannot be overemphasized (Figure 9.2)
- *Chemical.* Irritant substances may be applied directly to an exposed pulp or, more rarely, may diffuse through the dentine after placement of a restorative material. The chemical properties of restorative materials play a major role in

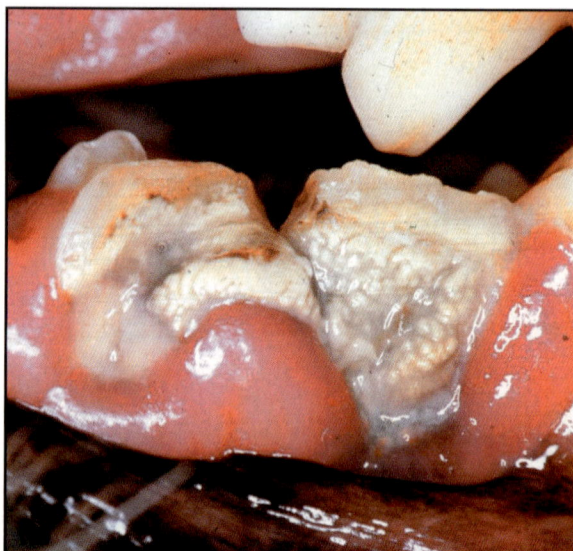

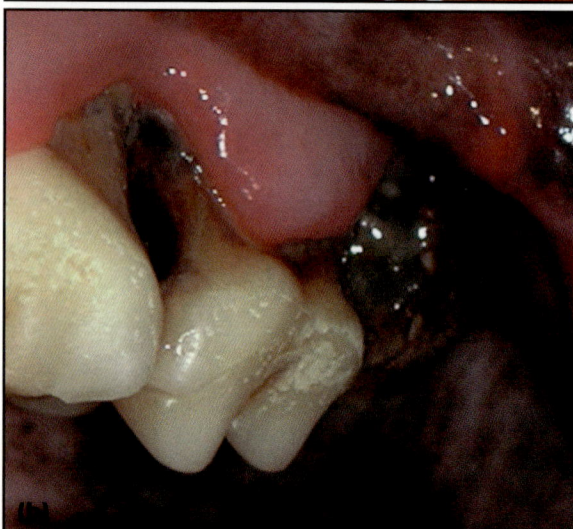

9.1 **(a)** The pulp is rapidly infected after complicated fractures (fractures exposing the pulp). **(b)** In moderate to severe marginal periodontitis lateral openings (canals) may allow bacteria to invade the pulp.

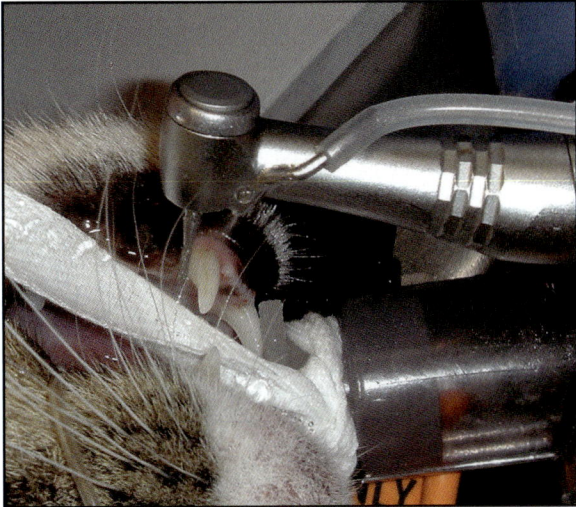

9.2 Spray irrigation with copious volumes of water gives the best cooling of dental structures. Cooling is mandatory during all cutting procedures using rotating instruments. Insufficient cooling will often cause pulp or osseous irritation and necrosis.

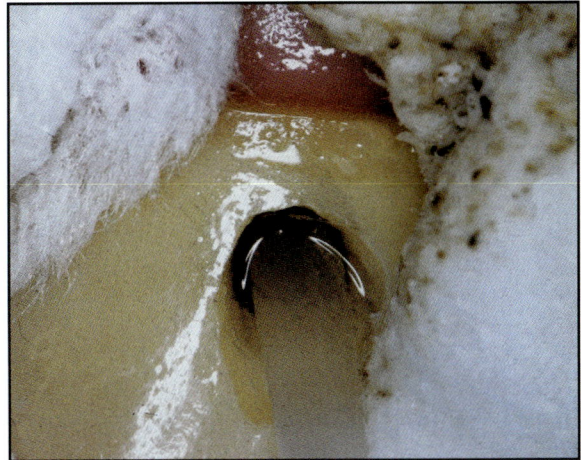

9.3 A necrotic pulp does not bleed after gentle probing and debris or dirt may be retrieved from the pulp chamber.

determining pulpal tissue compatibility. Depending on the severity of the pulpitis, the pulp may respond by forming reparative or tertiary dentine to protect the pulp, rather than the irritation leading to progression of the inflammation and pulp necrosis.

Pulpitis has been classified on a clinical and pathological basis into different types:

- Acute or chronic
- Partial or total
- Open or closed
- Exudative or suppurative.

However, these divisions seem somewhat artificial and confusing since inflammation of the pulp presents as a continuous spectrum of change and in animals it is almost impossible to ascribe an individual case clinically into such rigid groupings. In humans, pulpitis presents clinically as pain, which can be used to classify the pulpal pathology. However, investigations have shown that there is little or no correlation between the clinical features and the type or extent of pulp inflammation as shown by histological examination. An absence of symptoms is not evidence of a normal pulp as pulp death following pulpitis may occur with no previous history of pain.

For treatment purposes it is necessary to determine whether the pulp is necrotic or vital. In fractured teeth with exposed pulp chambers this is usually not difficult since a necrotic pulp presents with debris in the pulp chamber and an absence of bleeding on probing (Figure 9.3). The critical decision that has to be taken is whether a vital pulp is inflamed to a reversible or irreversible extent. Pulpitis is seldom diagnosed in animals and the patient usually presents with a necrotic pulp. Therefore, the decision is usually based on radiographic evidence and observations during operative procedures. Some animals present with discoloured

teeth as a consequence of pulpitis, where bleeding has occurred into the pulp chamber and canal.

Pulp healing

In animals it may be assumed that a large proportion of pulpitis is as a result of pulp exposure. Pulp vitality may be maintained by covering the pulp with a restoration (i.e. pulp capping). The longer the pulp has been exposed and the larger the defect, the more likely it is that the pulp has become irritated and inflamed or necrotic. Pulpal bleeding is usually considered to be associated with a vital pulp. However, an irreversibly inflamed pulp will often bleed more intensely, and haemorrhage is sometimes difficult to control. Pulp capping is considered in cases where the exposure is small, has recently occurred and haemostasis is readily attainable by direct pressure.

Ideally the capping agent should be non-irritant, antibacterial and stimulate formation of a calcific barrier. Calcium hydroxide preparations are widely used as pulp-capping agents (Figure 9.4). A necrotic zone

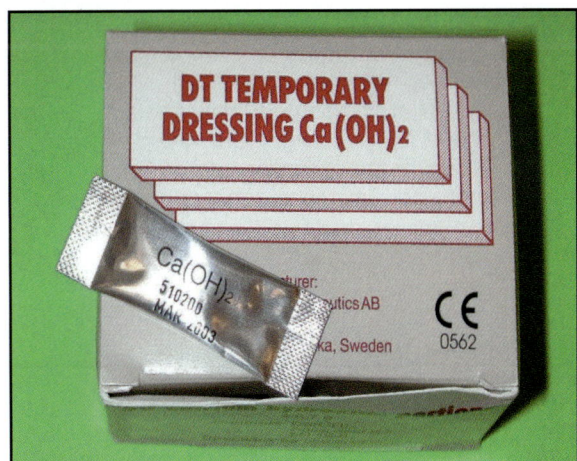

9.4 Calcium hydroxide for direct pulp capping is conveniently available in small sterile aqueous aliquots. Calcium hydroxide should not be kept in large quantities since exposure to air causes it to convert to calcium carbonate, which does not stimulate odontoblasts to form reparatory dentine.

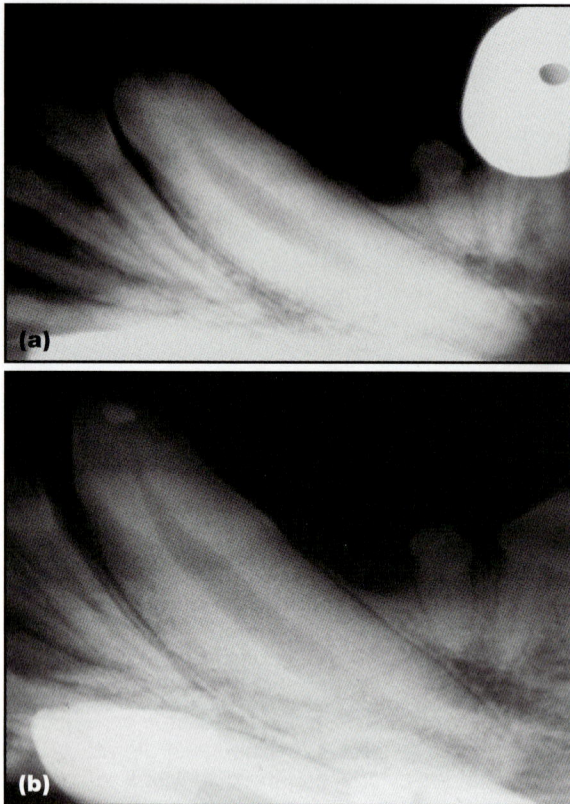

9.5 **(a)** Mandibular left canine (304) in a German Shepherd Dog, approximately 1 year after partial pulpectomy and direct pulp capping. Restoration with glass ionomer cement has been recently lost. Apical to the restoration a broad zone of reparatory dentine can be seen (dentinal bridge). **(b)** Mandibular right canine (404) in a German Shepherd Dog approximately 1 year after partial pulpectomy and direct pulp capping. Restoration is intact and apically reparatory dentine can be seen, although more discrete than in the left canine in (a). This radiograph has been orientated as in (a) for comparative reasons.

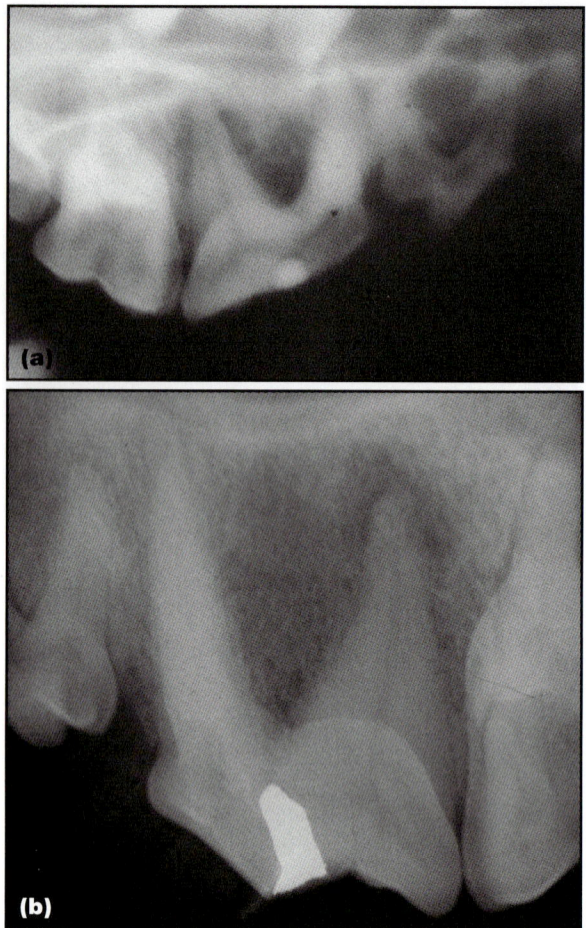

9.6 **(a and b)** Radiographs showing periapical periodontitis as a result of an amalgam restoration being used without any cavity liner or pulp protection. Note the pulp necrosis and periapical pathology.

develops beneath the calcium hydroxide layer shortly after it is applied to the exposed pulp. After approximately two weeks a zone of dense fibrous tissue is formed over a layer of odontoblast-like cells and following a further two weeks a dentine-like calcification of the zone beneath the fibrous layer begins to form (Figure 9.5).

In order to suppress pulp inflammation, corticosteroids have been incorporated into pulp-capping agents. However, the response is so variable that the use of corticosteroid preparations for pulp capping in general cannot be supported and is considered by some as a contraindication.

Periapical pathology

Aetiopathogenesis

Periapical periodontitis (Figure 9.6) describes inflammation of the periapical part of the periodontium and can be as a result of:

• Untreated pulpitis and pulp necrosis
• Trauma
• Endodontic treatment.

Untreated pulpitis and pulp necrosis

In time, untreated pulpitis and subsequent pulp necrosis results in inflammation, which extends along the root canal to the apex of the tooth. Bacteria or inflammatory mediators may then extend through the apical delta, causing periapical inflammation.

Trauma

Trauma to a tooth may extend to the periapical periodontal ligament, causing fibre damage and localized inflammation.

Endodontic treatment

Endodontic treatment may lead to periapical inflammation if contaminated instruments or chemicals are forced through the apex during operative procedures.

Clinical signs

Clinical signs of periapical lesions may be completely absent or may be obvious with intraoral or facial swelling (Figure 9.7), with or without the presence of draining sinus tracts.

Acute periapical periodontitis is characterized histologically by vascular dilation, oedema and neu-

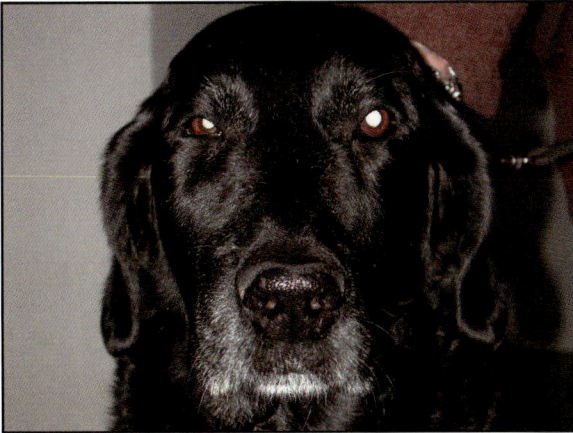

9.7 The most acute presentation of periapical pathology is seen as diffuse facial swelling, fever and pain. This is usually an acute exacerbation of a chronic condition and not considered a surgical emergency. Narrow spectrum antibiotics and NSAIDs will usually lead to rapid improvement. However, dental treatment is required.

trophil leucocyte infiltration. The lesion may become chronic with resorption of alveolar bone and suppuration. This type of lesion is called an acute periapical abscess and can result in osteomyelitis or cellulitis. Periapical abscesses may drain through the root canal (if this is open), through bone to form a sinus tract to the skin (Figure 9.8), the oral mucosa (Figure 9.9), the nasal cavity or maxillary recess (Figure 9.10), depending on the position of the apex.

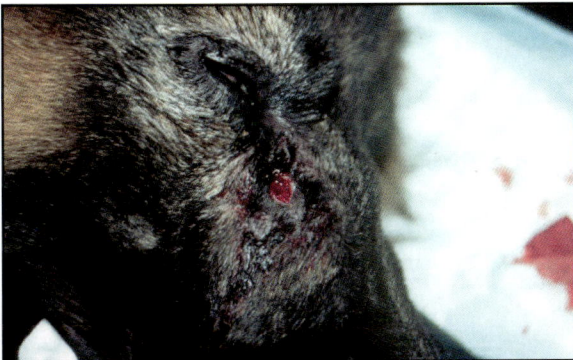

9.8 A typical draining tract secondary to a periapical abscess at the upper carnassial (108) tooth.

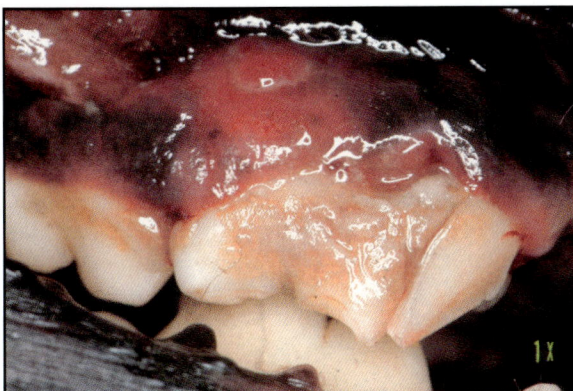

9.9 Draining sinus tracts from periapical abscesses may also open into the oral cavity, often at the mucogingival junction.

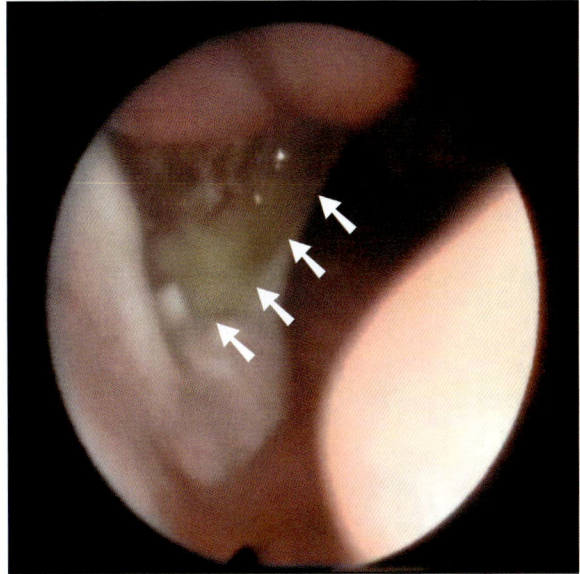

9.10 Rhinoscopic view of the rostral nasal cavity, showing a periodontal probe (arrowed) entering the nasal cavity through a deep periodontal pocket related to the palatal surface of a maxillary canine. Such lesions are often associated with perio-endodontic lesions.

A proportion (up to 20% in humans) of nasal discharge or sinus empyema cases may be associated with periapical abscessation. If the initial lesion is infiltrated by lymphocytes, plasma cells and macrophages with resultant production of granulation tissue, it is termed chronic periapical periodontitis or periapical granuloma (Figure 9.11). A periapical granuloma can be the origin of an acute periapical abscess. Proliferation of the epithelial cell rests of Malassez may transform periapical granulomas into fluid-filled periapical or radicular cysts (Figure 9.12).

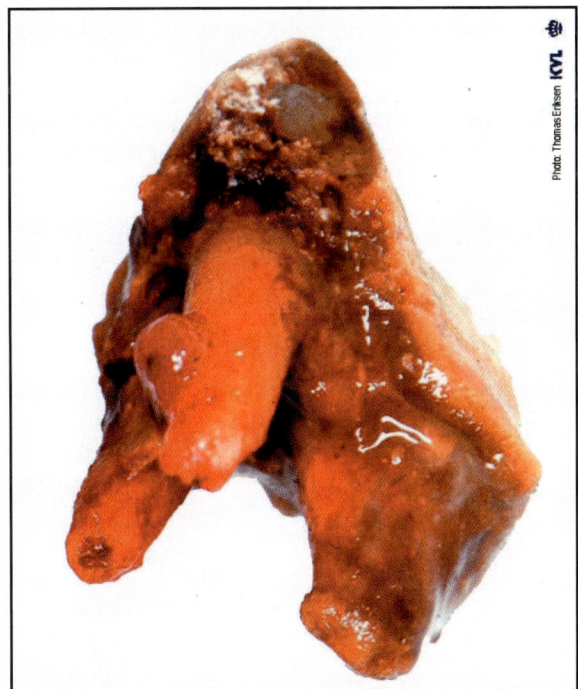

9.11 Extracted first molar tooth. Note the granulation tissue around one of the roots.

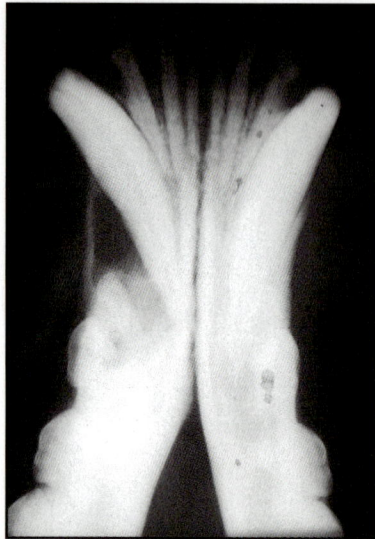

9.12 Periapical granulomas may be transformed into periapical or radicular cysts after proliferation of the epithelial cell rests of Malassez from within the periodontal ligament.

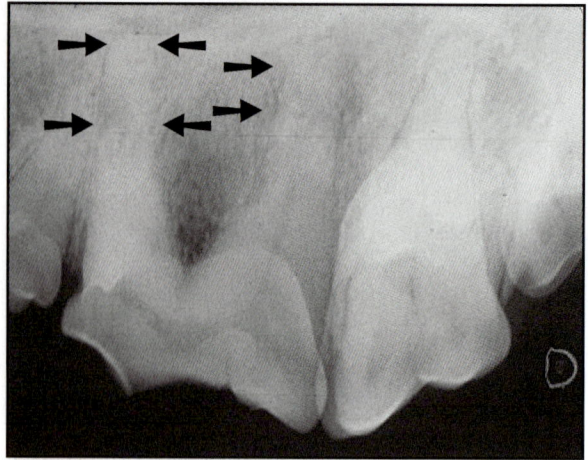

9.14 Radiograph of a fractured upper carnassial (208) tooth clearly showing signs of periapical pathology. Circular radiolucencies (arrowed) are seen at the apices of the three roots.

Diagnosis

Acute periapical periodontitis and periapical abscesses are painful. The regional lymph nodes may be enlarged and fever may be present. Periapical granulomas are usually asymptomatic and are often incidental findings on radiographic examination. Acute periapical periodontitis is very difficult to identify on radiographs. Early radiographic evidence of pathology is seen as a slight widening of the periodontal space or thinning of the lamina dura (Figure 9.13). If the inflammation persists, bony destruction occurs and the periapical abscess, granuloma or cyst is seen radiographically as a periradicular radiolucency (often circular in shape) (Figure 9.14). It is impossible to differentiate these lesions on radiographs alone. Clinical examination and histopathology are required, although the latter is rarely carried out in general veterinary dentistry.

However, care must be taken when viewing periapical rarefactions on radiographs as not all these radiolucencies will be due to pathology. For example, permanent canines often exhibit physiological periapical radiolucencies that are triangular in shape. To determine whether these lesions are pathological,

similar teeth in the same animal should be compared. A chronically inflamed or necrotic pulp can also result in periapical sclerosis being visible radiographically.

Treatment

Once the diagnosis of periapical pathology has been made, treatment must be initiated, even in the absence of symptoms. Treatment will involve either endodontic treatment by a specialist practitioner or extraction of the affected tooth.

Tooth loss or loss of tooth substance

Aetiopathogenesis

Apart from normal physiological shedding of deciduous teeth and alveolar bone resorption in periodontitis, loss of tooth substance may be caused by:

- Abnormal wear
- Resorption
- Fractures
- Luxation or avulsion.

During the life of an animal, teeth will be worn due to grooming, mastication, play and work. This is a situation that normally does not cause pathological changes to the pulp or periodontal tissues.

Any lesion associated with tooth loss or loss of tooth substance should be thoroughly examined under general anaesthesia using a dental explorer (Figure 9.15) and any involved tooth, and often the entire dentition, radiographed.

Abnormal wear

Abnormal wear may be defined as either attrition, abrasion or erosion. Attrition is the loss of tooth substance as a result of tooth-to-tooth contact. The most common cause of attrition in dogs and cats is as a result of malocclusion, following the selection of abnormal

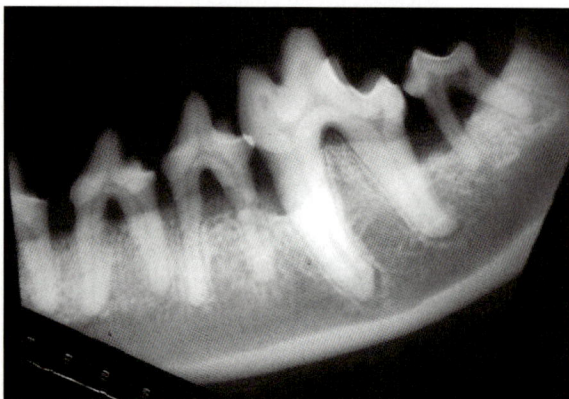

9.13 Slight widening of the periodontal space and thinning of the lamina dura may indicate periapical pathology. However, the lamina dura in dogs and cats without dental disease may also appear interrupted on radiographs.

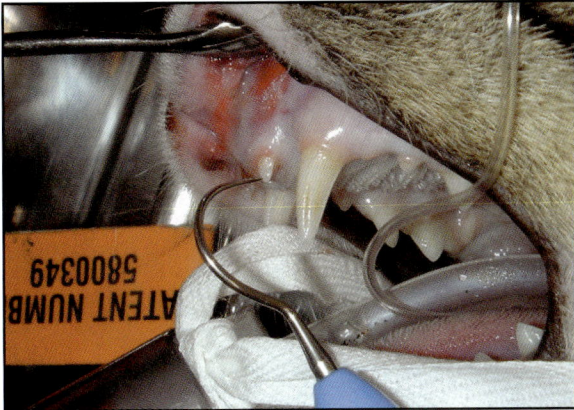

9.15 Any loss of tooth substance or increased tooth mobility should be thoroughly examined under general anaesthesia with the gentle use of a dental explorer.

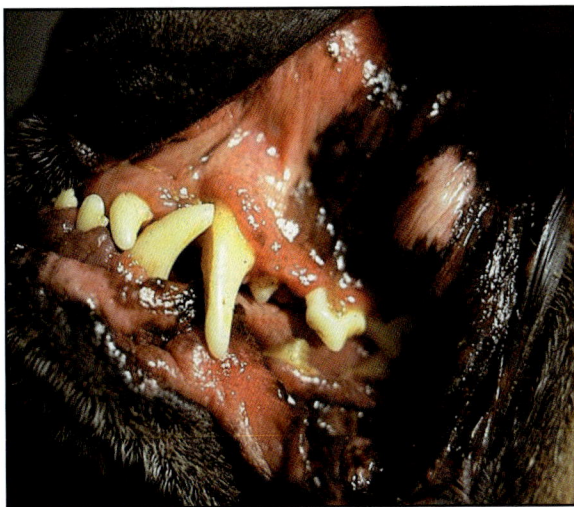

9.16 A Boxer with severe malocclusion and pronounced attrition of the upper canine (204).

skull shapes during breeding (Figure 9.16). Malocclusion can also occur as a result of tooth loss due to disease and trauma. If extensive extractions are being performed the resultant occlusion should be assessed.

Attrition is a physiological process that occurs in all animals to varying degrees and is more commonly seen in the incisor and canine region. The abnormal wear exposes the dentine, which can become discoloured (i.e. dark yellow or brown), mainly as a result of staining due to dietary substances. Exposure of the dentinal tubules by attrition leads to formation of reactionary dentine on the pulp surface, which protects the tooth against pulp exposure. Deposition of reparative dentine usually occurs at the same rate as loss of tooth substance and therefore pulpal exposure is rare under normal circumstances. The formation of translucent zones and dead tracts within reparative dentine leads to changes in extracellular osmolality in the dentinal tubules. This may lead to hypersensitivity of the exposed dentine. Humans sometimes complain of hypersensitive dentine in those teeth affected by attrition, but this is unusual as tooth substance loss by attrition tends to be a slow process.

Abrasion is the pathological wearing away of tooth substance by the friction of a foreign body, independent of occlusion (Figure 9.17). The most common causes of abrasion in dogs are stone chewing, working and cage biting. The pathogenesis of abrasion is similar to attrition but can be more rapid than the formation of reactionary (reparative) dentine, thereby resulting in pulp exposure. Furthermore, fractured teeth are often identified in a dentition exhibiting abrasions. For example, cage biting can lead to fracture of a tooth and often to pulp exposure. Attrition and abrasion are uncommon in cats.

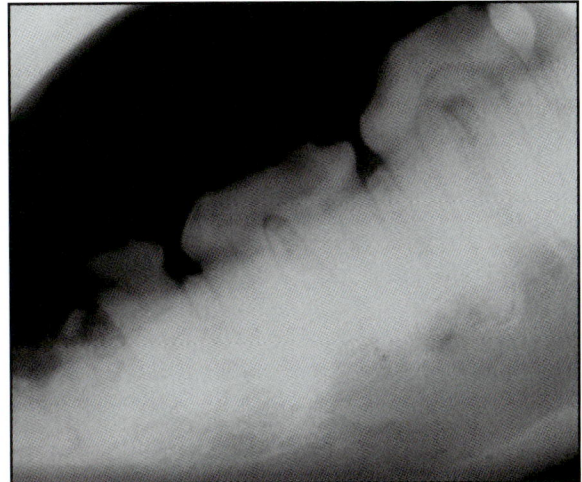

9.17 Moderate to severe abrasion of the lower premolars in a dog. Note the concurrent fractured second premolar. Fractures are often seen concurrently in dogs with abrasions, thus, careful dental examination is important.

Erosion is the loss of tooth substance by a chemical process that does not involve known bacterial action and is not relevant in dogs and cats. Erosion of the palatal aspect of maxillary incisors is often seen in bulimic people as a result of frequent gastric acid regurgitation.

Diagnosis: Dentitions with signs of abnormal wear should be examined for concurrent dental fractures or fracture lines, as well as pulpal and periapical pathology. Thorough clinical examination and exploration with a dental explorer, and a complete set of dental radiographs should be obtained. The surface of an abraded tooth is usually smooth and the dental explorer will not detect any irregularities.

Resorption

Resorption is very common and can be seen microscopically as areas of superficial resorption on the roots of permanent teeth. Microscopic resorptions are usually repaired by the apposition of cementum or bone. Resorption that can be seen and diagnosed radiologically is always pathological (Figure 9.18). Resorption is usually associated with some attempt at repair by cementum or bone production, often leading to ankylosis of the tooth (Figure 9.19) and surrounding alveolar bone. This is mainly seen in geriatric patients.

153

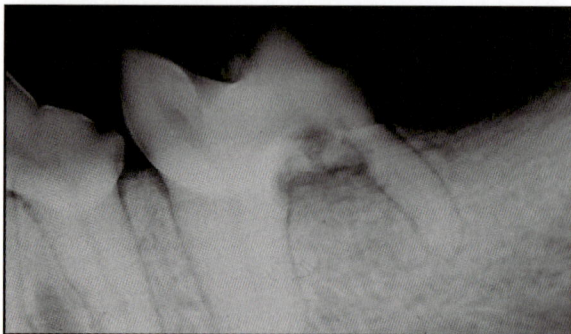

9.18 Teeth with external resorptions, such as a feline odontoclastic resorptive lesion (FORL) at the furcation of a lower carnassial, are (when involving exposed tooth substance) painful and should be extracted. Note the accumulation of calculus in this area.

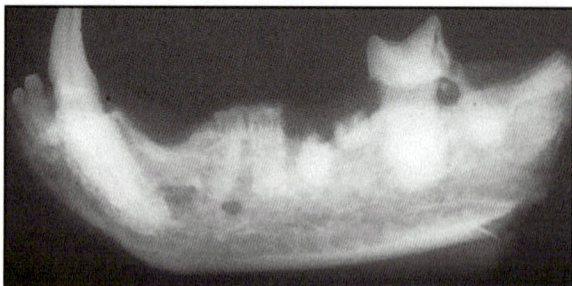

9.19 The lamina dura and periodontal space are lost in this case of severe resorption. Note that there are several fractures, indicating that the teeth and root remnants involved may be ankylosed.

Pathological resorption starting on the root surface (external resorption) may be as a result of:

• Periapical inflammation
• Cysts or neoplasia
• Unerupted teeth
• Re-implanted teeth
• Orthodontic treatment
• Periodontitis
• Idiopathic (e.g. feline odontoclastic resorptive lesions (FORLs)).

Pathological resorption starting from the pulpal surface (internal resorption) is usually caused by pulpitis (Figure 9.20). When the coronal dentine is involved the

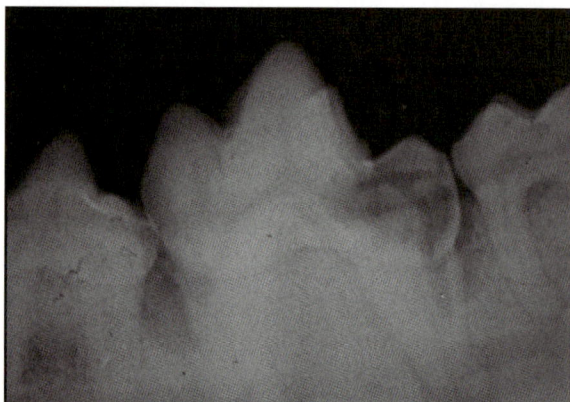

9.20 Severe internal resorption, most obviously seen at the distal pulp chamber. A peri-radicular radiolucency can be seen on the distal root.

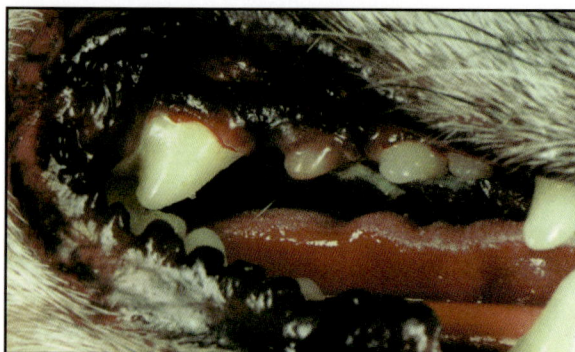

9.21 Internal resorption may be observed clinically as a so-called 'pink spot' when pulp tissues are visible through the resorbing enamel and dentine. In advanced cases (as in 107) the whole tooth can take on a translucent appearance and appear pink due to the destruction of dentine and the resulting superficial position of the pulp.

resorption may present clinically as a pink spot as a result of the vascular pulp being visible through the overlying enamel (Figure 9.21).

Diagnosis: Except for those involving areas that can be explored, resorptions are only detectable using radiography. Resorptions, in particular external resorptions, are often incidental findings in dogs. FORLs are covered in more detail in Chapters 8 and 10.

Fractures
Dental fractures are highly prevalent. They are traumatic in origin and are often associated with: traffic accidents, falling from height (especially in cats), chewing bones and hard toys, stone chewing and catching. Fractures may affect the tooth crown, root or both. Fractures are classified as uncomplicated or complicated, depending on whether the pulp is involved in the fracture line or not (Figure 9.22). Uncomplicated crown fractures, i.e. those not involving the pulp, may involve enamel alone or both enamel and dentine. The majority of uncomplicated fractures only involve the crown. 'Slab fractures' of the buccal cingulum of the upper carnassial teeth may involve both the crown and the root, and are often complicated (Figure 9.23).

Root fractures may be oblique or horizontal. Horizontal root fractures may be coronal (or cervical), mid-

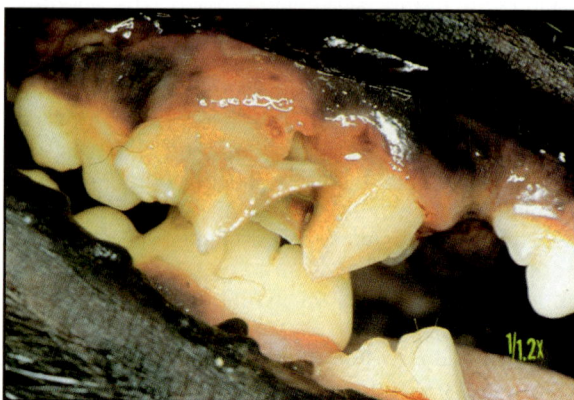

9.22 Complicated tooth fracture of an upper right carnassial (108) tooth in a dog. The pulp has been exposed.

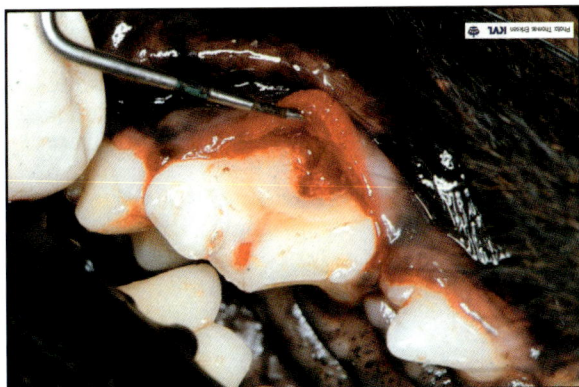

9.23 'Slab fracture' (sagittal fracture) of an upper carnassial tooth in a dog. Slab fractures are often complicated and may extend subgingivally. They are most commonly seen affecting the buccal cingulum of the maxillary carnassial tooth.

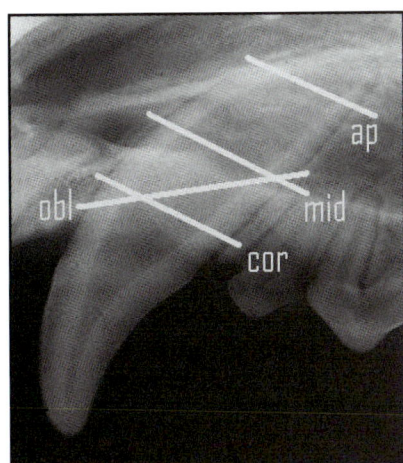

9.24 Radiographic diagram showing the typical location of oblique and horizontal (coronal, mid-root and apical) fractures.

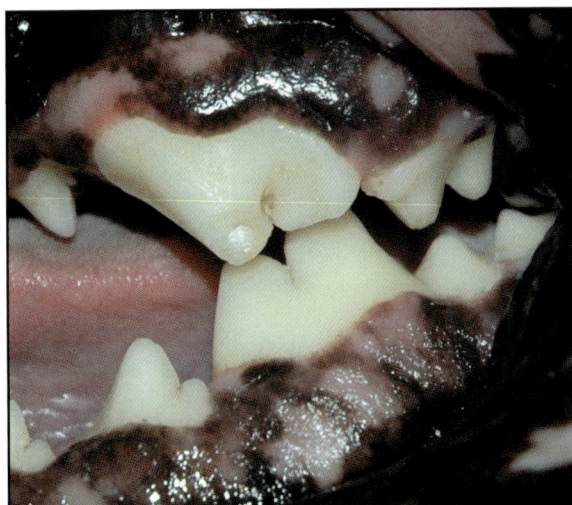

9.25 Uncomplicated fractures often need very little treatment. Sharp enamel edges should be smoothed with a bur and may be sealed with a varnish or sealant restoration. (Courtesy of C. Tutt)

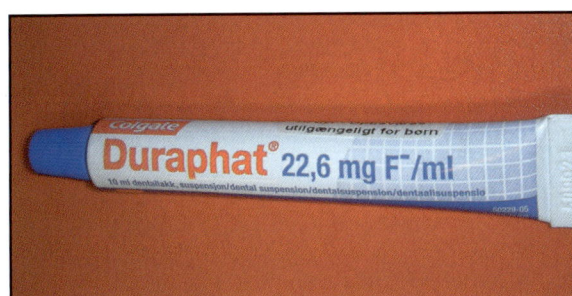

9.26 Exposed dentine may be treated with fluoride paste which desensitizes the dentine.

root or apical (Figure 9.24). Apical root fractures may heal without treatment. However, in general the presence of a root fracture indicates extraction of the affected tooth. Fractures along the long axis of a tooth are an absolute indication for extraction.

Diagnosis: Fractured teeth should be explored and radiographed, since fracture lines may be obscured by calculus. Root fractures, particularly coronal root fractures, result in increased tooth mobility.

Treatment: Uncomplicated tooth fractures often need very little treatment. Sharp enamel edges should be smoothed with a bur or polishing stone (Figure 9.25). Exposed dentine may be treated with a fluoride varnish (Figure 9.26) that desensitizes the dentine, or sealed with a dentine liner or restorative material to prevent further irritation of the pulp (Figure 9.27). Periapical status as an indicator of pulp vitality, should be reviewed and monitored radiographically at regular intervals.

Complicated fractures always need treatment. Deciduous teeth with complicated fractures require extraction to prevent damage to the adjacent developing permanent tooth. Complicated fractures of mature permanent teeth can be treated in a number of ways. Fractures not older than 1–2 days in younger dogs (<2 years old), with no other dental lesions and with a pulp

that appears vital on clinical examination, may be treated by means of partial pulpectomy and direct pulp capping. In an immature permanent tooth this treatment often retains a viable pulp, which is required for apexogenesis (continued root growth and closure of the root apex). The most coronal 8–10 mm of the pulp, which upon exposure, very quickly becomes inflamed, is amputated with a bur and the remaining healthy pulp is covered with a calcium hydroxide dressing.

The dressing comes in small sterile vials of 1 gram aqueous calcium hydroxide in airtight foil bags. This prevents the calcium hydroxide from being oxidized to calcium carbonate, which has no odontoblast-stimulating effect. The calcium hydroxide dissociates and stimulates the odontoblasts to form reparative dentine, sealing the pulp from the dressing. The cavity is restored with a permanent restoration. This procedure needs to be performed under aseptic conditions since contamination of the pulp by bacteria will lead to failure and pulp necrosis. The tooth should be monitored radiographically at approximately 3-month intervals. Dentinal bridge formation beneath the calcium hydroxide dressing and absence of periapical pathology indicate that the pulp has remained vital.

In the case of a necrotic pulp in an immature tooth, endodontic treatment should be performed with the aim of inducing apexification (treatment-induced root closure), or the affected tooth should be extracted.

155

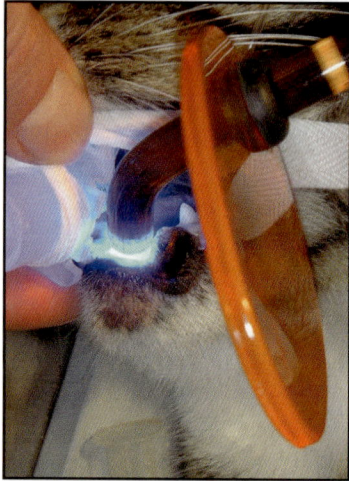

9.27

Treatment of an uncomplicated fracture. The lesion was restored with a light-cured composite. Patients must undergo regular radiographic monitoring of the treated teeth.

In animals >2 years of age with tooth fractures older than 1–2 days or where the chronicity of the fracture is unknown and in cases where severe pulp inflammation may be suspected, complete pulpectomy and root canal therapy or extraction is indicated. Severe pulpal inflammation should be suspected if bleeding is heavy and difficult to control. In conventional root canal therapy, the root canal is debrided, shaped, disinfected and filled with an antibacterial biocompatible root canal sealer. The access or fracture site is restored with an appropriate restoration (Figure 9.28). Root canal therapy and the overlying restoration must be performed carefully in order to completely debride and fill the root canal, and to create good apical and coronal seals. If this is not achieved bacteria and toxins in the pulp chamber or bacteria introduced via leakage from the coronal restoration will result in recurrent periapical pathology. If endodontic treatment cannot be performed the tooth should be extracted.

Teeth with oblique fractures extending below the gingival margin that are not extracted should be monitored at regular intervals since marginal periodontitis may develop more readily at these sites. Fractures extending less than approximately 2 mm below the gingival margin may be treated by smoothing with an appropriate bur or polishing stone, and sealing the fractured edges with a varnish or sealant. Crown elon-

gation techniques may be performed on teeth that have fracture lines which extend beyond 2 mm below the gingival margin, to facilitate exposure of the fracture margins supragingivally. These procedures should be performed by colleagues with experience in veterinary dental and oral surgery.

Teeth with or without fractures but with signs of pulp necrosis (discoloration) or periapical pathology should be treated endodontically or extracted. Asymptomatic teeth with periapical pathology require treatment as both periapical granulomas and radicular cysts can undergo acute exacerbation.

Fractured teeth with severe periodontitis should be extracted.

Treatment of horizontal root fractures is dictated by the level of the fracture. Teeth with apical root fractures have the best prognosis. The presence of a coronal root fracture indicates extraction of the affected tooth. Horizontal mid-root and apical fractures will heal if immobilized by means of dentinocemental callus, connective tissue union, fibrous union or osteofibrous union. If the pulp in the coronal portion of the root is necrotic then healing will not occur and endodontic treatment is required. The apical segment may be left *in situ* if no radiographic signs of apical pathology are present; however, if signs are present then the apical part of the root should be extracted via apicoectomy.

Luxation or avulsion

Luxation or avulsion of teeth is often associated with alveolar fractures. Trauma may cause damage to the periodontium, resulting in subluxation, luxation or avulsion of the tooth. In cases of subluxation, the tooth exhibits increased mobility within the alveolus but it is not dislocated. There may be bleeding from the gingiva and, in humans, the tooth is painful on percussion. Radiographic findings are generally unremarkable.

Displacement of the tooth may be seen as:

- Intrusion – the tooth is dislocated apically (Figure 9.29)
- Extrusion – the tooth is dislocated out of the alveolus
- Lateral luxation – almost always associated with fracture of the alveolar bone plate (Figure 9.30). Luxation results in the tooth crown being positioned

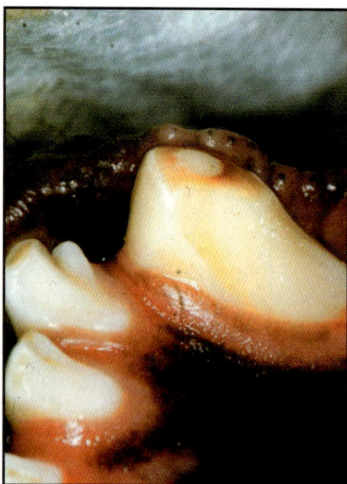

9.28

A restored lower canine (404) tooth in a dog after complete pulpectomy and root canal therapy.

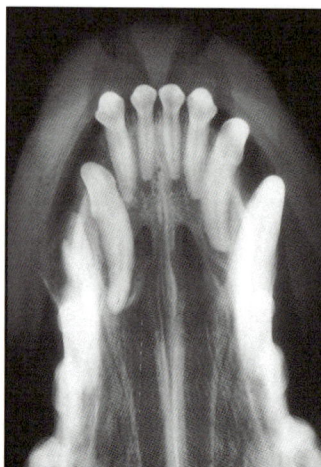

9.29

The upper lateral incisor (103) is displaced apically into the alveolus (intrusion). Intruded deciduous teeth will most likely cause damage to the permanent tooth germ, typically causing enamel defects.

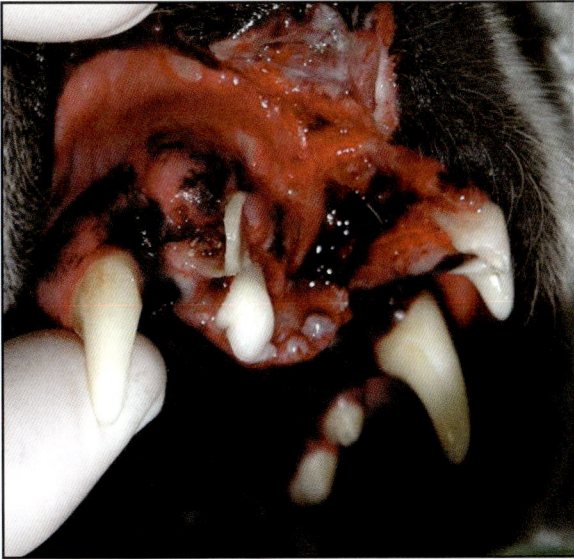

9.30 Alveolar fractures. Part of the fractured alveolus is exposed. One tooth has been displaced palatally while others have been avulsed. (Courtesy of C. Tutt)

palatally/lingually with the tooth root being labially/buccally or *vice versa*. Fracture of the alveolar bone plate allows the tooth to luxate rather than fracture. Avulsion causes complete displacement of the tooth out of the alveolus (Figure 9.31). Avulsion may or may not be associated with alveolar fractures. Both luxations and avulsions cause disruption of the dental neurovascular supply, resulting in pulp necrosis. These teeth require endodontic therapy if they are to be maintained in the dentition.

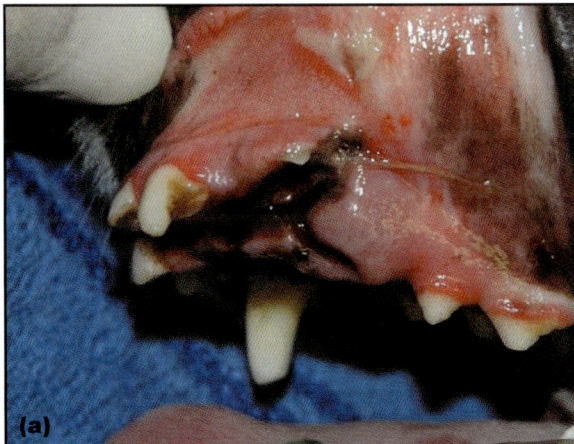

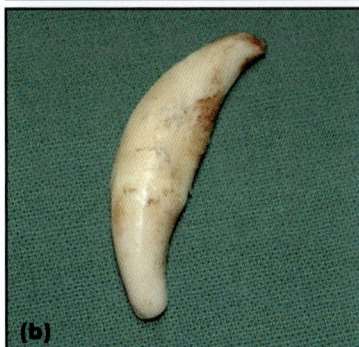

9.31

(a) The empty alveolus on presentation after the left maxillary canine was traumatically avulsed. **(b)** The avulsed tooth was presented 18 hours after avulsion, too late for replacement. (Courtesy of C. Tutt)

Treatment: Alveolar fractures are generally treated together with luxated or avulsed teeth. Subluxations result in damage to the periodontium but usually need no further treatment. Chewing activity should be kept to a minimum with soft food fed for approximately a week. The pulpal status should be reviewed periodically to check for signs of pulp necrosis.

Luxated teeth should be replaced and stabilized with interdental wiring and acrylic splinting. Luxated teeth will usually require endodontic treatment. Avulsed teeth should also be replaced into the alveolus. The extra alveolar time is the most crucial factor determining successful re-implantation. Teeth that have been avulsed for more than 30 minutes have a poor prognosis. The avulsed tooth must be kept moist and at body temperature, ideally in milk, until re-implantation. The root, if contaminated, should be cleaned very carefully (by flushing with large volumes of polyionic fluid) since removal of any remaining periodontal fibres will result in root resorption. Following re-implantation the avulsed tooth requires stabilization and endodontic treatment. Endodontic treatment is usually performed 18–20 days post re-implantation. Since most avulsed teeth are contaminated the animal should be treated with antibiotics for 2–3 days. Luxated or avulsed teeth with severe periodontitis, caries, resorptive lesions or periapical pathology and deciduous teeth should not be replaced.

Electrical, chemical and radiation injuries

Electrical injuries are uncommon. This type of lesion occurs mainly in young animals after playing with electrical cords. Chemical burns are rare in dogs and cats. However, ulceration of the oral mucosa, tongue and oesophagus is occasionally seen after ingestion of corrosive chemicals. Although stomatitis or facial dermatitis may be seen as a sequel to radiation therapy, bone necrosis (radio-osteonecrosis) is uncommon in dogs and cats.

Aetiopathogenesis
The effect of electrical injuries may be local (Figure 9.32) or systemic. Acute pulmonary oedema may be life-threatening. Local lesions are similar to those lesions

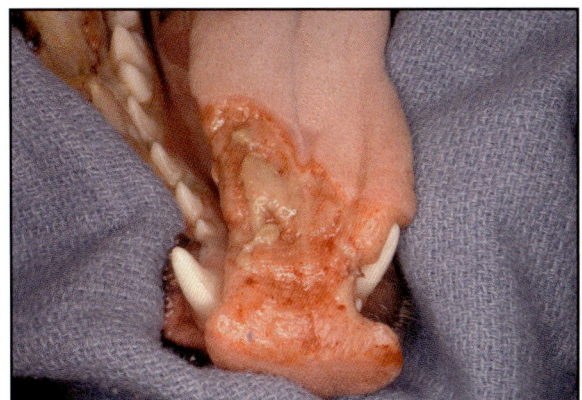

9.32 Localized tongue lesion after electrical burn. The lesion has commenced healing but harbours only little granulation tissue and some necrosis. Scarring is usually extensive in such lesions. © Frank JM Verstraete.

157

seen after burns but are usually dominated by early necrosis of the oral tissues (Figure 9.33), which may include the dental pulp and mandibular or maxillary bone (Figure 9.34). Chemical injuries are usually seen as ulcerations with pseudomembranes of necrotic debris (Figure 9.35). Stomatitis or dermatitis secondary to radiation therapy may include erythema, desquama-

tion (dry and later moist) and finally necrosis. Stomatitis usually begins to occur 2–3 weeks after initiation of radiation. Healing begins 1–2 weeks after cessation of radiation. Chronic facial radiation dermatitis may occur several years after radiation therapy.

Diagnosis and treatment

Chemical burns may be very difficult to diagnose since the owner may not have observed the animal drinking or licking at the solution. Since lesions, especially from ingesting caustic lye, may be profound and also involve the oesophagus, thorough examination is recommended. Chemical burns to the oesophagus may cause severe complications such as perforations and strictures, and result in an increased risk of developing oesophageal cancer. Treatment is symptomatic and aimed at palliation. Lesions should be debrided and necrotic tissue removed. Oral discomfort may be reduced with anti-inflammatory drugs, mainly corticosteroids. This may also help animals to maintain normal oral feeding. If normal oral feeding cannot be maintained, assisted feeding should be considered at an early stage. Naso-oesophageal, oesophageal, ventricular or enteral feeding tubes are options depending on the needs of the patient, which are mainly determined by the expected length of the healing period.

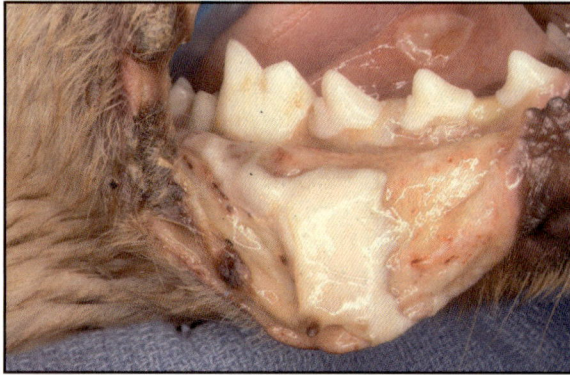

9.33 Severe necrosis of the labial mucosa following an electrical burn. © Frank JM Verstraete.

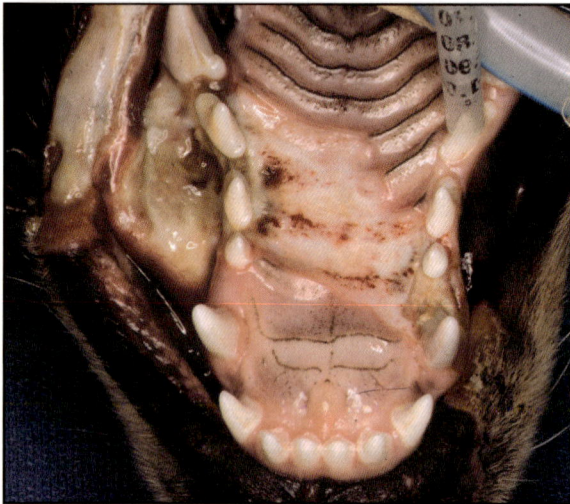

9.34 Exposure of the maxillary alveolar bone around teeth 105 and 207, following an electrical burn. Note the large necrotic defect of the left labial mucosa and commissure. © Frank JM Verstraete.

Jaw fracture and dental complications

Fractures of the mandible and maxilla account for only 5–7% of fractures in the dog and cat. However, jaw fractures are often complex since they can be open and commonly present with associated dental complications (Figure 9.36). The most common complications found in association with jaw fractures are dental fractures and the involvement of periodontally compromised teeth in fracture lines. The majority of jaw fractures present as alveolar fractures and, to a lesser degree, are affected by severe periodontitis. Repair of pathological (i.e. spontaneous) fractures due to bone loss in severe periodontitis is a challenge, since both the affected teeth and bone are chronically and severely diseased. Pathological fractures often occur at the level of the lower first molar as the carnassial tooth

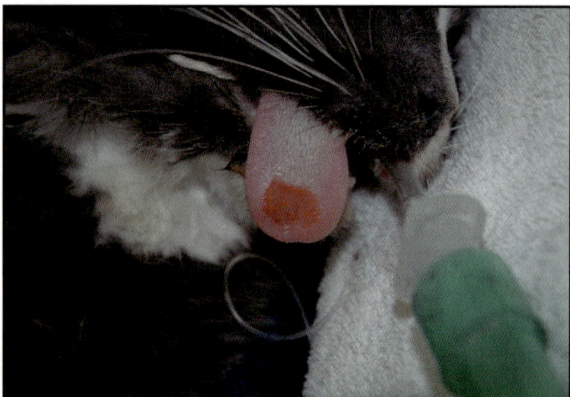

9.35 Chemical injury to the tongue of this cat was confirmed on histopathology, although the cause of the ulceration was not found. Injuries due to lye or other alkaline substances are usually more profound and serious than those caused by acids. © Cedric Tutt.

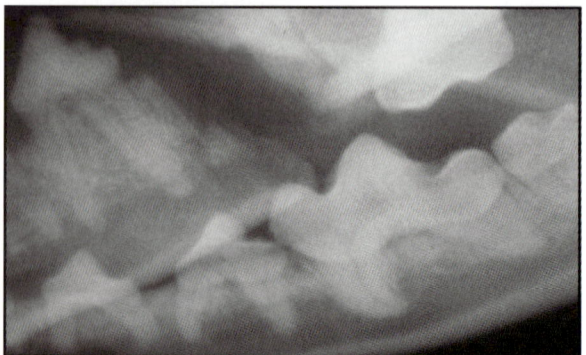

9.36 Complicated oblique jaw fracture with the rostral limit dorsal and the caudal limit ventral. This fracture line orientation leads to instability due to distraction by the digastric muscle.

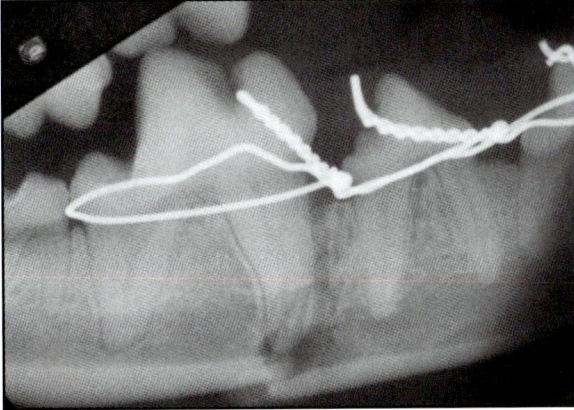

9.37 Fixation of a mandibular fracture using interdental wiring (Stout wiring). Note that the fracture ends overlap, which may delay healing. Frequent radiographic monitoring of 409 is essential as the vascular supply to the mesial root may have been disrupted. Subsequent periapical radiolucencies at both apices will indicate pulp involvement.

comprises the major substance of the mandible at this site, and since severe periodontal or periapical pathology is often found here. Diagnosis is based on history, clinical examination and radiography.

Treatment: With the advancement in endodontic therapy and better fracture management, it is no longer always necessary to extract teeth involved in jaw fracture lines. With the development of intraoral wiring and splinting techniques, teeth in fracture lines may be used for jaw stabilization (Figure 9.37). Teeth with long axis fractures, horizontal coronal fractures, fragmented teeth and teeth with severe displacement of segments should be extracted. Periodontally diseased teeth with periodontal ligament necrosis will often result in impaired fracture healing and should be extracted. Orthopaedic jaw fixation using implants, such as pins, screws and plates, and interosseous circlages should be used under strict consideration so as not to damage root structures or disrupt the dental vascular supply.

References and further reading

Bojrab MJ and Tholen MA (1990) *Small Animal Oral Medicine and Surgery*, ed. MA Tholen and MJ Bojrab, pp. 248–252. Lea & Febiger, Philadelphia

Gorrel C (2004) *Veterinary Dentistry for the General Practitioner*. WB Saunders, London

Harvey CE and Emily PP (1993) *Small Animal Dentistry*. Mosby, St. Louis

Soames JV and Southam JC (1985) *Oral Pathology, 2nd edn*, ed. JV Soames and JC Southam, pp. 32–59 and 60–65. Oxford University Press, Oxford

10

Other oral and dental conditions

Simone Ostermeier

Oral mass lesions

The oral cavity is the fourth most common site of neoplasia in dogs and cats. It is also a common site for hyperplastic and cystic lesions (Figure 10.1). Clinically, these various lesions can look deceivingly similar and the distinction between neoplasia, be it benign or malignant, and non-neoplastic lesions can rarely be made on clinical presentation alone. In the majority of cases, biopsy and histopathological examination are required.

General principles for diagnosing oral mass lesions

- The accurate location of lesions must be detailed and specified in relation to adjacent teeth, where applicable. For example: 'mass right maxilla' is not sufficient; instead 'mass on gingiva at mesial aspect of 104' should be specified (see Chapter 2 for details on dental charting and the modified Triadan system).
- Radiography should be used to gain more information about: (i) the lesion, and to clarify whether bone involvement is present; and (ii) concurrent conditions such as periodontal disease. Absence of detectable radiographic bony changes does not rule out malignancy (Frew and Dobson, 1992).
- Biopsy samples for histopathological evaluation should be taken. The type of biopsy method used should be chosen according to the order of probability of differential diagnoses. For example, a deep incisional biopsy if malignancy is suspected, or an excisional biopsy if a lesion is more likely to be benign. (Refer to the *BSAVA Manual of Canine and Feline Oncology* for details on the principles of taking biopsy samples.)
- An evaluation for metastatic disease should be included in the diagnostic work-up if malignant neoplasia is part of the differential diagnosis. The World Health Organization (WHO) TNM classification for tumours of the oral cavity is a useful tool in establishing the degree of severity of the disease (see Figure 10.21).

Group	Lesions
Oral hyperplastic lesions	Gingival hyperplasia: • focal • multiple focal • generalized • combined focal and generalized Cheek chew lesions Hyperplasia of caudal sublingual mucosa Peripheral giant cell granuloma Pyogenic granuloma
Oral cystic lesions and mucoceles	Odontogenic: • radicular cysts • dentigerous cysts (eruption cysts and follicular cysts) • odontogenic keratocysts (primordial cysts) Soft tissue: • ranula
Oral proliferative inflammatory lesions	Feline eosinophilic granuloma complex (see Chapter 8) Leishmanial stomatitis in dogs (see Chapter 7)
Oral hamartomas (odontomas)	Complex odontoma Compound odontoma
Benign oral neoplasia	Odontogenic: • peripheral odontogenic fibroma • acanthomatous ameloblastoma • ameloblastoma (central or intraosseous) • ameloblastic fibroma • amyloid-producing odontogenic tumour Non-odontogenic: • viral papillomatosis • others (e.g. fibroma, neurofibroma, haemangioma, lipoma, chondroma, osteoma) Malignant potential: • mast cell tumour • plasmacytoma
Malignant oral neoplasia	Odontogenic: • rare (odontogenic sarcoma) Non-odontogenic: • malignant melanoma • squamous cell carcinoma • fibrosarcoma • osteosarcoma • lymphosarcoma • others (e.g. haemangiosarcoma, neurofibrosarcoma, spindle cell sarcoma, canine transmissible venereal tumour, leiomyosarcoma)

10.1 Oral mass lesions in dogs and cats affecting the oral mucosa and/or gingiva.

Gingival hyperplasia

Gingival hyperplasia is a common condition in dogs but less common in cats. It represents a variation in host tissue response to the accumulation of plaque. Other causative factors are breed predisposition, drug therapy with ciclosporin, calcium channel blockers or phenytoin and chronic irritation (Figure 10.2). The extent of gingival hyperplasia varies and can be described as:

- Focal lesions
- Multiple focal lesions
- Generalized hyperplasia
- Combinations of the above.

Group	Examples
Breed predisposition	Boxer, Border Collie, Labrador, German Shepherd Dog
Drug-induced	Phenytoin
Ciclosporin
Calcium channel-blocking agents
Chronic irritation	Accumulation of dental plaque
Odontoclastic resorptive lesions (see Figure 10.29)
May be part of gingivitis (Chapter 7) and gingivostomatitis (Chapter 8)
May be present on the *surface* of an area infiltrated by a neoplasm
Mechanical irritation (e.g. malocclusion with frequent contact of an occluding tooth against gingival tissues)
Systemic conditions	Infectious systemic disease. One report published on disseminated cryptococcosis and an associated proliferative gingival lesion (Odom and Anderson, 2000)
Non-infectious systemic conditions causing gingival hyperplasia reported in humans, e.g. Crohn's disease (Galgut *et al.*, 2001)

10.2 Causative factors of gingival hyperplasia.

The involvement of chronic inflammation within the hyperplastic lesions varies and is clinically expressed in presentations ranging from firm, pink (where not pigmented) and smooth lesions to soft, hyperaemic and ulcerated lesions. Histologically, there is a spectrum of change varying from relatively non-inflamed and avascular masses of dense collagen fibres to chronically inflamed richly cellular granulation tissue. The lesions may have varying degrees of pigmentation, usually reflecting the general degree of pigmentation of the oral mucosa. The crowns of the teeth may be partially or nearly completely covered by the hyperplastic gingiva (Figures 10.3 and 10.4). The space created between the crown and the hyperplastic gingiva is termed a pseudo-pocket and is an area of potentially increased plaque retention (Figure 10.5).

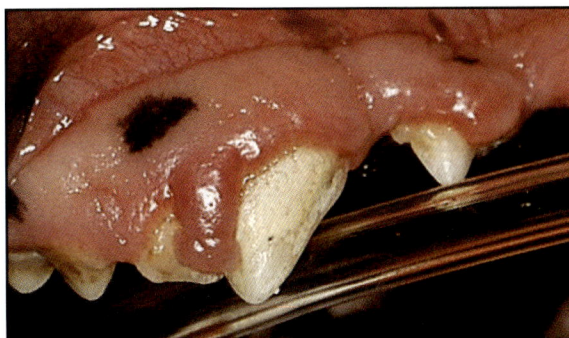

10.3 Generalized gingival hyperplasia in an English Springer Spaniel with multiple focal hyperplastic gingival lesions. Note the presence of calculus deposits and plaque on the third and fourth maxillary premolar teeth.

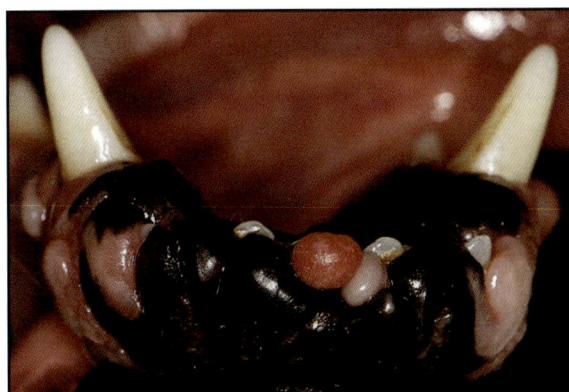

10.4 Generalized gingival hyperplasia combined with focal hyperplastic gingival lesions in an English Springer Spaniel. Rostral view of the mandibular incisor teeth. Note that some teeth are completely covered by excess gingival tissue.

Clinical significance

The presence of gingival hyperplasia in the oral cavity should be viewed as a symptom of an imbalance in the plaque/host tissue response and underlying causes must be addressed. The most common causative factor is lack of plaque control and initiation of an oral hygiene protocol, such as daily tooth brushing, will be an essential part of most treatment regimes. Pseudo-pockets form recesses that are inaccessible for routine oral home care and will encourage more plaque accumulation, increasing the risk of periodontitis (see Figure 10.5). The covering of crowns with hyperplastic gingiva can render some teeth non-functional. Focal prominent lesions may be bitten during normal mastication, resulting in pain and slight to moderate haemorrhage. This can give rise to the occasional emergency presentation.

Diagnosis and differential diagnoses

Generalized gingival hyperplasia can often be diagnosed by history, signalment and clinical presentation. Oral radiographs should be taken to diagnose or rule out additional conditions. A common concurrent condition in particular, is periodontitis. Alveolar bone loss is seen radiographically and is often associated with increased probing depths (true pockets). Full dental charting should be performed, with special attention given to periodontal pocket depths.

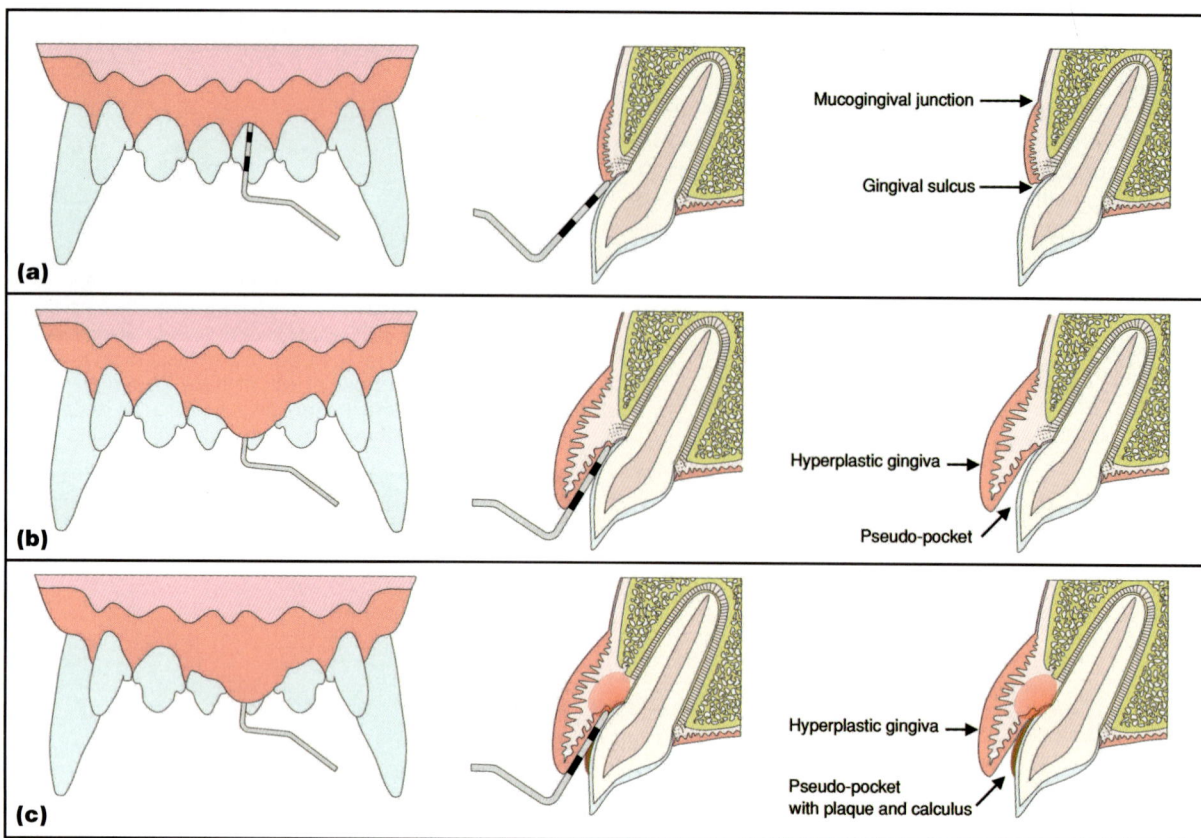

10.5   **(a)** Healthy gingiva with normal sulcus depth (1–3 mm). **(b)** Gingival hyperplasia. Periodontal probe used to measure depth of pseudo-pocket. **(c)** Subgingival plaque and calculus, leading to inflammation.

Biopsy samples should be taken of any areas of hyperplastic gingiva that present with clinical signs of inflammation, with softer than expected tissue texture, or with radiographic findings indicating bone involvement. Histopathology samples must be accurately labelled so the appropriate treatment can be implemented after the result is known, if required.

The *focal gingival hyperplastic lesion*, as well as any prominent focal lesion in a patient with generalized gingival hyperplasia, can only be definitively diagnosed on histopathological examination. Oral radiography should be performed on all focal gingival lesions. The temptation to extrapolate a diagnosis from one focal mass lesion to all other gingival mass lesions present in the same oral cavity should be resisted, as several different types of lesion may well be present concurrently (Sitzman, 2000). Figure 10.6 gives differential diagnoses for the focal lesion.

Treatment

The majority of patients with gingival hyperplasia will need a multimodal treatment strategy for improved plaque control. Under general anaesthesia, and following complete diagnostics as outlined above, gingivectomy and gingivoplasty procedures should be performed if clinically significant pseudo-pockets exist. These procedures help to eliminate pseudo-pockets and re-establish near-normal anatomy of the affected gingiva. *Gingivectomy* (Figures 10.7 and 10.8) is the excision of gingival tissue to create a new gingival margin, aiming at pocket reduction or elimination. *Gingivoplasty* is the

Group	Types
Neoplasia	Benign, odontogenic Benign, non-odontogenic Malignant
Non-neoplastic dental disorders	Embedded or impacted tooth
Non-neoplastic osteoproliferative disorders	Cysts Inflammatory exostosis of alveolar bone
Anatomical structures	Lingual molar salivary gland in cats (see Chapter 1)

10.6   Differential diagnoses for focal hyperplastic gingival lesions.

Dental radiographs (see Chapter 2)
Periodontal probe (or a specific periodontal pocket depth marker)
No. 11 or No. 15 scalpel blades with handle
Gauze swabs
Equipment for scaling and polishing (see Chapters 5 and 7)

Note: In human periodontal surgery, special cutting hand instruments, such as a Kirkland gingivectomy knife, an Orban interproximal gingivectomy knife and a specially angled scalpel blade holder (Blake's handle), are commonly used. These instruments can be used by the veterinary dental surgeon, depending on availability and operator preference

10.7   Equipment required for the gingivectomy procedure (cold-steel technique).

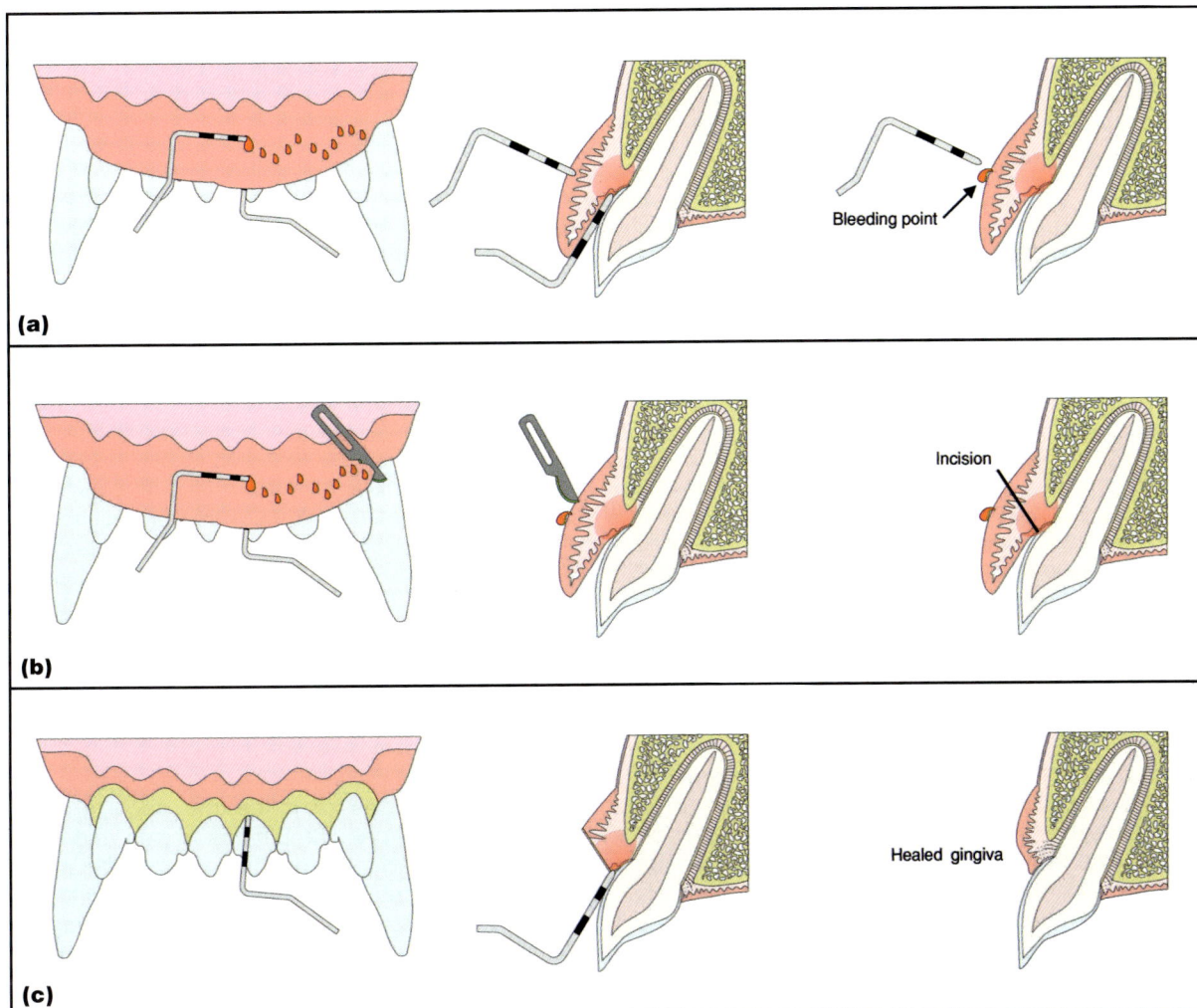

10.8 Gingivectomy procedure. **(a)** Use the periodontal probe to establish pseudo-pocket depth. Withdraw the periodontal probe from the pocket, hold it against the gingiva with its tip indicating the floor of the pseudo-pocket (i.e. the pseudo-pocket's most apical extent at that precise location), then angle the probe perpendicular to the gingiva while maintaining contact with the tip, and press the tip into the gingival tissue. This creates a 'bleeding point', which serves as a guide for the gingivectomy incision. Create bleeding points every few millimetres along the teeth that require gingivectomy, both on their buccal and lingual aspects. Note that this will result in a scalloped pattern because the bleeding points represent the contour of gingival attachment around the teeth. **(b)** Use a No. 15 scalpel blade to start the incision 1–3 mm apically to the line created by the bleeding points, and directing the incision coronally towards the bleeding point. This should result in an external bevel of about 30–45°. A No. 11 scalpel blade may be useful in connecting the buccal and lingual incisions at the proximal aspects, especially in teeth such as the incisors that have very narrow interproximal spaces. *This is not a procedure suitable for a surgeon who is unaccustomed to operating in the oral cavity: a fair amount of cutting pressure is required to cut through the tough hyperplastic gingival tissue, and cutting on convex surfaces can easily lead to unintentional slippage of the blade. Cutting with the blade must be controlled millimetre by millimetre.* **(c)** Use a dental scaler to cut and remove the excised gingival collarette around the tooth. Finish by scaling and polishing all treated teeth.

term used to describe corrective gingival surgery that does not alter the gingival margin; its aim is to recreate a correct anatomical shape (Harty, 1994).

Contraindications

- Gingivectomy procedures are contraindicated in cases where less than 2 mm of attached gingiva is present. Measure the distance between the bleeding point and the mucogingival junction, and ensure that it is at least 2 mm wide.
- Gingivectomy procedures are not suitable for infrabony pockets.

Electrosurgery and laser surgery

Alternatives to gingivectomy performed with cold-steel cutting instruments are electrosurgery and laser surgery. Caution must be exercised when using electrosurgery for gingivectomy: any contact of the electrodes with the crowns of teeth must be avoided to prevent heat damage to the pulp, which may lead to irreversible pulpitis and pulp necrosis. Experience with the use of the electrosurgery unit is important, to ensure efficient cutting with the lowest possible setting and a light touch. A combination of the use of electrosurgery and cold-steel cutting instruments is often chosen, as this combines speed (electrosurgery) and precision (cold-steel cutting instrument).

Gingival surgery performed with laser is a novel approach that has found application in human periodontal surgery and some veterinary specialist centres (Bellows, 2001; Holmstrom *et al.*, 2004). However, the cost of laser surgery units thus far has made their use prohibitive in general veterinary practice.

Analgesia

Adequate analgesia must be administered pre-, peri- and postoperatively (see Chapter 3), as some discomfort is to be expected following surgery. Periodontal dressings, containing local anaesthetic agents, are routinely used in the postoperative care of human patients, but are not tolerated by dogs or cats.

Other procedures

It is important to remember that gingivectomy should never be a stand-alone procedure. Firstly, tooth extractions may be indicated where moderate to advanced periodontitis is present. Secondly, complete plaque control has to be achieved by a combination of professional scaling and polishing of all teeth and effective oral home care (see Chapter 7). If the gingival hyperplasia is drug-induced, alternative medications may have to be considered according to a risk:benefit ratio. In focal hyperplastic gingival lesions, the underlying cause must be addressed where it can be identified (e.g. if an odontoclastic resorptive lesion or a malocclusion is the cause). The excised focal lesion should be treated as an excisional biopsy and be submitted for histopathological examination. Where the clinical examination or radiographic evidence of a focal lesion give rise to consideration of a malignant neoplastic lesion as a potential differential diagnosis, an incisional biopsy may be preferred.

Prognosis, prevention and follow-up

Following surgical excision and histopathological confirmation, the prognosis following treatment for gingival hyperplasia is good, although local recurrence is possible. The incidence of local recurrence can be reduced by implementation of an efficient oral home care regimen. The patient should be re-examined at least every 6 months to review the clinical situation and to monitor the efficacy of oral home care.

The term 'epulis'

Controversy exists regarding whether a focal gingival hyperplastic lesion may be termed an 'epulis'. The term appears firmly entrenched in both human and veterinary dental and pathology literature, but its use for reactive hyperplastic gingival lesions and also for certain tumours of odontogenic origin has been the source of confusion.

Some authors would prefer the use of the term epulis exclusively as a descriptive term, meaning 'a mass arising from the gingiva' (Verstraete *et al.*, 1992). Veterinary pathologists may choose to use the term epulis in a histopathological diagnosis in combination with other descriptive terms. It is by review of the histopathological description or by the pathologist's comment that the veterinary clinician can determine whether the lesion was found to be reactive, hyperplastic, or neoplastic.

Other oral hyperplastic lesions

Lesions of oral soft tissue

Cheek chew lesions

The most common non-gingival sites of hyperplasia affecting the oral mucosa in dogs are caused by mastication and entrapment of mucosa between the teeth. These are commonly termed cheek chew lesions if they are located at the occlusal level of the caudal buccal mucosa. They have also been found along the caudal sublingual tissue (sublingual (tongue) chewing lesions). In the author's experience, these lesions have not been observed in cats.

Clinically, differentiation from oral neoplastic lesions is made by observing the symmetry of the cheek chew lesions. The definitive differentiation is made by histopathological examination, and is usually described as granulomatous. Depigmentation of the lesions is common. There should be no ulceration of the lesions, except where a direct explanation is at hand, such as trauma by a sharp enamel margin of an adjacent tooth due to crown fracture or caries. Following treatment and elimination of sharp dental margins, ulceration of a cheek chew lesion should heal within days.

Granulomas

Occasional reports describe the occurrence of *peripheral giant cell granulomas* in cats and dogs. These lesions are of a reactive hyperplastic nature and can occur anywhere on the gingiva or alveolar mucosa (if located on the gingiva, the lesion may be called giant cell epulis in some texts). They present as pedunculated or sessile swellings of varying size and may have an ulcerated surface. Radiographs may reveal superficial erosion of the margin of the alveolar bone.

Another rare occurrence is the *pyogenic granuloma*, which presents as a soft, deep red swelling on the gingiva or on other sites of oral mucosa. In some texts, it is called a vascular epulis.

Hyperplastic pulpitis

Chronic hyperplastic pulpitis is a recognized condition in humans, also called pulp polyp (Soames and Southam, 1998). Hyperplastic pulpitis can only occur when caries or a complicated tooth fracture has previously created a communication between the pulp chamber and the oral cavity, and the newly formed hyperplastic tissue has an opening through which to expand. Not many reports identifying pulpal hyperplasia exist in the veterinary literature. In the author's clinical observation, where occasional cases of dogs with carious lesions, complicated crown fractures or teeth with odontoclastic resorptive lesions have been found, tissue resembling the clinical description of epithelialized chronic hyperplastic pulpitis has been seen protruding from the pulp chamber (Figures 10.9 and 10.10). Histopathology had not been performed on the cases in Figures 10.9 and 10.10, and published studies of clinical cases including histopathological reports are required to determine whether such cases truly represent pulpal hyperplasia.

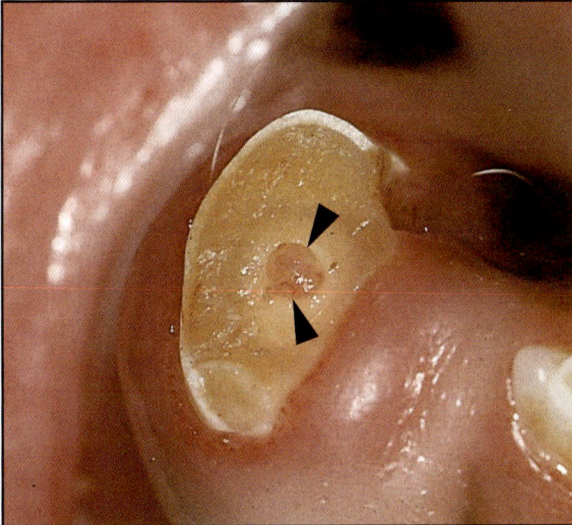

10.9 Iatrogenic pulp exposure in the mandibular right canine tooth of a Bulldog. An unethical attempt at 'disarming' by crown amputation without the necessary subsequent vital pulp therapy had been performed several months prior to presentation. The exposed pulp had reacted with the formation of slightly prominent soft tissue with a smooth pale pink surface (arrowheads). The clinical presentation resembled epithelialized chronic pulpal hyperplasia in humans. Histopathology on the presumed pulpal lesion had not been performed but radiography confirmed continuity of the lesion with the pulp chamber.

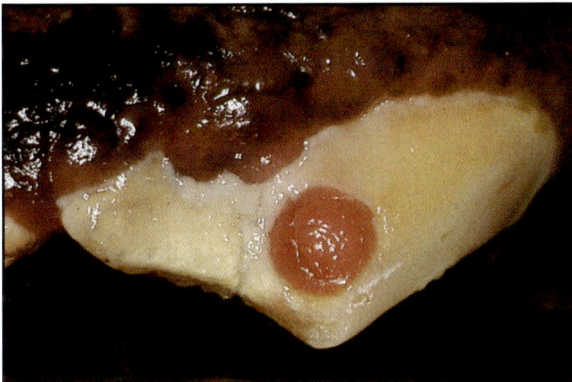

10.10 Canine odontoclastic resorptive lesion with protruding soft tissue in a German Shepherd Dog. The tissue was protruding from the side of the crown of a maxillary right fourth premolar tooth that was affected by a resorptive lesion. Histopathology on the lesion was not performed; however, the clinical presentation of the prominent pink to pale-pink tissue with a smooth surface resembled that of epithelialized chronic hyperplastic pulpitis in humans.

The underlying cause needs to be addressed and treatment will usually consist of endodontic therapy or extraction.

Hypercementosis

Hypercementosis occurs commonly in dogs and cats and the incidence increases with age (Soames and Southam, 1998). To an extent, incremental thickening of the apical part of cementum with increasing age is a physiological adaptive process. Its thickness and the presence of incremental lines may form part of

forensic and archaeological dental investigations to determine age.

In certain reactive circumstances, however, cemento-genesis may be abnormally increased and thus can be classified as hypercementosis (Figure 10.11). Some cases of hypercementosis are idiopathic, but others may be associated with mechanical forces, such as high bite forces, over a period of time. It is interesting to note that excessive mechanical forces applied to a tooth may produce root resorption, but, if applied below a certain threshold, may instead stimulate hyper-cementosis. In humans, a number of other causes for hypercementosis have been identified. Hypercemen-tosis may occur adjacent to periapical inflammation; it may also occur in unerupted teeth, and in teeth of patients with Paget's disease (Soames and Southam, 1998).

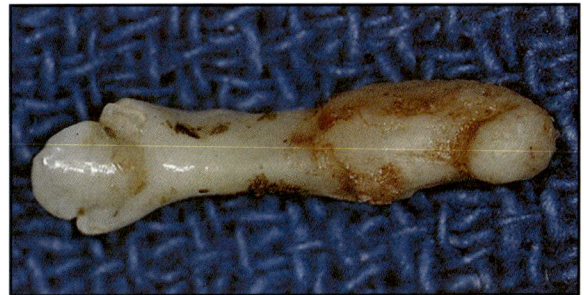

10.11 A central maxillary incisor tooth (palatal aspect) of a 7-year-old Shetland Sheepdog, exhibiting hypercementosis of the root. Note that cementum *per se* is avascular; blood on the specimen originates from the periodontal ligament.

Hypercementosis is diagnosed radiologically. Par-ticular attention should be paid to the evaluation of the periodontal ligament space, as hypercementosis can be associated with root ankylosis. It can also be asso-ciated with concrescence of roots (see Chapter 6).

The clinical significance of hypercementosis is that its presence increases the degree of difficulty of an extraction procedure, should this be indicated for an-other reason. *Hypercementosis in itself is not an indi-cation for extraction.* If hypercementosis is present in conjunction with root ankylosis, and the extraction of the tooth in question is indicated, the surgeon should be prepared for a very challenging and time-consum-ing surgical extraction (see Chapter 11).

Oral hamartomas

Hamartomas (odontomas) of the oral cavity deserve separate mention, as they represent a group of lesions that are tumour-like but are classified as non-neoplastic (see Figure 10.1). Generally, hamartomas consist of an overgrowth of normal cells and tissues in their normal anatomical location but in a disordered ar-rangement. They will reach a point of maturity at which stage they will stop growing.

Oral hamartomas are derived from dental formative tissue, and are found occasionally in young dogs but appear to be rare in cats (Walsh *et al.*, 1987; Stebbins *et al.*, 1989; Poulet *et al.*, 1992; Hale and Wilcock, 1996; Eickhoff *et al.*, 2002; Felizzola *et al.*, 2003). They can also be called odontomas and may have been classified under 'odontogenic tumours' in some veterinary textbooks.

Clinical signs of oral hamartomas depend on their size, location and degree of eruption. Some patients can experience pain from inflammation of the mass itself or from self-trauma to adjacent soft tissue structures during mastication. Partial eruption can result in secondary infection, causing pain and halitosis. Masses can vary in size from small to those involving nearly the whole length of a jaw quadrant and aggressively replacing normal jaw bone structure. The growth rate can be rapid or slow, and clinical signs may warrant surgical treatment even though the mass is non-neoplastic and destined to reach a final mature size and state.

Treatment of smaller odontomas by surgical enucleation is usually successful, but there may be local recurrence. For larger odontomas, or if avoidance of recurrence is a priority, the surgeon may opt for a more aggressive surgical resection.

Complex odontoma

The complex odontoma is a disorderly array of dentine, enamel, ameloblastic epithelium and odontoblasts. Although most components of a tooth are present, there is no structure that resembles a tooth. It can be a coincidental finding during radiographic evaluation, or it can be sufficiently large to cause expansion of the alveolar bone. Radiographic signs of a complex odontoma are those of an amorphous radiopaque mass of mainly dentine and enamel opacity.

Compound odontoma

This type of odontoma has been reported more frequently than the rarer complex odontoma. In the compound odontoma, multiple structures resembling small teeth are present, so-called denticles. They can be unerupted, or partially or fully erupted. Compound odontomas are mostly unilateral, though reports of bilateral lesions exist. Radiographically, a compound odontoma shows radiopaque dental material including abnormally shaped tooth-like structures within the mass. The denticles may be surrounded by radiolucent cystic areas.

Other odontomas

The invaginated odontoma (dens invaginatus, or *dens in dente*) and the enamel pearl can be classified as oral hamartomas. They mainly affect the hard tissues of a single tooth.

Odontogenic tumours

Odontogenic tumours originate from dental formative tissues and may be classified according to the origin of the neoplastic cells (Figure 10.12). Some odontogenic tumours, in particular the malignant forms, are exceedingly rare. The following paragraphs describe the more common odontogenic tumours.

Benign	Malignant
Epithelial tumours without odontogenic mesenchyme: • ameloblastoma • amyloid-producing odontogenic tumour Epithelial tumour with odontogenic mesenchyme [a]: • acanthomatous ameloblastoma (formerly acanthomatous epulis) • feline inductive odontogenic tumour • ameloblastic fibro-odontoma • ameloblastic fibroma Mesenchymal tumours: • peripheral odontogenic fibroma (formerly fibromatous or ossifying epulis)	Odontogenic carcinomas (very rare) Odontogenic sarcomas (very rare): • odontogenic fibrosarcoma Odontogenic carcinosarcomas (none reported in cats or dogs)

10.12 Classification of odontogenic tumours. [a] The compound and complex odontomas are listed here as well and this has to be understood with the definition 'tumour' pertaining to the description of a 'swelling' or 'mass lesion'. Using the term 'tumour' does not automatically attribute a neoplastic origin of the mass.

Peripheral odontogenic fibroma

This benign tumour arises from the periodontal ligament and is the most common type of benign tumour found in the oral cavity in dogs (Figure 10.13). In cats, it is somewhat rarer but presented as the third most common diagnosis of oral tumours in one survey (Harvey and Emily, 1993). It was commonly called fibromatous epulis and ossifying epulis, the distinction between the two being merely the grade of mineralization. The term peripheral odontogenic fibroma is now preferred by many authors (see 'The term 'epulis'', above).

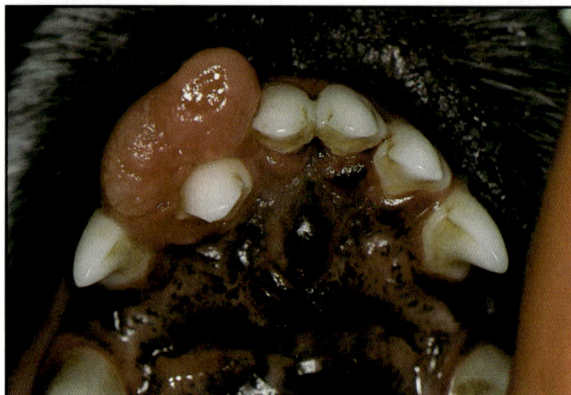

10.13 Peripheral odontogenic fibroma of the rostral maxilla in a dog. Note the displacement of the second incisor tooth and the small ulcerated mark on the tumour surface that was caused by traumatic occlusion against the lower incisor teeth.

Clinical presentation and diagnosis

Peripheral odontogenic fibromas present as firm, smooth, often sessile swellings of the gingiva. They may be clinically indistinguishable from focal gingival hyperplastic lesions, except when displacement of the teeth occurs. Diagnosis requires radiographs (to differ-

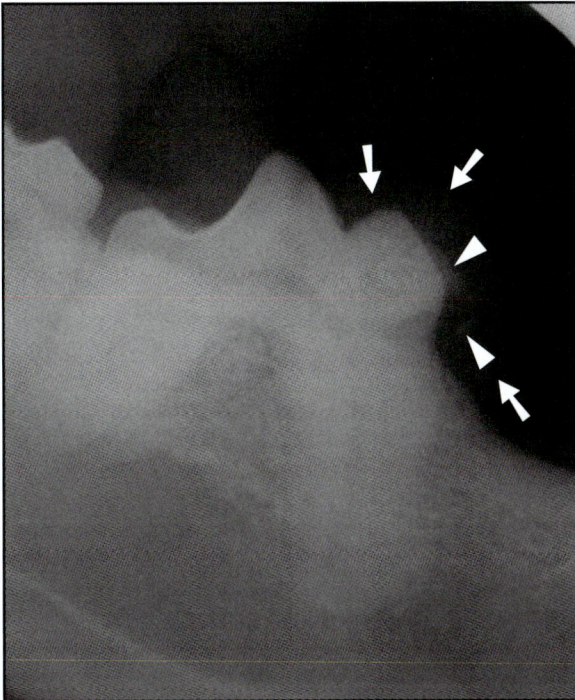

10.14 Radiograph of a peripheral odontogenic fibroma (arrowed) with foci of mineralization (arrowheads) mesial to the mandibular first molar tooth in a dog.

entiate from malignant or locally aggressive lesions and hence determine that an excisional biopsy is appropriate). The radiograph of a peripheral odontogenic fibroma shows a soft tissue swelling in the region of the gingiva with varying degrees of mineralization, but no signs of bone invasion (Figure 10.14). Radiographically, the distinction between a hyperplastic gingival lesion and a peripheral odontogenic fibroma cannot be made, and a biopsy should therefore be performed.

Treatment and prognosis
Treatment is by excision, the depth of which should be determined by the exact location of the neoplastic origin within the periodontal ligament. Typically, this cannot be determined and the surgeon has the option of an excision at gingival level, or a deep resection including surrounding tissue. This involves extraction of the affected tooth and curettage of the alveolar socket to remove any remnants of periodontal ligament. The excision at gingival level will often be chosen if histopathology is still required to differentiate it from focal gingival hyperplasia. The more aggressive resection may be chosen when the diagnosis is known, or if the lesion causes displacement of a tooth (see Figure 10.13). The prognosis following surgical resection is good, though recurrence following incomplete excision is common.

Acanthomatous ameloblastoma
The acanthomatous ameloblastoma is a benign but locally invasive tumour (Figures 10.15 and 10.16), which is a fairly common oral tumour in dogs, but only a few occurrences have been reported in cats.

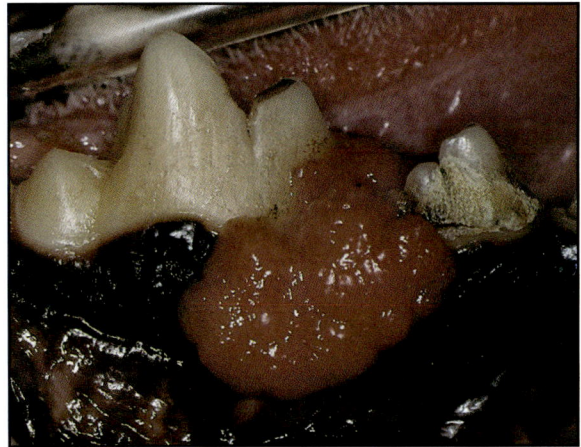

10.15 Acanthomatous ameloblastoma in a mixed-breed dog, emerging from the gingiva between the mandibular fourth premolar and the first molar teeth.

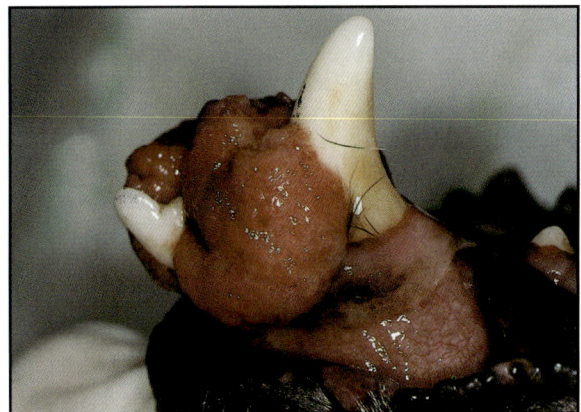

10.16 Acanthomatous ameloblastoma of the rostral mandible of an American Pitbull Terrier. Note the rostral displacement of the lateral incisor tooth.

Terminology used to describe acanthomatous ameloblastoma has varied and includes acanthomatous epulis, peripheral ameloblastoma, basal cell carcinoma and adamantinoma. The latter term is now no longer used.

Clinical presentation and diagnosis
The acanthomatous ameloblastoma appears in the gingiva, often surrounding and sometimes displacing one or more teeth. The lesions are often raised, sessile and have a soft cauliflower-like surface. Radiographically they can show lytic invasion of the underlying alveolar bone. They are slow growing, and, if left untreated, can become grotesque in size with extensive jaw bone involvement, and thereby mimic advanced stages of oral malignancies. These tumours do not metastasize. The diagnosis is made radiographically and by histopathology.

Treatment and prognosis
Treatment is by surgical resection with wide margins (at least 1 cm) and the prognosis following complete excision is good. Radiation therapy has proved to be a very successful treatment modality for the acanthomatous ameloblastoma, but there is a fairly high risk (1:8 in one study) (Thrall *et al.*, 1981) of malignant

transformation at a later stage, which may occur at the site of the previous lesion. Radiation therapy should be considered in those cases where surgical resection with wide margins is not an option.

Ameloblastoma (central ameloblastoma)

This fairly rare tumour of dogs and cats is slow growing and locally invasive. In contrast to the acanthomatous ameloblastoma, it often grows in the depth of the alveolar bone without gingival involvement, although gingiva and alveolar mucosa are likely to be secondarily expanded with increasing size of the tumour. Ameloblastomas do not tend to metastasize.

Clinical presentation and diagnosis

The ameloblastoma is an expansive intrabony lesion, and displacement of teeth may be present. Radiographically, ameloblastomas can be cystic or solid, and may present with osteolysis around associated tooth roots. The latter may have a similar radiographic appearance to a dentigerous cyst, and only histopathological evaluation may differentiate the two (Dubielzig, 1982; Anderson and Fong Revenaugh, 2000).

Treatment

Surgical resection with wide margins has been reported to be successful. Radiation therapy has been employed for the treatment of ameloblastomas in a small number of reported cases, with a 1 in 4 success rate (Dubielzig and Thrall, 1982). The number of reported cases is too small, however, to draw any firm conclusions about the usefulness of radiotherapy in the treatment of ameloblastomas.

Amyloid-producing odontogenic tumour

This tumour has often been called a calcifying epithelial odontogenic tumour, a term used for a common epithelial odontogenic tumour in humans. However, histological differences have led to the proposal of the term amyloid-producing odontogenic tumour (Gardner *et al.*, 1994). Although generally fairly rare in dogs and cats, it is one of the more common odontogenic tumours found in cats (Figure 10.17).

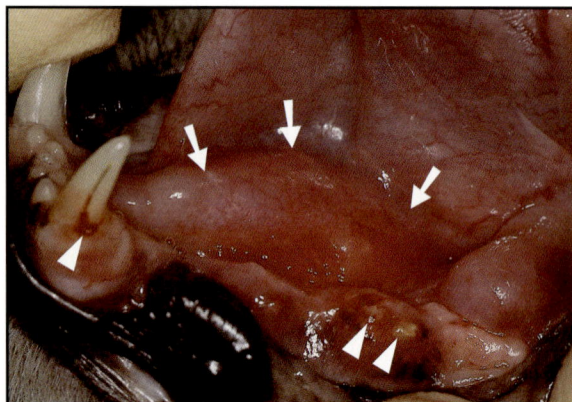

10.17 Amyloid-producing odontogenic tumour in a Domestic Shorthair cat. The tongue has been lifted upwards for the photograph. Note the expansion and swelling of the tumour extending towards the left sublingual area (arrowed). The coincidental finding of resorptive lesions of two teeth is indicated by arrowheads.

Clinical presentation and diagnosis

Clinical presentation can be similar to the squamous cell carcinoma, with a friable, ulcerated surface. Some amyloid-producing odontogenic tumours are melanotic, making them difficult to distinguish clinically from malignant melanoma. The amyloid-producing odontogenic tumour appears histologically fairly well demarcated from the surrounding tissue but is not encapsulated. It does not infiltrate bone but can erode bone and appears to grow by expansion, though some authors consider it locally invasive. Radiographs may show mineralization within the mass, and marked periosteal reactions may occur (Figure 10.18).

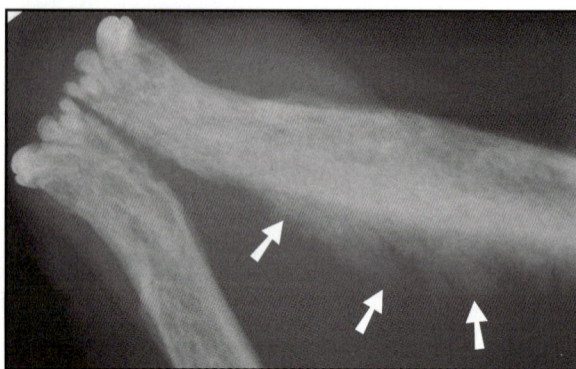

10.18 Radiograph of an amyloid-producing odontogenic tumour in the mandible of a cat. Note the marked periosteal reaction on the lingual aspect, which takes on a 'sun-burst' pattern in places (arrowed).

Treatment

According to the histological description, surgical excision with a narrow margin would appear to be appropriate surgical management, but detailed reviews of surgical treatment of these tumours are lacking in the literature. Recurrence following incomplete excision is possible, and radiation therapy should be considered as an adjunct following incomplete surgical resection.

Feline inductive odontogenic tumour

This tumour has been found mainly in cats aged 14 months or younger. It has also been described as inductive fibroameloblastoma and as ameloblastic fibroma.

Clinical presentation and diagnosis

The tumour appears to occur primarily in the rostral maxilla or mandible, and tends to show varying growth rates. It may be locally invasive, but metastasis has not been reported. Radiographically, lysis of the underlying bone is common and occasionally areas of mineralization within the tumour may be seen. Teeth may be missing in larger lesions and the tumour may invade the nasal cavity.

Treatment

Surgical resection with margins of normal tissue would appear to be the appropriate treatment. Radiation therapy as an adjunct to surgery may be considered in cases where complete surgical resection cannot be achieved.

Benign oral neoplasia (non-odontogenic)

Viral papillomatosis

Viral papillomas occur mostly in young dogs and are caused by a papovavirus (Figure 10.19). Their clinical presentation is very typical, with a pale grey and filiform surface. They are usually self-limiting and do not tend to cause interference with normal function except in rare cases, where multiple lesions cover extensive areas of the oral cavity and may cause severe halitosis and functional problems. Treatment in these rare, extreme cases consists of surgical resection, but recurrence is common.

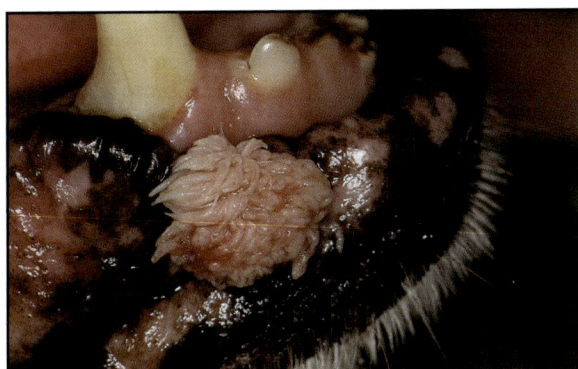

10.19 Viral papilloma in a Labrador Retriever. This dog was 13 years old but the majority of viral papillomas occur in young dogs.

Fibroma

Fibromas may occur on the lips and surrounding facial areas in cats. Surgical resection is usually successful. Caution should be exercised in dogs with a diagnosis of oral fibroma, because fibrosarcomas can appear histologically benign but be biologically aggressive (Ciekot *et al.*, 1994).

Other

Lipomas, haemangiomas, neurofibromas, chondromas and osteomas occur occasionally in the oral cavity. Some tumours are classified as neither benign nor malignant, as they represent solitary lesions with malignant potential, e.g. mast cell tumours and plasmacytomas (Figure 10.20).

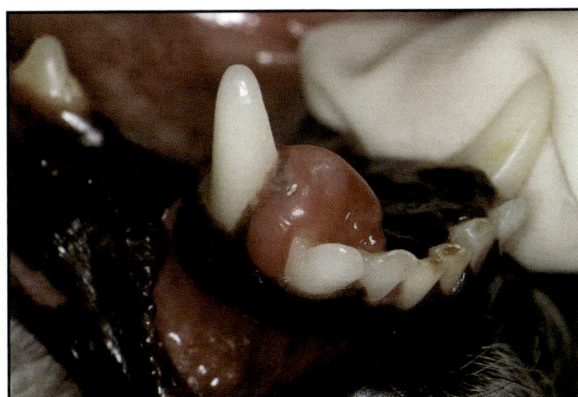

10.20 Plasmacytoma in the rostral mandible of a Cairn Terrier. Note the resemblance in clinical appearance to many other oral tumours.

The management of benign oral tumours follows general principles of oral and oncological medicine and surgery. For more detail, please refer to the *BSAVA Manual of Canine and Feline Oncology*.

Malignant oral neoplasia (non-odontogenic)

The oral cavity is a common site of malignant neoplasia in both dogs and cats. Early lesions can be confused with benign lesions, just as advanced benign lesions can mimic malignant tumours. Biopsy is therefore required to form a diagnosis and prognosis for the patient. It must be remembered that highly inflamed

Group code	Group	Stage code	Stage
T	Primary tumour	TIS	Pre-invasive carcinoma (carcinoma *in situ*)
		T1	Tumour 2 cm or less maximum diameter: (a) without bone involvement (b) with bone involvement
		T2	Tumour 2–4 cm or less maximum diameter: (a) without bone involvement (b) with bone involvement
		T3	Tumour more than 4 cm maximum diameter: (a) without bone involvement (b) with bone involvement
N	Regional lymph nodes	N0	Regional lymph nodes not palpable
		N1	Movable ipsilateral nodes: (a) Nodes not considered to contain growth (b) Nodes considered to contain growth
		N2	Movable contralateral or bilateral nodes: (a) Nodes not considered to contain growth (b) Nodes considered to contain growth
		N3	Fixed nodes
M	Distant metastasis	M0	No evidence of distant metastases
		M1	Distant metastases present

Stage Grouping	
I	T1; N0, N1a or N2a; M0
II	T2; N0, N1a or N2a; M0
III	T3; N0, N1a or N2a; M0; *or* any bone involvement, *or* any T, N1b
IV	Any T; N2b or N3; M0; *or* any T, any N, M1

10.21 WHO staging system for tumours of the oral cavity (World Health Organization, 1984).

tissue at the surface may only represent reactive tissue, while the neoplastic lesion itself may be located deeper within the jaw. Deep incisional biopsies or small *en bloc* resections including jaw bone are therefore recommended. For details on treatment modalities for malignant oral neoplasia, refer to the *BSAVA Manual of Canine and Feline Oncology*.

Once an oral malignancy has been diagnosed, staging according to the TNM classification can be meaningful (Figure 10.21). Herring *et al.* (2002) proposed that parotid, mandibular and medial retro-pharyngeal lymph nodes should be excised completely and submitted for histopathological evaluation, because all of the named lymph nodes receive drainage from the oral cavity and the maxillofacial region. Serial sectioning of lymph nodes by the pathologist provides additional information for metastatic detection (Herring *et al.*, 2002).

Malignant melanoma

The malignant melanoma is the most common oral malignancy in dogs; it is rarer in cats. Amelanotic malignant melanomas may look similar to many other oral lesions (Figure 10.22). Conversely, if a black lesion is found in the oral cavity, it is not pathognomonic of malignant melanoma, as other oral lesions can become melanotic as well. Most malignant melanomas appear on the gingiva and alveolar mucosa in older dogs and cats, but have also been found on the buccal mucosa, the palate and tongue. Radiographically, irregular bone destruction may be seen.

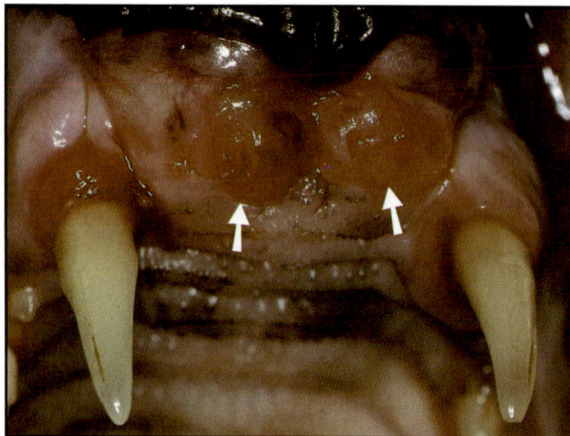

10.22 Amelanotic malignant melanoma (arrowed) on the rostral maxilla in a cat.

Treatment

Of major concern in oral malignant melanomas is that in a high percentage of cases metastases to regional lymph nodes and lungs are present at the time of diagnosis. Multimodular treatment may therefore result in longer survival times compared with surgery or radiation therapy alone. In a study by Rassnick *et al.* (2001), there was an indication that carboplatin may be considered an appropriate adjunct to local treatment, and activity against macroscopic tumours had been noted. The study included 27 dogs with spontaneously occurring malignant melanoma; of these, 25 were oral malignant melanomas and two were dermal malignant

melanomas. One dog with oral malignant melanoma and regional lymph node metastases responded with 100% tumour size reduction and no recurrence at the time of euthanasia for unrelated reasons 950 days after initiation of treatment. Six dogs had a partial response with tumour size reduction of < 100% but > 50% for a median duration of 165 days. A report by Bergman *et al.* (2003) indicated that immunotherapy may play an important role in adjunct treatment of malignant melanoma in the future.

Successful local control of the tumour may be improved by wide marginal or radical excision, or by radiation therapy.

Squamous cell carcinoma

Squamous cell carcinoma is the most common oral tumour in cats (60–70% of all oral tumours) (Figures 10.23 and 10.24) and it is the second most common oral malignancy in dogs (Figure 10.25) (Stebbins *et al.*, 1989; Harvey and Emily, 1993). It is a fast-growing oral mass that can arise from any mucosal surface, including the tonsils. Its surface is often ulcerated. The oral squamous cell carcinoma tends to show varying degrees of malignancy based on the location in the oral cavity. More rostral locations carry relatively better prognoses, as they tend to be more amenable to surgical resection with wide margins, and they are slower to metastasize. In more caudal locations, lesions appear to show a faster growth rate and metastasize quicker, and surgical options may be more limited.

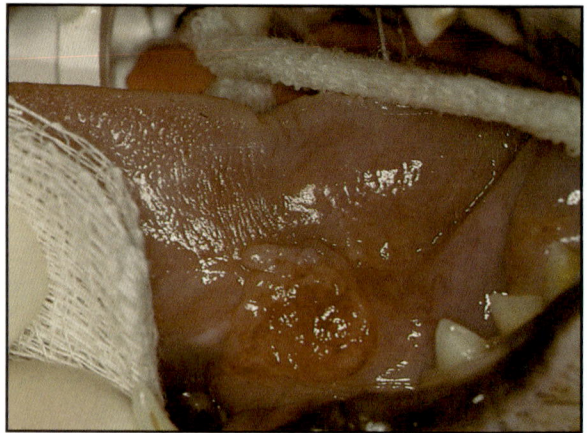

10.23 Sublingual squamous cell carcinoma in a cat.

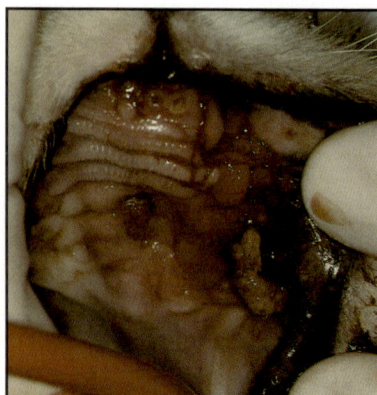

10.24 Squamous cell carcinoma of the caudal maxilla in a cat. Note the predominantly destructive growth pattern.

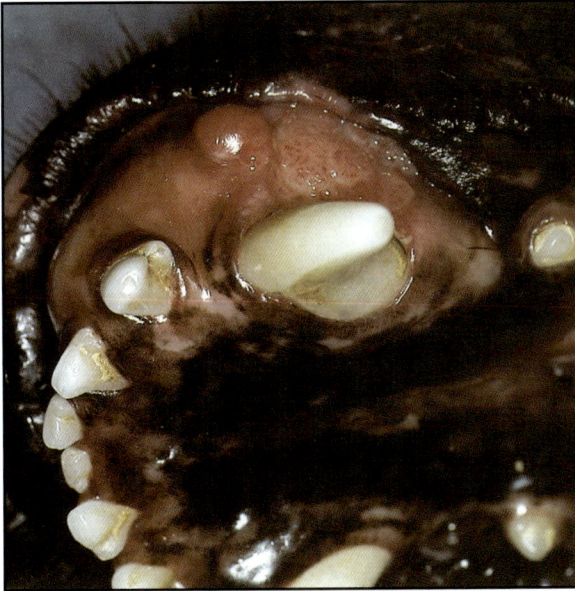

10.25 Squamous cell carcinoma of the rostral mandible in a mixed-breed dog. Note the swelling with partially ulcerated surface on the labial aspect of the right mandibular canine and lateral incisor teeth.

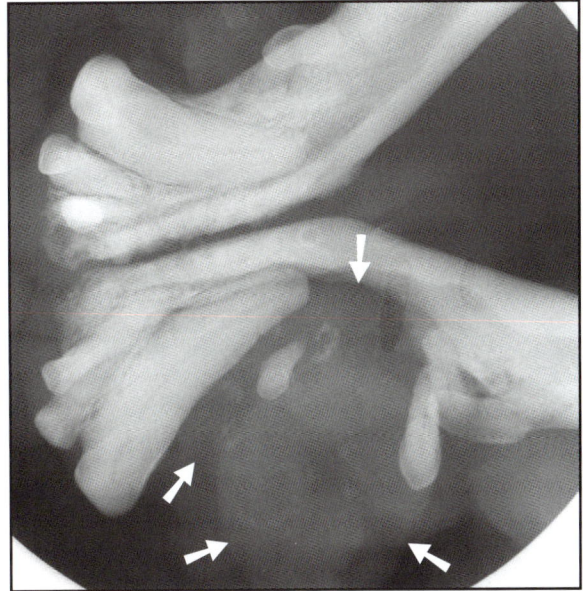

10.26 Radiograph of the rostral mandible of a Boxer with squamous cell carcinoma (arrowed). Note the aggressive bone destruction.

Special considerations in cats

Squamous cell carcinoma commonly presents in a sublingual location in cats. However, on presentation of an undiagnosed sublingual mass lesion, it must be remembered that not all sublingual lesions are squamous cell carcinomas (see Figure 10.17) (Kapatkin *et al.*, 1991). Another particular feature of the oral squamous cell carcinoma in cats is that lesions in more caudal locations may be predominantly destructive and lytic (see Figure 10.24). Death due to distant metastasis is unusual, and most cats die due to complications from local tumour growth and invasion. A retrospective study of treatment modalities for oral squamous cell carcinoma in 52 cats found survival rates in the region of 2–3 months for surgery or radiation therapy alone, or with a combination of radiation therapy and chemotherapy or local hyperthermia (Postorino-Reeves *et al.*, 1993). A study of seven cats with mandibular squamous cell carcinoma described the use of surgery (mandibulectomy and mandibular lymph node resection) followed by radiation therapy and reported a median survival time of 14 months (Hutson *et al.*, 1992). The results of these studies and many other reports on the treatment of feline squamous cell carcinoma suggest that a very guarded prognosis must be given. However, treatment options should be considered for each individually.

Treatment

Radiographically, oral squamous cell carcinomas tend to show aggressive bone destruction (Figure 10.26). Treatment consists of surgical excision with a wide margin (at least 1 cm), and multimodular treatment methods may be chosen to help to improve survival times if complete excision cannot be achieved. Radiation therapy has proved to be a useful adjunct in the treatment of canine gingival squamous cell carcinoma.

Piroxicam, a non-steroidal analgesic, has been shown to have a potential palliative effect on oral squamous cell carcinomas in dogs. In some cases, partial and total remission of the lesion can be achieved, and in addition it has analgesic properties (Frimberger, 2000; Schmidt *et al.*, 2001). Piroxicam has not been evaluated in cats.

Papillary squamous cell carcinoma: Papillary squamous cell carcinomas may occur in young dogs, often in the first year of life. Early lesions may look similar to viral papillomas. They are locally invasive, and recurrence following incomplete excision is common. Surgical resection with wide margins of at least 1 cm should be performed, or a combination of surgery and radiation therapy may be used if wide surgical resection is not an option.

Fibrosarcoma

Fibrosarcomas are the second most common malignant tumour of the oral cavity in cats and the third most common in dogs (Figure 10.27). They tend to occur at a younger age compared with other oral malignancies. They are firm, often flat masses that are deeply attached to the underlying tissue. Ulceration is not as common as in other oral tumours. Radiologically, a brush-border periosteal reaction may be seen. Fibrosarcomas show aggressive local infiltration to such a degree that radical surgical excision with at least 2 cm margins has to be recommended. Recurrence following conservative surgery is common. The metastatic potential is variable. Histologically low grade fibrosarcomas have less metastatic potential than high grade lesions. However, particular attention should be paid to the potential of a fibrosarcoma to present as a histologically low grade lesion yet behave as a biologically high grade lesion (Ciekot *et al.*, 1994).

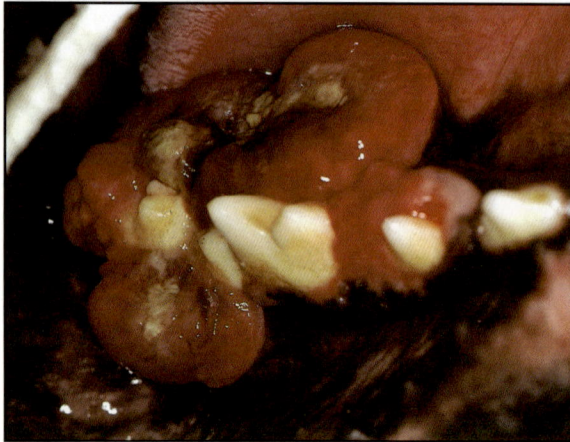

10.27 Fibrosarcoma of the mandible in a 4-year-old Labrador Retriever.

Osteosarcoma

Six percent of osteosarcomas in dogs are located in the mandible and maxilla. The prognosis following surgery with appropriate margins is more favourable for oral osteosarcoma than for those of other skeletal locations. Radical surgery may produce better local control than conservative surgery.

Lymphoma (malignant lymphoma, lymphosarcoma)

Lymphomas can occur anywhere on the oral mucosa. They may present as flat or raised pink masses. Lymphosarcoma of the oral cavity represented 3.4% of oral tumours in the cat in one survey (Harvey and Emily, 1993). The feline leukaemia virus (FeLV) status should be checked in all cases, although in recent years a decrease in FeLV-positive cats with lymphoma has been noted. The incidence of FeLV-positive cats with lymphoma is higher in the younger age group (Nelson and Couto, 1998). Lymphoma of the oral cavity is slightly less common in dogs. Oral lymphosarcoma is most often part of disseminated lymphosarcoma, and therefore may present as only a minor part of the clinical syndrome. About a third of canine lymphoma cases are of T-cell origin and carry a far worse prognosis than lymphoma derived from B-cells.

Specific forms of lymphoma in the dog that can affect the oral cavity as well are the epitheliotropic cutaneous lymphoma (also known as mycosis fungoides) and the non-epitheliotropic cutaneous lymphoma. Clinically, these forms of lymphoma can present as solitary or multiple nodules and plaques. Immunophenotyping of histopathological samples will be required to obtain a definitive diagnosis in these cases (Moore *et al.*, 2000). Refer to the *BSAVA Manual of Canine and Feline Oncology* for more information on lymphoma.

Special surgical considerations

En bloc resections of jaw bone

Techniques are described in many surgical publications. Refer to the *BSAVA Manual of Canine and Feline Oncology*. These surgeries are performed with observation of tumour-free margins if complete local control is to be achieved. The surgeon first designs and performs the resection, and then has to design appropriate closure of the created defect with the aid of mucogingival flap techniques (see Chapter 11), sometimes with flaps drawn from the facial and cervical skin (Pavletic, 1993). Particular attention should be paid to the tension-free closure of the wound margins. To achieve this, the flap must be sufficiently undermined and mobilized, the cut bone margins smoothed and rounded, and sufficiently large bites of tissue taken with a reverse cutting needle during closure, in a double layer when possible. Suture lines, in particular in maxillectomy sites, should be positioned over bony support to help prevent wound dehiscence, though some surgeons have good results without the placement of suture lines over bony support as long as tension-free suturing can be achieved (Salisbury, 2003). An adequate blood supply must be maintained to the mucosal flap. This can best be achieved by designing the flap with a broad base and maximum thickness. Avoidance of the use of electrocoagulation along the wound edges is important for successful wound healing.

Another factor that may contribute to wound dehiscence following *en bloc* jaw bone resections is the movement of the jaws and tongue by the patient. Soft food that is easily swallowed should be offered for one month postoperatively, and toys and chews should be withdrawn. Restriction of jaw movements can be achieved by cheiloplasty or by placement of a tape-muzzle (Harvey and Emily, 1993).

Partial wound dehiscence may occur in as many as one-third of maxillectomy cases (Schwarz *et al.*, 1991) and, depending on the extent of the resectional surgery, may result in oronasal or oroantral fistulas.

Another potential complication of ostectomy of the jaw bones is damage to adjacent teeth. Tooth roots that are transected during ostectomy must be extracted at the time of surgery. If the alveolus of a tooth root is entered so that the tooth root is partially exposed but not visibly damaged, and the tooth is seated firmly in its alveolus, it may be left in place. The owner must be warned that the tooth may develop problems with its periodontium and/or its pulp, and may require treatment at a later date.

Tumours of the tongue

The tongue is the site of 4% of non-odontogenic oropharyngeal tumours. Surgical resection of up to 60% of the tongue is well tolerated by dogs (Carpenter *et al.*, 1993). Partial glossectomy techniques involve preplacement of sutures, wide simple interrupted sutures for wedge glossectomy and horizontal mattress sutures for transverse glossectomy (Dunning, 2003). Care must be exercised to avoid tying down the tongue when operating in a sublingual location.

Cats only tolerate minimal lingual resections, such as wedge glossectomy. Though technically possible, transverse glossectomy of most of the free part of the lingual body results in high morbidity after surgery, and oral feeding may not be re-learned.

Conditions of the salivary glands pertaining to oral mass lesions

Salivary sialoceles

A sialocele is an accumulation of saliva in the subcutaneous tissue next to a salivary gland or duct. Mucoceles are sialoceles that also contain a mucus component (see Chapter 1; the parotid gland produces serous secretion only, while the other major salivary glands produce seromucus secretions). They are lined with inflammatory connective tissues and can thus be differentiated from cysts, which have epithelial linings. The aetiology is predominantly traumatic but can also be idiopathic. The major salivary glands are located caudal to the oral cavity, and a common site for the formation of a sialocele is the intermandibular cervical area (cervical mucocele) (see *BSAVA Manual of Head, Neck and Thoracic Surgery* for more details). The ducts of the mandibular and sublingual salivary glands and the polystomatic part of the sublingual salivary gland are located in the sublingual space. A mucocele of these salivary systems will cause a sublingual swelling or ranula.

Diagnosis and treatment

Diagnosis is by paracentesis of the swelling. If fluid can be aspirated, cytology can be used to confirm the presence of a mucus component by the use of special staining, such as the periodic acid–Schiff (PAS) technique.

Definitive treatment is removal of the salivary gland. Treatment of ranulae by marsupialization has been described. A portion of the overlying sublingual mucosa is removed with an elliptical incision. The pocket of saliva is emptied and the rim of oral mucosa is sutured to the adjacent connective tissue lining. Marsupialization may not provide satisfactory long-term results, because the lining of the mucocele is comprised of fibrous or inflammatory tissue.

Sialoliths

A sialolith is a salivary stone formed within a salivary duct. It can cause obstruction, swelling or rupture of the affected gland. Sialoliths are rare in dogs and have been reported only in the parotid duct. They must be differentiated from odontogenic tumours and other oral tumours with foci of mineralization. Diagnosis is by palpation, radiography, ultrasonography or sialography. Treatment involves incision of the parotid duct over the sialolith and its removal. The duct should be subsequently cannulated and flushed to ensure patency. Closure of the duct incision is not necessary.

Salivary gland tumours

Tumours of the salivary gland are rare in dogs and cats, and are most commonly found in the parotid and mandibular glands. Adenocarcinoma and carcinoma are the most common types of neoplasia diagnosed in salivary glands. Distant metastasis may occur. Sialoceles may form part of the clinical presentation of a salivary gland tumour. Careful differentiation is therefore warranted.

Other causes of swellings of salivary glands

Sialadenosis is an idiopathic non-inflammatory, non-neoplastic enlargement of salivary glands, which has been reported in dogs and cats (Sozmen *et al.*, 2000).

Salivary gland necrosis has been described in dogs and is characterized by enlarged, hard, painful salivary glands, which, depending on the location of the glands, may also be accompanied by laryngopharyngeal complaints (retching, regurgitation). In a retrospective study of 19 cases, 16 presented with associated conditions, most of which affected the oesophagus. In those cases where successful treatment of the associated condition was possible, the salivary gland necrosis resolved as well (Schroeder and Berry, 1998).

Lipomatous infiltration of the parotid or mandibular salivary gland in dogs has been reported (Brown *et al.*, 1997). It carries a good prognosis following surgical excision.

Idiopathic external tooth resorption

Feline odontoclastic resorptive lesions

Feline odontoclastic resorptive lesions (FORLs) are very common in cats (Figures 10.28 and 10.29). Epidemiological data on prevalence vary depending on whether the group of cats were presented to the veterinary hospital for dental reasons or for any other reasons, or whether museum skull specimens were examined. It appears that up to around 30% of cats presented for any reason to veterinary hospitals have FORLs. This figure increases to around 60% prevalence of FORLs in cats presented for dental disease. The disease can occur from about 2 years of age onwards, and its prevalence increases with increasing age (van Wessum *et al.*, 1992). All teeth can be affected, and a patient with FORLs of one tooth has a high risk of developing FORLs in multiple teeth. The teeth most commonly affected are the maxillary and mandibular third premolars, the maxillary fourth premolar and the mandibular first molar teeth (Reiter and Mendoza, 2002).

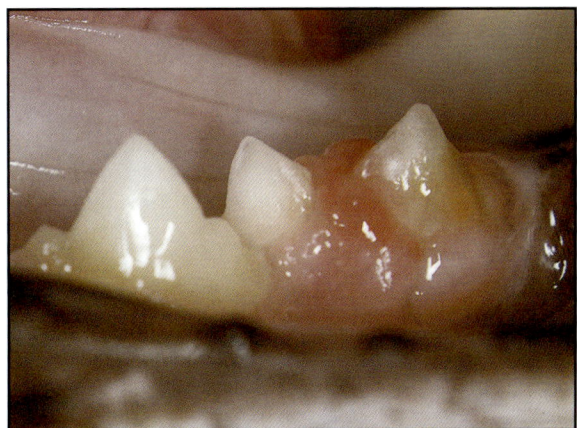

10.28 FORL of the mandibular left first molar tooth. Central parts of the crown are missing. Note the relatively low grade inflammation of the granulation tissue, which is forming a small focal hyperplastic gingival lesion.

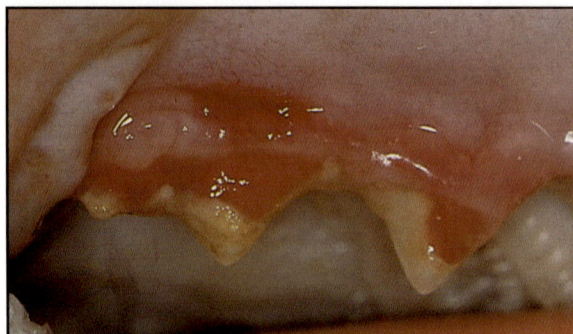

10.29 Multiple FORLs and associated multifocal gingival hyperplasia in a Domestic Shorthair cat.

Aetiology and pathogenesis

The aetiology of FORLs is still unknown. There is evidence in one study (Reiter, 2003) of an association between high levels of 25-hydroxyvitamin D and presence of FORLs. As some commercial cat foods contain concentrations of vitamin D that exceed the recommended concentration of 250 IU/kg dry matter, there is a possible link between excessive vitamin D intake and FORLs (Reiter, 2003). Further studies are required to investigate this possible link.

The pathogenesis of FORLs is fairly well understood. Resorptive lacunae are formed on the surface of dental hard tissue, in which odontoclasts are attached to the cementum or dentine surface and continue their clastic activity (Gauthier *et al.*, 2001). This process can be found in the physiological shedding of deciduous teeth, but any such activity in the permanent dentition is pathological. It has been suggested that the periodontal ligament has an inherent protective function against clastic resorption of the tooth root. One study showed loss of the periodontal ligament architecture and narrowing of the periodontal ligament space in what might have been early FORLs (Gorrel and Larsson, 2002). Once the odontoclastic activity has begun, it progresses into the root and/or crown of the tooth. According to the depth of the resorptive lesion, the following classification has been suggested (Reiter and Mendoza, 2002):

- Stage 1 lesion: cementum only affected
- Stage 2 lesion: cementum and crown or root dentine affected; lesions are likely to become painful once dentinal tubules are exposed
- Stage 3 lesion: dental pulp is affected as well; these lesions are assumed to be painful
- Stage 4 lesion: extensive structural damage has occurred, dentoalveolar ankylosis may have occurred
- Stage 5 lesion:
  - 5a: the crown is lost, and only root remnants or 'ghost roots' are left
  - 5b: the crown is present, but almost all root structure is lost.

Complete staging of FORLs therefore always requires radiography. Many authors propose that any cat presented for dental disease should undergo full-mouth dental radiography, to help to detect FORLs

subgingivally (amongst other disorders that are only revealed radiographically) (Verstraete *et al.*, 1998). A study by Heaton *et al.* (2004) proposed a rapid screening technique for the FORL status in cats. By evaluating the radiographs of the mandibular left and right third premolar teeth (307 and 407), this study was able to determine, with a sensitivity of 78.5%, whether or not a cat had odontoclastic resorptive lesions.

Clinical presentation

The resorptive lesion may not be visible on oral examination, if its activity is contained subgingivally. Once it has extended into the dentine and enamel of the crown it becomes clinically visible in the form of punched-out, often triangular defects (see Figure 10.28) filled with highly vascular granulation tissue.

The tooth crown may already be partially or completely lost as a result of being weakened and undermined by the destructive process. Occasionally, less inflamed and slightly more prominent granulation tissue can fill the defects and forms a subcategory of focal gingival hyperplastic lesions in cats (see Figures 10.2 and 10.29). A fine sharp explorer (Figure 10.30) helps in the clinical evaluation of teeth in the anaesthetized cat, and may detect FORLs if they are positioned just at, or below, the level of the gingival margin. Rather than finding a smooth transition from very smooth and hard enamel to slightly rougher cementum (the explorer tip will transmit a tactile sensation to the examiner's hand), a defect may cause the tip of the explorer to sink in, as though it 'falls over the edge'. It is important to differentiate this finding from the tactile sensation transmitted by the tooth furcation and subgingival calculus. This is easily determined by performing subgingival scaling on any questionable area, and then repeating the exploration. A gentle constant puff of air from a three-way syringe, directed along the crown of the tooth, will inflate the free gingival sulcus (or pocket wall) sufficiently to allow subgingival visualization.

Radiographically, FORLs may show notched radiolucencies with sharp or scalloped margins (Figure 10.31). The root may be ankylosed, which means that the periodontal ligament space around the root is lost

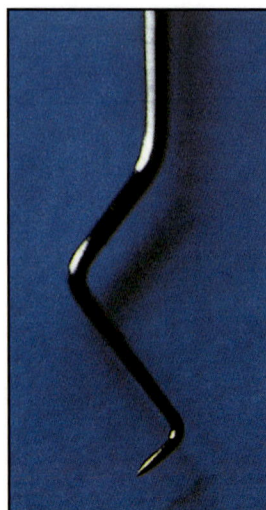

10.30 The tip of a fine sharp explorer. This instrument is used with a light touch for subgingival exploration in cats' teeth and should be held so that the working tip is at an angle of nearly 90 degrees to the surface that it explores.

and the tooth root appears to continue into alveolar bone without any demarcation between them. Another radiographic presentation is that of root replacement resorption, in which the root appears to become bone-like. This leads to the appearance of 'ghost roots', or in some cases the roots may not be visible radiographically at all. Resorptive lesions in the canine teeth of cats often show slightly different radiographic changes in that the pattern of root dentine lysis often appears longitudinally, oriented to the long axis of the tooth, giving the root a striated appearance.

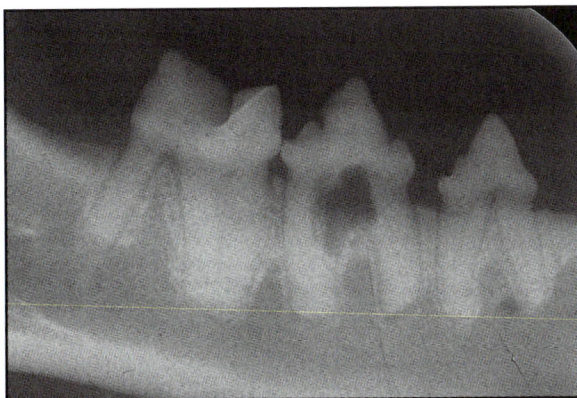

Radiograph of a FORL of the mandibular right fourth premolar tooth.

Treatment

Treatment of FORLs consists of extraction of the affected teeth. This is performed under the assumption that the patient is likely to experience discomfort or pain from the affected tooth at least during some of the stages of disease progression. Unfortunately, the evaluation of dental pain in cats with FORLs is not straightforward. Resentment of the dental examination can be interpreted as pain in some cases, but may be behavioural in others. Anorexia or inappetence may be a presenting complaint that suggests dental pain in the absence of other common causes of anorexia in cats. In many cases of coincidental diagnosis of FORLs during a routine physical examination of the cat, the owner may report that the cat has a good appetite and no obvious signs of pain. There are multiple anecdotal reports, however, that the behaviour of the cat following a dental procedure is improved to such an extent that owners feel retrospectively that the cat may have been in discomfort and pain prior to the procedure. Another indication for extraction of teeth with FORLs is that lesions may predispose periodontal disease, which can progress to presentations of combined multiple FORLs and severe periodontal disease.

Research results suggest a possible medical alternative to extraction or a possible preventive medication for FORLs. Alendronate, a bisphosphonate used extensively in postmenopausal women for the treatment of osteoporosis, has been shown to bind to periodontal bone and tooth root surfaces in cats (Mohn *et al.*, 2003). It is hypothesized that it may exert a protective or anticlastic effect in this location, and a pilot study showed encouraging results. Some cats treated with oral alendronate appeared to show less progression of FORLs in terms of size of the lesions, and it arrested further lesion development in some cases (Harvey, 2003). Further studies are required to investigate the therapeutic potentials of alendronate in cats.

Special considerations

Extraction of teeth with FORLs is commonly difficult for two reasons: (i) the extensive damage to tooth structure predisposes to fragmentation of the roots during extraction; and (ii) root ankylosis can make regular luxation and elevation impossible. Some authors therefore suggest the use of the crown amputation technique with intentional root retention (Du Pont, 1995, 2002; Harvey, 2003).

> **WARNING**
> **This technique must not be misused as a blanket replacement for proper extraction technique. It has very specific indications and contraindications. It should always be accompanied by thorough dental diagnostics, including dental radiographs.**

- *Indications.* Ankylosed roots and 'ghost roots' (usually stage 4 and 5 lesions).
- *Contraindications.* Clinical or radiographic evidence of endodontic disease, periodontal pocketing or generalized stomatitis and improper technique of mucogingival flaps for closure over the resected roots.
- *Complications.* Oral pain and development of painful sinus tracts associated with chronic infection of root remnants, sometimes leading to osteomyelitis.

The gingival tissue is reflected and the tooth is resected with a dental bur to below the alveolar margin, then the gingiva is sutured over the remaining 'root' segment. Some of these deliberately retained roots will be completely resorbed and some will stay in place for the life of the cat, without clinical consequences.

Regular postoperative examinations are necessary to monitor the healing following intentional root retention. Any foci of inflammation of the gingiva at the site of crown amputation that are present after healing is expected to be complete (2–6 weeks postoperatively, which may depend on the choice of suture material) may indicate chronic infection of the retained root segment, and complete removal is indicated. Follow-up radiographic examination of these cases is mandatory.

> **WARNING**
> **This approach remains a controversial issue, as the outcome is not always favourable and because of the risk of misuse of the technique. Even with good technique, the question of the fate of the remaining pulp in the root segment remains unanswered. It is possible that the patient may be in considerable pain from pulpitis for some time after the procedure. The benefits of a shortened procedure under general anaesthetic have to be carefully weighed against the risk of possible complications.**

Canine odontoclastic resorptive lesions (CORLs)

Odontoclastic resorptive lesions occur rarely in older dogs (see Figures 10.10 and 10.32). They often present as coincidental findings, and dogs tend not to show obvious signs of pain associated with affected teeth. Similar to the equivalent phenomenon in cats, it is difficult to understand how lesions that expose dentinal tubules and cause communications of dental pulp with the oral cavity can exist without the presence of very obvious signs of pain. Due to the difficulty in evaluation of chronic pain in animals, however, one has to assume that some form of discomfort and chronic pain will be associated with affected teeth. Therefore extraction of teeth with CORLs is recommended.

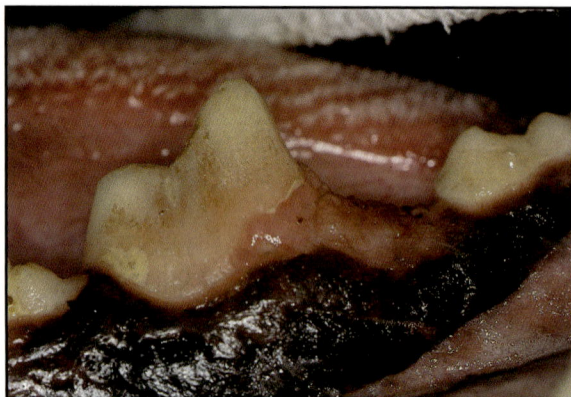

10.32 CORL of a mandibular left first molar tooth. Note the extensive damage to the crown structure and presence of granulation tissue, which appeared firmer and less vascularized than the equivalent tissue in cats. (Same dog as in Figure 10.10.)

References and further reading

Anderson JG and Fong Revenaugh A (2000) Canine oral neoplasia. In: *An Atlas of Veterinary Dental Radiology*, eds DH DeForge and BH Colmery, pp. 89–99. Iowa State University Press, Ames, Iowa

Bellows J (2001) Laser use in veterinary dentistry. *Proceedings of the 15th Annual Veterinary Dental Forum 2001*, pp. 221–228

Bergman PJ, McKnight J, Novosad A, Charney S, Farrelly J, Craft D, Wulderk M, Jeffers Y, Sadelain M, Hohenhaus AE, Segal N, Gregor P, Engelhorn M, Riviere I, Houghton AN and Wolchok JD (2003) Long-term survival of dogs with advanced malignant melanoma after DNA vaccination with xenogeneic human tyrosinase. A phase I trial. *Clinical Cancer Research* 9, 1284–1290

Brown PJ, Lucke VM, Sozmen M, Whitbread TJ and Wyatt JM (1997) Lipomatous infiltration of the canine salivary gland. *Journal of Small Animal Practice* 38, 234–236

Carpenter LG, Withrow SJ, Powers BE, Ogilvie GK, Schwarz PD, Straw RC, LaRue SM and Berg J (1993) Squamous cell carcinoma of the tongue in 10 dogs. *Journal of the American Animal Hospital Association* 29, 17–24

Ciekot PA, Powers BE, Withrow SJ, Straw RC, Ogilvie GK and LaRue SM (1994) Histologically low-grade, yet biologically high-grade, fibrosarcomas of the mandible and maxilla in dogs: 25 cases (1982–1991). *Journal of the American Veterinary Medical Association* 204(4), 610–615

Dhaliwal R, Kitchell BE and Manfra Maretta S (1998) Oral tumour in dogs and cats. Part I: Diagnosis and clinical signs. *Compendium on Continuing Veterinary Education* 20, 1011–1021

Dubielzig RR (1982) Proliferative dental and gingival diseases of dogs and cats. *Journal of the American Animal Hospital Association* 18, 577–584

Dubielzig RR and Thrall DE (1982) Ameloblastoma and keratinizing ameloblastoma in dogs. *Veterinary Pathology* 19, 596–607

Dunning D (2003) Tongue, lips, cheeks, pharynx, and salivary glands. In: *Textbook of Small Animal Surgery, 3rd edition*, ed. D Slatter, p. 554. Saunders, Philadelphia

Dupont G (1995) Crown amputation with intentional root retention for advanced feline resorptive lesions – a clinical study. *Journal of Veterinary Dentistry* 12(1), 9–13

Dupont G (2002) Crown amputation with intentional root retention for dental resorptive lesions in cats. A step-by-step contribution. *Journal of Veterinary Dentistry* 19(2), 107–110

Eickhoff M, Seeliger F, Simon D and Fehr M (2002) Erupted bilateral compound odontomas in a dog. *Journal of Veterinary Dentistry* 19, 137–143

Felizzola CR, Trierveiler Martins M, Stopiglia A, Soares de Araujo N and Orsini Machado de Sousa S (2003) Compound odontoma in three dogs. *Journal of Veterinary Dentistry* 20, 79–83

Frew DG and Dobson JM (1992) Radiological assessment of 50 cases of incisive or maxillary neoplasia in the dog. *Journal of Small Animal Practice* 33, 11–18

Frimberger AE (2000) Anticancer drugs: new drugs or applications for veterinary medicine. In: *Kirk's Current Veterinary Therapy XIII Small Animal Practice*, pp. 474–478. Saunders, Philadelphia

Galgut PN, Dowsett SA and Kowolik (2001) *Periodontics: Current Concepts and Treatment Strategies*, ed. PN Galgut *et al.*, pp. 78–79. Martin Dunitz Ltd., London

Gardner DG, Dubielzig RR and McGee EV (1994) The so-called calcifying epithelial odontogenic tumour in dogs and cats (amyloid-producing odontogenic tumour). *Journal of Comparative Pathology* 111, 221–230

Gauthier O, Boudigues S, Pilet P, Aguado E, Heymann D and Daculsi G (2001) Scanning electron microscopic description of cellular activity and mineral changes in feline odontoclastic resorptive lesions. *Journal of Veterinary Dentistry* 18, 171–176

Gorrel C and Larsson A (2002) Feline odontoclastic resorptive lesions: unveiling the early lesion. *Journal of Small Animal Practice* 43(11), 482–488

Hale FA and Wilcock BP (1996) Compound odontoma in a dog. *Journal of Veterinary Dentistry* 13, 93–95

Harty FJ (1994) *Concise Illustrated Dental Dictionary, 2nd edn*. Wright, Oxford

Harvey CE (2003) Odontoclastic resorptive lesions (ORL) in cats. *Proceedings of Hill's European Symposium on Oral Care*, pp. 42–48

Harvey CE and Emily P (1993) *Small Animal Dentistry*. Mosby, St Louis, Missouri

Harvey CE, Mohn KL, Jacks TM, Schleim KD, Miller B and Feeney WP (2003) Alendronate inhibits progression of feline odontoclastic resorptive lesions. *Proceedings of the 12th European Congress of Veterinary Dentistry 2003*, p. 13

Heaton M, Wilkinson J, Gorrel C and Butterwick R (2004) A rapid screening technique for feline odontoclastic resorptive lesions. *Journal of Small Animal Practice* 45, 598–601

Herring ES, Smith MM and Robertson JL (2002) Lymph node staging of oral and maxillofacial neoplasms in 31 dogs and cats. *Journal of Veterinary Dentistry* 19, 122–126

Holmstrom SE, Frost Fitch P and Eisner ER (2004) *Veterinary Dental Techniques for the Small Animal Practitioner, 3rd edn*. Saunders, Philadelphia

Hutson CA, Willauer CC, Walder EJ, Stone JL and Klein MK (1992) Treatment of mandibular squamous cell carcinoma in cats by use of mandibulectomy and radiotherapy: seven cases (1987–1989). *Journal of the American Veterinary Medical Association* 201(5), 777–781

Kapatkin AS, Manfra Maretta S, Patnaik AK, Burk RL and Matus RE (1991) Mandibular swellings in cats: prospective study of 24 cats. *Journal of the American Animal Hospital Association* 27, 575–580

Mohn KL, Jacks TM, Schleim KD, Halley B and Feeney WP (2003) Alendronate binds to periodontal bone and tooth root surfaces in cats. *Proceedings of the 12th European Congress of Veterinary Dentistry 2003*, p. 12

Moore PF, Affolter VK and Vernau W (2000) Immunophenotyping in the dog. In: *Kirk's Current Veterinary Therapy XIII Small Animal Practice*, ed. JD Bonagura, pp. 505–509. Saunders, Philadelphia

Nelson RW and Couto CG (1998) *Small Animal Internal Medicine, 2nd edition*. Mosby, St Louis, Missouri

Odom T and Anderson JG (2000) Proliferative gingival lesion in a cat with disseminated cryptococcosis. *Journal of Veterinary Dentistry* 17(4) 177–181

Pavletic M (1993) *Atlas of Small Animal Reconstructive Surgery*. Lippincott, Philadelphia

Postorino Reeves NC, Turrel JM and Withrow SJ (1993) Oral squamous cell carcinoma in the cat. *Journal of the American Animal Hospital Association* 29, 438–441

Poulet FM, Valentine BA and Summers BA (1992) A survey of epithelial odontogenic tumors and cysts in dogs and cats. *Veterinary Pathology* 29, 369–380

Rassnick KM, Ruslander DM, Cotter SM, Al-Sarraf R, Bruyette DS, Gamblin RM, Meleo KA and Moore AS (2001) Use of carboplatin for treatment of dogs with malignant melanoma: 27 cases (1989–2000). *Journal of the American Veterinary Medical Association* **218**(9), 1444–1448

Reiter AM (2003) The role of calciotropic hormones in the etiology of feline odontoclastic resorptive lesions (FORL). *Proceedings of the 12th European Congress of Veterinary Dentistry 2003*, pp. 14–15

Reiter AM and Mendoza KA (2002) Feline odontoclastic resorptive lesions: an unsolved enigma in veterinary dentistry. *The Veterinary Clinics of North America: Small Animal Practice* **32**, 791–837

Salisbury KS (2003) Maxillectomy and mandibulectomy. In: *Textbook of Small Animal Surgery, 3rd edn*, ed. D Slatter, p. 563. Saunders, Philadelphia

Schmidt BR, Glickman NW, DeNicola DB, de Gortari AE and Knapp DW (2001) Evaluation of piroxicam for the treatment of oral squamous cell carcinoma in dogs. *Journal of the American Veterinary Medical Association* **218** (11), 1783–1786

Schroeder H and Berry WL (1998) Salivary gland necrosis in dogs: a retrospective study of 19 cases. *Journal of Small Animal Practice* **39**, 121–125

Schwarz PD, Withrow SJ, Curtis CR, Powers BE and Straw RC (1991) Partial maxillary resection as a treatment for oral cancer in 61 dogs. *Journal of the American Animal Hospital Association* **27**, 617–624

Sitzman C (2000) Simultaneous hyperplasia, metaplasia, and neoplasia in an 8-year-old boxer dog: a case report. *Journal of Veterinary Dentistry* **17**, 27–30

Soames JV and Southam JC (1998) *Oral Pathology, 3rd edn*. Oxford University Press, Oxford

Sozmen M, Brown PJ and Whitbread TJ (2000) Idiopathic salivary gland enlargement (sialadenosis) in dogs: a microscopic study. *Journal of Small Animal Practice* **41**, 243–247

Stebbins KE, Morse CC and Goldschmidt MH (1989) Feline oral neoplasia: a ten-year survey. *Veterinary Pathology* **26**, 121–128

Thrall DE, Goldschmidt MH and Biery DN (1981) Malignant tumor formation at the site of previously irradiated acanthomatous epulis in four dogs. *Journal of the American Veterinary Medical Association* **178**, 127–132

Van Wessum R, Harvey CE and Hennet P (1992) Feline dental resorptive lesions. prevalence patterns. *The Veterinary Clinics of North America: Small Animal Practice* **22**, 1404–1416

Verstraete FJM, Kass PH and Terpak CH (1998) Diagnostic value of full-mouth radiography in cats. *American Journal of Veterinary Radiology* **59**(6), 692–695

Verstraete FJM, Ligthelm AJ and Weber A (1992) The histological nature of epulides in dogs. *Journal of Comparative Pathology* **106**, 169–182

Walsh KM, Denholm LJ and Cooper BJ (1987) Epithelial odontogenic tumours in domestic animals. *Journal of Comparative Pathology* **97**, 503–521

11

Dental surgical procedures

Alexander M. Reiter

Extraction of teeth (*exodontics*) is one of the most frequently performed procedures in small animal practice (Harvey and Emily, 1993). It should not be treated lightly, as 'extraction' is final. Utilizing good instrumentation and applying proper techniques can help to provide a stress-free and controlled procedure for the operator with minimal trauma to the patient, faster recovery and healing, and more dependable long-term results (Kertesz, 1993).

Indications

The most common indications for tooth extraction in dogs are periodontal disease and tooth fracture, and in cats tooth resorption (FORL) and gingivostomatitis. If any disease process is too advanced for the teeth to be saved, extraction is necessary. Financial and other considerations may lead the client to request extraction (Harvey and Emily, 1993). Indications for extraction include:

- *Periodontal disease.* Teeth affected by periodontal disease are usually extracted if periodontal health cannot be restored, or if the client is unwilling to commit to a combination of oral home and periodic professional care
- *Tooth resorption.* About one-third of domestic cats (Reiter and Mendoza, 2002) suffer from idiopathic resorption of multiple permanent teeth. Extraction of the affected teeth is the current recommended treatment of choice
- *Tooth crown or root fracture with pulp exposure.* A tooth fractured beyond repair, or beyond the owner's financial constraints to preserve the tooth, must be extracted
- *Endodontic or periapical disease.* Teeth with pulpitis, pulp necrosis or periapical disease for which endodontic treatment is inappropriate, or is declined by the owner, must be extracted
- *Caries.* Maxillary and mandibular first and second molars in dogs are most commonly affected. These teeth must be extracted if restoration or endodontic treatment are not feasible
- *Persistent deciduous teeth.* Two homologous teeth should never be in the mouth at the same time and at the same location (i.e. permanent tooth has erupted and corresponding deciduous tooth has not yet exfoliated). Persistent deciduous teeth interfere with the normal

eruption pathway of their permanent successors. They can then compete for the same space in the mouth, which may result in malocclusion and crowding, predisposing to periodontal disease
- *Malocclusion.* Maloccluding teeth should be extracted if they interfere with masticatory function, cause trauma to other tissues or lead to periodontal disease and if orthodontic treatment, occlusal equilibration or other corrective techniques are not feasible or are declined by the client
- *Supernumerary teeth.* Extra teeth can cause crowding and may interfere with normal occlusion and periodontal health
- *Non-functional malformed teeth.* Malformed teeth may interfere with normal occlusion and periodontal health. Restoration is often not feasible because of the extent or type of malformation or for economic reasons
- *Unerupted (retained) teeth.* If no cause can be identified for a tooth to remain unerupted, it is termed an embedded tooth. Embedded teeth must be periodically evaluated radiographically. An unerupted tooth is considered impacted if the path of eruption is blocked or impaired. Unerupted teeth in adult animals must be removed using surgical extraction principles to prevent infection, pressure necrosis and the potential formation of a dentigerous cyst and/or neoplasia
- *Fractured and retained roots.* These must be extracted if they communicate with the oral cavity or are associated with periodontal, endodontic or periapical disease. Roots may also be identified radiographically following radical jaw resections
- *Teeth in areas of osteomyelitis and osteonecrosis.* Antimicrobial therapy is supported by extraction of involved teeth and aggressive debridement of infected tissues
- *Teeth involved with or surrounded by oral neoplasia.* Teeth in biopsy sites and those interfering with normal occlusion and mastication (as a result of neoplasia) should be extracted
- *Diseased teeth in a jaw fracture line.* Those with moderate to severe periodontitis should always be extracted. A multi-rooted tooth may be sectioned and the loose crown-root segment removed, while the solid crown-root segment(s) surrounded by reasonably healthy periodontium may be retained. Endodontic treatment must be performed on the remaining tooth segment(s) Reiter *et al.*, 2003).

The general opinion that teeth in fracture lines must always be extracted, regardless of health, should be rejected, as they may be used as anchor points during jaw fracture repair and provide stability to the fracture repair (see Chapter 9)
- *Traumatically displaced teeth.* Luxated teeth should be extracted if they cannot be repositioned and treated endodontically. Nasally intruded teeth must be extracted to prevent chronic secondary rhinitis and intermittent epistaxis
- *Client preference.* Extraction is performed when the client desires less expensive but definitive treatment. Alternative treatments for strategic teeth (i.e. canines and carnassials) should be recommended if the periodontium is sound.

Tooth extraction is to be encouraged rather than leaving pathology untreated.

Contraindications
Tooth extraction is contraindicated (Holmstrom *et al.*, 1998) in:

- Patients that cannot be anaesthetized due to health concerns
- Patients undergoing radiation therapy involving the jaws that would inhibit healing
- Patients with uncontrolled bleeding disorders
- Patients on medications that may cause prolonged bleeding times or prevent healing.

Preparation

Client
Alternative treatments should always be discussed with the client, as extraction is final. The client's approval must be obtained for the extent of treatment, the cost anticipated by the clinician and a plan of action in the event that an unexpected problem requiring further treatment is discovered during the extraction procedure (Holmstrom *et al.*, 1998). This is essential to avoid the potential for future litigation.

Patient
Reasonable health, determined by physical examination and laboratory tests, is required when an animal is to undergo general anaesthesia.

- An endotracheal tube with inflated cuff and an oropharyngeal pack will prevent blood, calculus and other debris from entering the trachea or oesophagus.
- The jaws should be securely propped open without unnecessary strain on the temporomandibular joints. The use of sprung gags is to be avoided.
- A towel beneath the patient's head will cushion it from pressure during the procedure.
- Ophthalmic lubricating ointment will protect eyes from drying and a cloth covering the face will prevent skin and fur soiling.
- The anaesthetized animal should be placed in a comfortable position that allows easy access to the side of the mouth being operated on.

Veterinary dentists are fortunate to work with tissues that have an abundant blood supply and an epithelial surface constantly bathed by saliva, a fluid rich in antimicrobial properties. Healing of incisional wounds in oral mucosa is more rapid than in skin, with superior phagocytic activity and earlier epithelialization. Infections after oral surgery procedures are rare despite preoperative preparation of the oral mucosa being more difficult than skin, and despite the inability to isolate the affected area postoperatively.

Extractions should ideally be performed in a clean mouth. Scaling and polishing the teeth followed by preoperative rinsing with dilute chlorhexidine gluconate (0.12%) aids in reducing bacteraemia and prevents calculus and other debris from contaminating the alveolar sockets and interfering with normal wound healing. Perioperative broad-spectrum antibiotics are given in selected cases, such as:

- Debilitated and immunocompromised patients
- Patients suffering from organ disease, endocrine disorders, cardiovascular disease and severe local and systemic infection
- Patients having permanent implants and transplants.

Dental radiographs should be obtained prior to tooth extraction to evaluate alveolar bone health and variations in root anatomy, and to determine the presence of dentoalveolar ankylosis or replacement resorption of roots that could potentially complicate the extraction procedure (see Chapter 2). Additional pain control is achieved by nerve blocks and field/infiltration blocks using longer-lasting local anaesthetics intraoperatively (see Chapter 3).

Technician
Laws vary with regard to extraction of teeth performed by registered veterinary nurses or technicians. The law in most countries forbids them from performing surgery. However, closed extractions are often referred to as 'non-surgical', thus presenting a potential conflict for the veterinary nurse or technician (Holmstrom, 2000).

The American Veterinary Dental College (AVDC) developed a position statement regarding veterinary dental health care providers (adopted 5 April, 1998): 'Only veterinarians shall determine which teeth are to be extracted and perform extraction procedures ...' In the United Kingdom at present Schedule 3 does not allow veterinary nurses to perform open (surgical) extractions, but they may extract loose teeth under the direct supervision of the veterinary surgeon who has made the diagnosis requiring this treatment option.

Operator
Practice on a cadaver and familiarity with dental anatomy are mandatory prior to performing new techniques on a patient (Figure 11.1). Safety measures during extraction procedures include the wearing of safety glasses, masks and gloves (see Chapter 4). Adequate lighting, magnification, suction, use of an air/water syringe, and relative position of the clinician and patient are all factors affecting visibility.

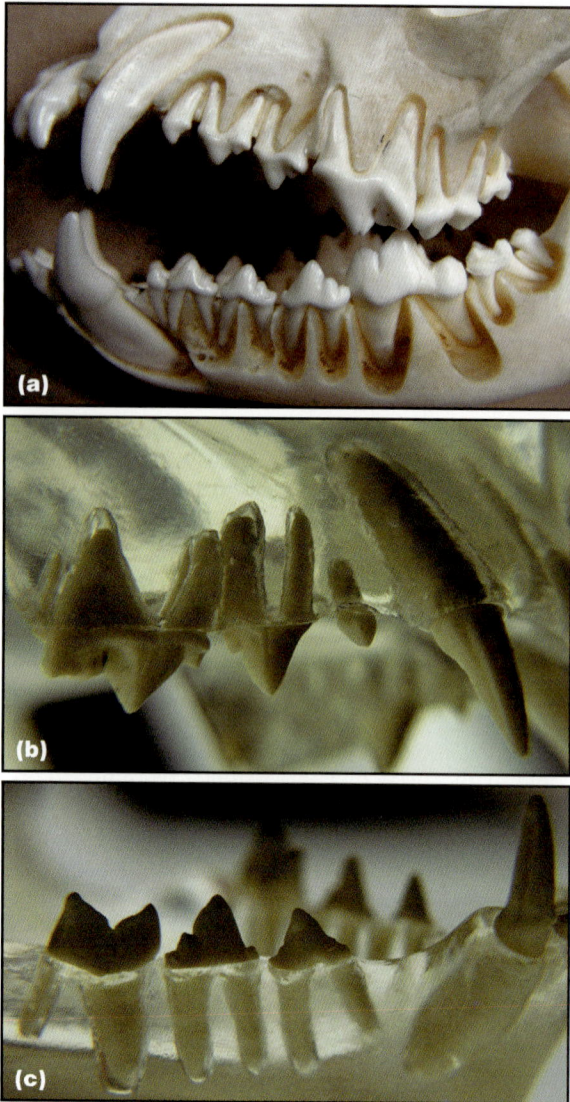

11.1 Study models. **(a)** Buccal alveolar bone has been removed in this dog skull to show the buccal aspects of the roots of these teeth. **(b and c)** Transparent plastic models are also available to review root anatomy of upper and lower teeth in cats and dogs.

During maxillary tooth extractions, the patient's head is cradled with the palm of the free hand over the bridge of the maxilla. During mandibular tooth extractions, the lower jaw can be cradled in the palm of the free hand, or the individual side can be grasped between the thumb and forefinger. These positions help to prevent jaw fracture by neutralizing pressure applied to the bone during extraction. Luxators and elevators are grasped with the butt of the handle seated in the palm and the index finger extended along the blade of the instrument to act as a stop should the instrument slip. Used in this way, iatrogenic damage is prevented (Harvey and Emily, 1993).

Mechanics

Teeth are anchored to the alveolar bone of the mandibles, incisive bones and maxillae by soft tissue components of the periodontium, the gingiva and periodontal ligament. During the extraction process, these tissues must be severed (junctional epithelium and gingival connective tissue) or stretched and torn (periodontal ligament) to allow delivery of the tooth being extracted. Gentle tissue handling is important to minimize trauma and to allow rapid healing of both soft and hard tissues.

Carnivores' incisor roots are often curved and flattened oval in cross-section, providing anti-rotational retention. The canine tooth of the dog has a curved root with an oval cross-section. Its maximum bulbosity (circumference) is not at the cementoenamel junction or the alveolar margin, but at some distance apical to them. Through this feature, alveolar bone locks the root into the jaw. Divergence of premolar and molar roots is another important retention aid. The mesial roots of mandibular carnassial teeth in dogs have indentations (developmental grooves) with a corresponding alveolar ridge for additional anti-rotational retention (Figure 11.2). Cheek teeth in cats

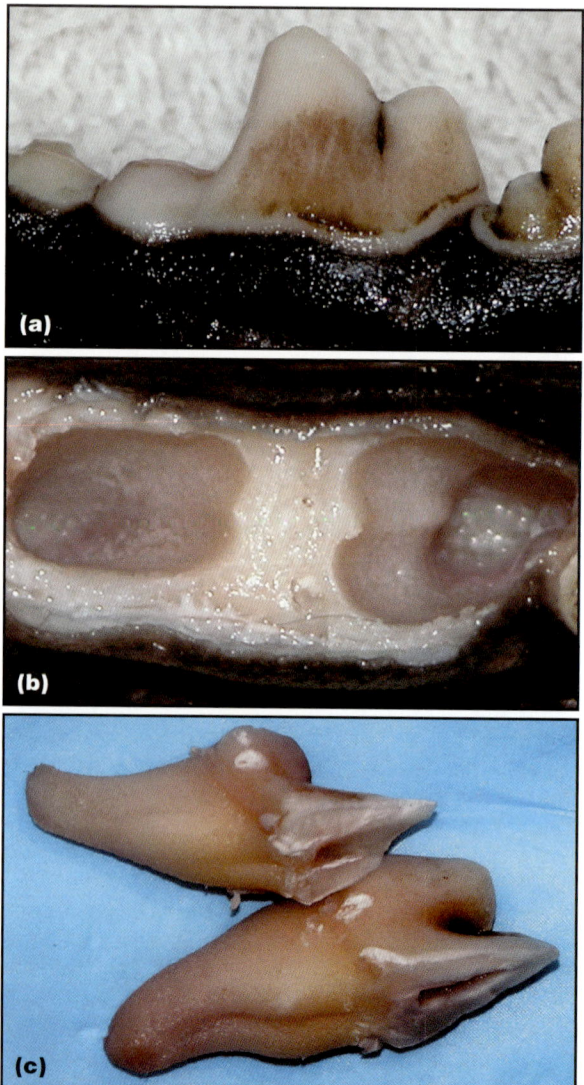

11.2 The mesial (and to some extent the distal) roots of lower carnassial teeth in dogs have indentations (developmental grooves) with a corresponding alveolar ridge for anti-rotational retention. **(a)** Lower first molar. **(b)** Occlusal view of both alveoli; note alveolar ridges. **(c)** Extracted crown-root segments; note indentations along root surfaces.

often have bulbous apices due to hypercementosis, which increases retention. Cheek teeth in small dogs may have apically curved roots reaching into the ventral mandibular cortex. Both of these clinical scenarios can make extraction of the teeth a challenging process (Kertesz, 1993). In the dog the incisors, canines, first premolars and mandibular third molars are single-rooted teeth; in the cat, the incisors, canines and commonly the maxillary second premolars are single-rooted. The cat's maxillary first molars may be treated as single-rooted teeth; even though they have more than one root, these roots are usually fused together.

Three basic types of lever (Figure 11.3) are involved in tooth extraction (Holmstrom *et al.*, 1998):

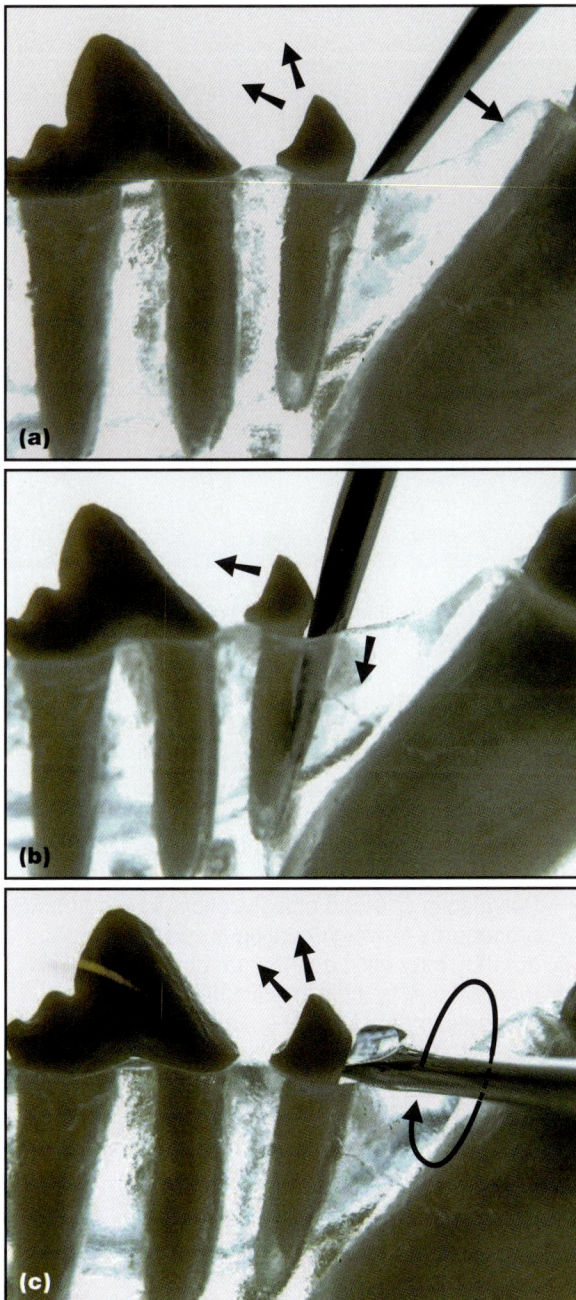

11.3 Three basic types of lever. **(a)** First-class. **(b)** Wedge. **(c)** Wheel and axle.

- A first-class lever, with a fulcrum between the resistance and the force
- A wedge lever
- A wheel and axle lever.

Instrumentation

Extraction is considered a surgical procedure and since the instruments will enter tissue they must be sterile.

- Dental radiographic equipment
- High-speed dental turbine with water irrigation
- Non-surgical-length and surgical-length dental burs: cross-cut fissure (701, 702), round ($1/4$, $1/2$, 1, 2, 4) and pear-shaped (330, 331, 332)
- Number 3 scalpel handle with blades (11, 15, 15c)
- Small periosteal elevators
- Dental elevators
- Dental luxators
- Small extraction forceps
- Root tip picks/forceps
- Small spoon curettes
- Irrigation solutions (sterile polyionic fluid, dilute chlorhexidine)
- Gauze sponges
- Gingival scissors
- Small Metzenbaum scissors
- Bone implant materials
- Needle holders
- Fine tissue forceps
- Absorbable suture material (4/0, 5/0) with swaged-on needle
- Small Mayo scissors

11.4 Ideal instrumentation required for tooth extraction.

Luxators
Dental Luxators® (DirectaDental, Sweden) have sharp and often thin-tipped blades designed to penetrate into the narrow periodontal space and cut periodontal ligament fibres (wedging force). Luxators are made of softer steel and should not be used with a leverage technique for large teeth or root fragments, as they can easily bend or break.

Elevators
The size of dental elevators should closely approximate the size of the tooth or root segment being elevated. Most are made of hard steel. The relative thickness of some elevator tips often makes them unsuitable for wedging between the tooth and alveolar bone (unless space has been created by a luxator). Luxating elevators are now available with thin, sharp tips.

The blade of the instrument is gently worked into the space between the tooth and the alveolar bone. A well controlled rotational motion around the shank's long axis between the root and a fulcrum point (vertical rotation) (Figure 11.5) is performed to create a slow, gentle and steady pressure on the tooth. This pressure is held for at least 10 seconds to break down the periodontal ligament fibres. The elevator can also be

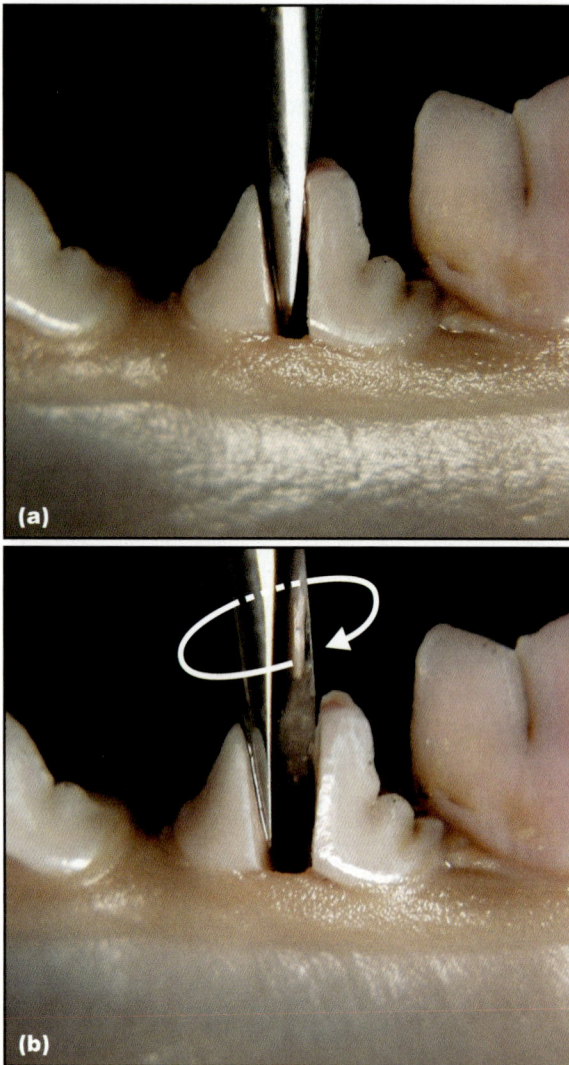

11.5 Vertical rotation. **(a)** The elevator is inserted parallel to and between two crown segments. **(b)** The elevator is rotated around its long axis.

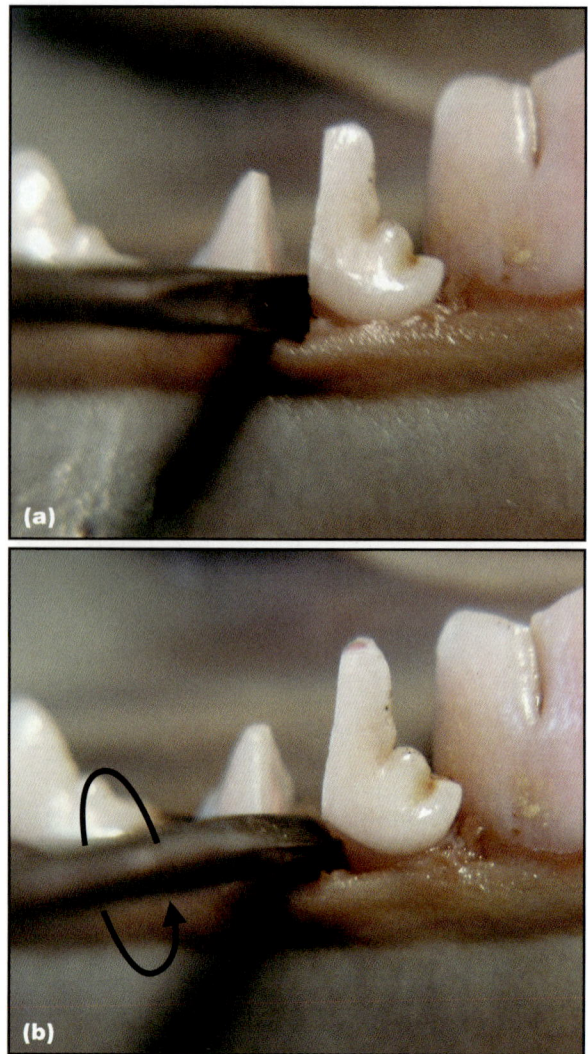

11.6 Horizontal rotation. **(a)** The elevator is inserted perpendicular to and between two crown-root segments. **(b)** The elevator is rotated around its long axis.

placed perpendicular to the tooth or root segment to lever it out of the alveolus through the line of least resistance, with a fulcrum point preferably on alveolar bone (horizontal rotation) and not on adjacent teeth (unless the tooth used as a fulcrum is to be extracted as well) (Figure 11.6).

Ideally both dental luxators and elevators should be used and sharpened frequently.

Extraction forceps

Extraction forceps should have a narrow beak, fit the tooth as closely as possible and be applied as far apically on the tooth as possible to reduce the chances of root fracture. They should only be applied when the tooth is very loose. Forceps can easily apply excessive or improper forces resulting in tooth fracture (Harvey and Emily, 1993).

Suture material

An absorbable suture material is preferred for wound closure in the oral cavity so that sedation or anaesthesia for suture removal can be avoided.

- Chromic catgut persists for 4–7 days and elicits the greatest inflammatory tissue reaction of all suture materials. Its use is not recommended. Therefore, a longer-lasting synthetic material is preferred in dogs and cats to avoid early wound breakdown.
- Polyglactin 910 and polyglycolic acid are good for procedures in which healing is relatively rapid, but they may elicit an inflammatory tissue reaction due to their multifilament nature.
- Synthetic monofilament sutures induce the least foreign body reaction in oral tissues.
- Polyglecaprone 25 is the preferred suture material for most oral surgeries (1.5 (4/0) for dogs; 1 (5/0) for cats and small dogs) and persists for about 3–5 weeks.
- The use of polydioxanone for closure of extraction sites is discouraged, due to its prolonged persistence.

Small swaged-on 3/8-circle reverse-cutting needles cause minimal tissue drag and are recommended for the suturing of oral tissues (Verstraete, 1999). When inflamed and friable soft tissues are sutured, a round tapered needle may be preferred to avoid severing the flap.

Techniques

The principles of tooth extraction (Figure 11.7) are to reduce or eliminate the retentive factors of the roots. Forceps should not be applied to teeth until such a level of mobility has been obtained that the instrument can be used solely for the delivery of the tooth or roots (Kertesz, 1993). It is best to slowly stretch, sever and tear the periodontal ligament fibres using luxators and elevators. Little benefit is achieved by working forcefully against the mechanical factors that retain the teeth. A rotational motion should be used and the tooth eased out of the socket rather than forced. The entire root must be removed. The key to effective tooth extraction is patience.

- Obtain preoperative dental radiographs
- Section multi-rooted teeth into single-rooted segments
- Perform surgical extraction where indicated
- Do not create incision lines over a future void
- Minimize thermal damage by water irrigation
- Avoid excessive alveolectomy
- Stretch and tear the periodontal ligament fibres
- Keep index finger close to the instrument tip
- Use free hand to support the jaw
- Do not use force, but use slow steady pressure
- Do not leave root fragments behind
- Smooth rough alveolar bone edges
- Provide fresh soft tissue margins
- Cover any exposed bone with soft tissue
- Do not suture flaps under tension

11.7 Principles of tooth extraction.

Extractions can be performed using the closed technique, i.e. without raising a mucoperiosteal flap, or using the open technique, i.e. raising a mucoperiosteal flap to expose alveolar bone (Gorrel and Robinson, 1995).

Closed extraction technique

Single-rooted teeth

1. Insert a scalpel blade into the gingival sulcus or periodontal pocket, direct it at 45 degrees to the long axis of the tooth to the depth of the alveolar margin, and incise the gingival attachment around the tooth.
2. Insert a luxator/elevator between the gingival margin and the crown or exposed root at an angle of 10–20 degrees to the long axis of the tooth.
3. Force the luxator/elevator apically between the alveolar bone and the root, using it as a wedge lever.
4. Once there is enough space created between the tooth and alveolar bone, the procedure may proceed with elevators only. Apply pressure while slowly rotating the elevator through a small arc. At the end of each rotation, hold the instrument firmly against the tissues for at least 10 seconds. Place a slow, gentle, steady pressure on the tooth rather than quick, rocking motions to fatigue and tear the periodontal ligament fibres. Haemorrhage into the widened periodontal space assists in tearing fibres through hydraulic pressure.
5. As the periodontal space widens, it is often helpful to change from smaller to larger instruments. Work not only in areas where progress appears to be made but return to more resistant sites. Move the elevator around the whole circumference of the tooth and gradually advance apically until the tooth begins to loosen. At this time the elevator may be used as a first-class or wheel and axle lever to elevate the tooth out of the socket (a notch may be made with a bur at the neck of the tooth for better instrument purchase).
6. When the tooth is sufficiently loose (i.e. it can move freely within its alveolar socket), forceps may be placed as far apically on the tooth as possible, and the tooth rotated slightly around its long axis with a steady pull and removed from its socket. Extraction forceps are to be used with extreme care because, if incorrectly applied or used with excessive force, their use will result in crown and/or root fracture.
7. Examine the extracted tooth, ensuring that the entire root has been extracted. Most roots have a smooth tip. Obtain a radiograph if there is any suspicion that a root fragment is retained in the alveolus.
8. If necessary, debride the alveolus with a spoon curette to remove granulation tissue, debris, pus and bony fragments.
9. Use a large diamond-coated round bur with water irrigation to reduce, shape and smooth the alveolar margin (alveoloplasty).
10. Gently lavage the extraction site, preferably with a polyionic solution (e.g. Ringer's lactate) (Buffa *et al.*, 1997). Air or air/water spray must not be blown into an extraction socket, as it may result in emphysema or air embolism.
11. Leave a blood clot (an essential part of socket healing) in the alveolus. If there is no bleeding into the socket, the socket should be curettaged with a curette to initiate bleeding and formation of a clot. Based on the belief that they aid haemostasis and healing of the extraction site and prevent the occurrence of infection, the alveolus may be packed with various materials, such as:
    - Autogenous bone grafts
    - Bioglass® and other synthetic osteopromotive materials
    - Materials made of gelatine, polysaccharides (e.g. cellulose), collagen and calcium alginate
    - Bone wax
    - Polylactic acid granules
    - Tetracycline powder.

12. Digitally compress the extraction area with a gloved finger or a damp gauze pack, and suture the gingiva using a simple interrupted tension-free pattern. Suturing may not be necessary when extracting very small teeth and if minimal damage has occurred to periodontal tissues. Suturing is required when packing the alveolus with the aforementioned materials.

Two- and three-rooted teeth

A radiograph should be taken prior to extraction to determine whether a mobile multi-rooted tooth can be extracted using the closed technique. If it can, the tooth is removed as one unit by severing its gingival attachment and loosening the roots with dental luxators and elevators. An elevator can sometimes be placed into an open furcation perpendicular to the long axis of the tooth to gain good purchase, and coronally directed pressure applied to remove the tooth, provided that the roots are not divergent or hooked. If extraction forceps are used, each root must be completely loosened before extraction, and minimal twisting used to remove the tooth. If little space exists between two teeth, a fissure bur can be used to remove the dental bulge at the mesial or distal surface of the tooth to be extracted to facilitate placement of the elevator during the leverage process (care must be taken to avoid damage to the tooth that will be retained) (Figure 11.8). In selected cases where one root of the tooth is severely affected by periodontitis but the periodontium of the other root is still relatively healthy, bisection and endodontic treatment of the remaining crown-root segment may be performed.

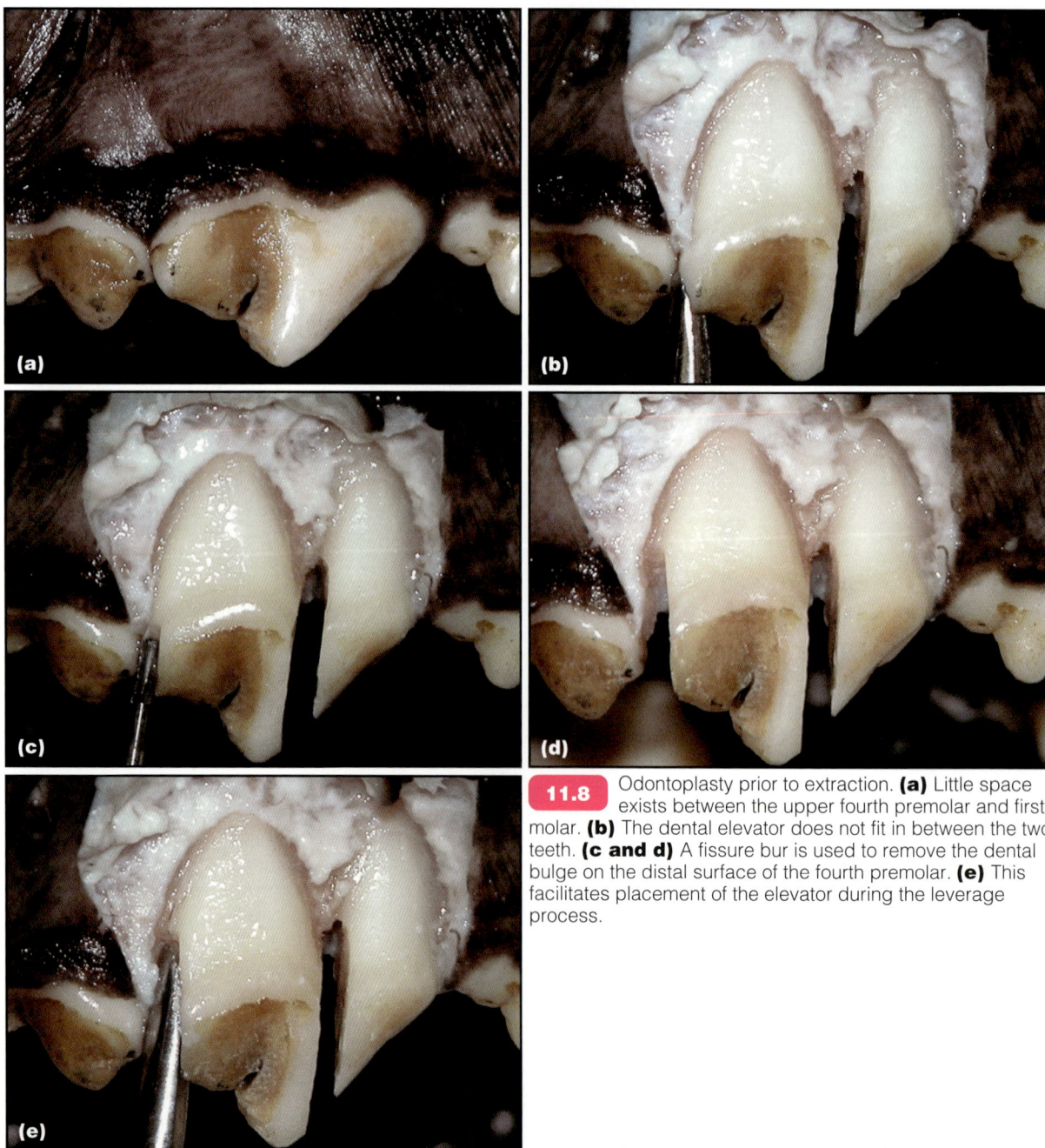

11.8 Odontoplasty prior to extraction. **(a)** Little space exists between the upper fourth premolar and first molar. **(b)** The dental elevator does not fit in between the two teeth. **(c and d)** A fissure bur is used to remove the dental bulge on the distal surface of the fourth premolar. **(e)** This facilitates placement of the elevator during the leverage process.

Firmly attached multi-rooted teeth must be sectioned prior to extraction to avoid root fracture. This provides multiple single-rooted segments, whose extraction is no more difficult than that of multiple single-rooted teeth (Figure 11.9).

1. Incise the gingival attachment around the tooth.
2. Reflect the gingiva to locate the furcation area(s).
3. Section the tooth into single-rooted segments using a cross-cut fissure bur in a high-speed handpiece with water irrigation. Sectioning is performed starting from the furcation through the tooth crown.
   (a) *Two-rooted teeth*: Separate the tooth into one mesial and one distal single-rooted segment.
   (b) *Three-rooted teeth*: Separate the tooth first into one two-rooted and one single-rooted segment. Then separate the two-rooted segment into two single-rooted segments.

4. Luxate and elevate each segment as in a closed single-rooted tooth extraction. The elevator can also be placed perpendicular to the long axis of the tooth between its segments (a notch may be made with a bur at the neck of the segments to gain additional purchase) (Figure 11.10). The

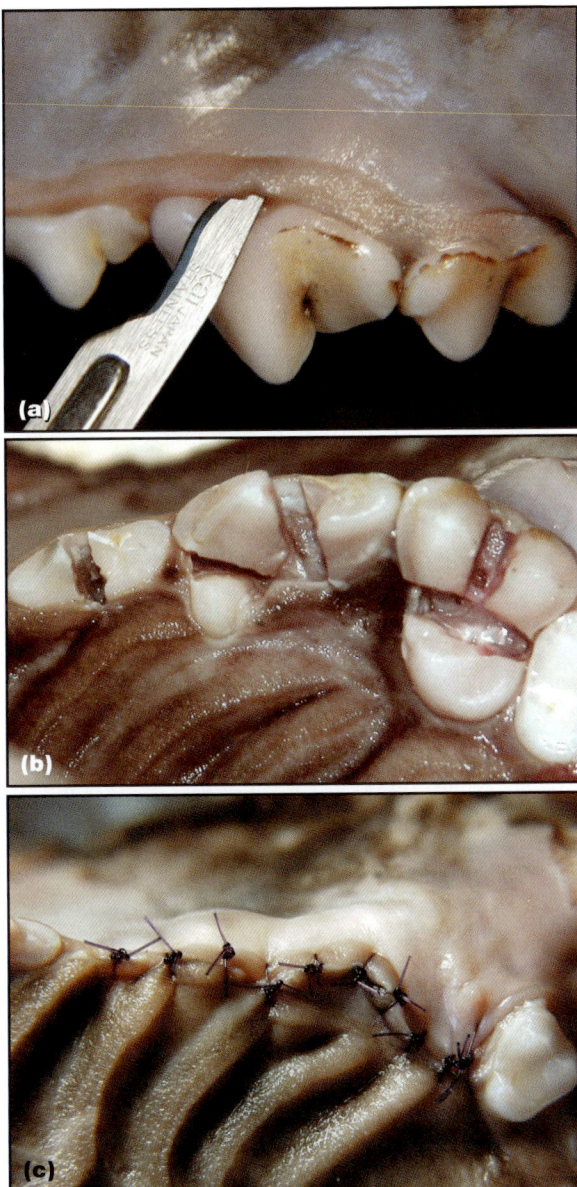

11.9 Closed extraction of the upper third premolar, fourth premolar and first molar in a dog. **(a)** Gingival attachment is incised. **(b)** Coronal view of sectioned crowns. **(c)** Extraction sites are sutured closed.

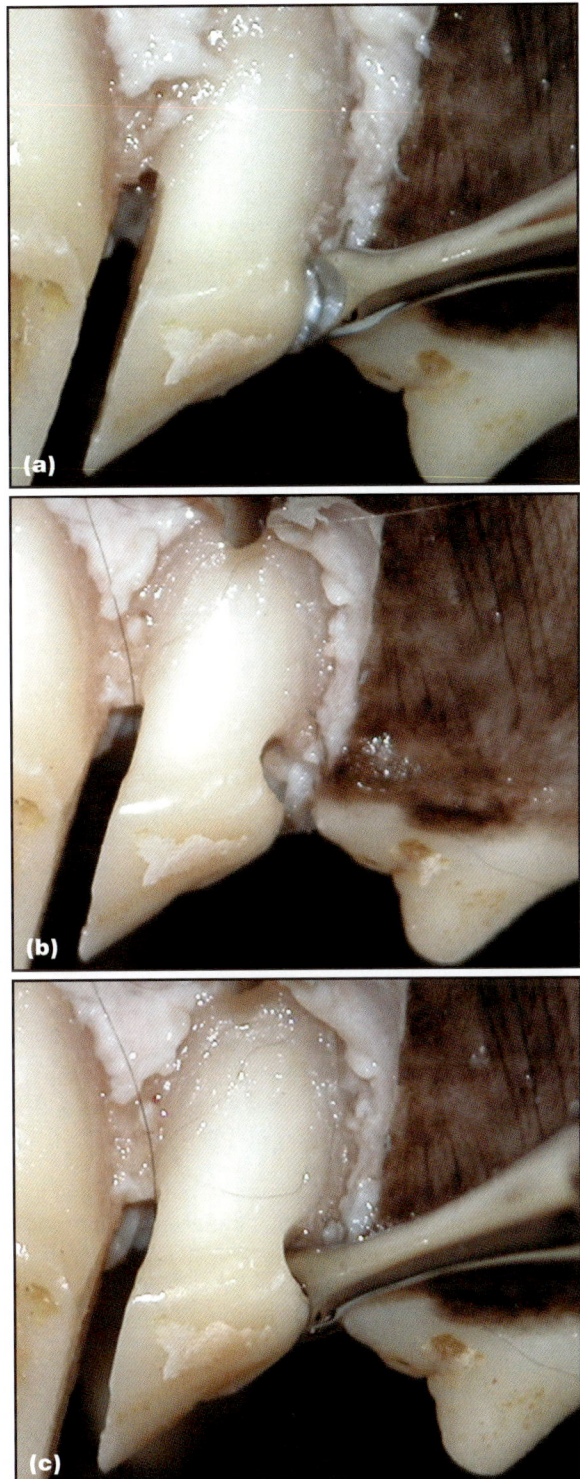

11.10 Wheel and axle. **(a)** The elevator is placed perpendicular to the long axis of the tooth between crown-root segments or two teeth that are both to be extracted. **(b)** A notch is created with a bur at the neck of the segment to be removed. **(c)** This provides additional elevator purchase.

elevator is rotated slightly. Hold the pressure for at least 10 seconds to loosen the root segment. This action elevates one segment (wheel and axle lever) while the other (used as a fulcrum) is slightly intruded and moved mesially/distally.

5. Loosen all segments progressively and extract them as if they were single-rooted teeth.
6. Once all segments are extracted, proceed as described for a closed extraction of a single-rooted tooth.

Open extraction technique

The open or surgical extraction technique is employed when a tooth resists appropriate elevation due to its size and root anatomy/pathology, or if the operator is unable to retrieve a fractured or retained root through the alveolar socket. It is futile, time-consuming and damaging to the surrounding tissues to continue the closed extraction process blindly. Raising mucoperiosteal flaps will improve visibility of and expedite access to any tooth or root that requires extraction.

1. Incise the gingival attachment around the tooth and extend horizontal gingival incisions to the midpoint between adjacent teeth if interdental spaces are wide.
2. Raise a mucoperiosteal flap.
   (i) Make one or two releasing incisions in the alveolar mucosa down to the bone, keeping in mind that future suture lines should not lie over a void, and connect them with the rostral and/or caudal end of gingival incisions. Releasing incisions must extend beyond the mucogingival line and diverge apically, permitting adequate blood supply to the flap. Near the infraorbital and middle mental foraminae, split-thickness flaps may be made to avoid neurovascular structures.
   (ii) Use a sharp periosteal elevator to free the attached gingiva and alveolar mucosa from the underlying bone. Care should be taken to keep the periosteal elevator close to the bone to raise a full-thickness flap and to avoid perforating the flap at the mucogingival line. The flap should be elevated beyond the end of the bony prominences (alveolar juga) covering the roots.
   (iii) Elevate the lingual or palatal gingiva as an envelope flap to expose the alveolar margin.
3. If the tooth is multi-rooted, section it appropriately. Retraction of the flap with a surgical retractor or the blunt end of a scalpel handle will protect it from iatrogenic damage during tooth sectioning.
4. Use a round bur with water irrigation to reduce the level of the alveolar bone overlying the roots buccally, mesially and distally by as much as one-third to two-thirds of the length of the root(s). Septal bone in the furcation area may also be reduced. Continuous water irrigation is required to: (a) cool the alveolar bone to prevent overheating and bone necrosis; (b) cool the bur to prevent overheating and loss of cutting

efficiency; (c) wash away bone chips that would clog the bur; and (d) maintain good visibility of the surgical site.

5. Luxate, elevate and extract the tooth or root segments. If progress is not achieved, remove further buccal alveolar bone rather than use excessive force. Slots can also be burred at mesial and distal aspects of the root(s) at the junction of the alveolar margin and the tooth to allow for better elevator purchase (consider proximity of the roots of adjacent teeth to avoid damaging them).
6. Proceed with debridement, alveoloplasty and lavage of the extraction site as described for closed tooth extractions.
7. Replace the mucoperiosteal flap.
   (i) Avoid tension on the closed flap. To increase its vertical dimension and elasticity, the flap is raised and held with tissue forceps. A scalpel blade is used on the exposed underside to incise the periosteum in a rostrocaudal direction across the entire base of the flap. The tissue will advance as the inelastic periosteum is cut. Releasing incisions may also be extended and further mucosa freed until tension-free closure can be accomplished.
   (ii) Smooth any sharp spicules and reduce projections of alveolar bone prior to positioning the flap over a freshly formed blood clot. The alveolar margin may be further reduced to facilitate repositioning of the flap without tension, prior to suturing.
   (iii) If required, freshen up and shape the gingival margins of the flaps with fine scissors.
   (iv) Appose the flap to the palatal/lingual gingiva by means of simple interrupted sutures. The corners of the flap are sutured first, and additional sutures are placed 2–3 mm apart and 2–3 mm from the flap edges.
   (v) Suture the releasing incision(s), ensuring that suture lines do not lie over a void.

Crown amputation with intentional root retention

Ankylosed teeth and those with roots undergoing replacement resorption are commonly encountered in cats and cannot be easily elevated and extracted, even when open extraction principles are applied. An alternative to complete extraction of such teeth and roots is crown amputation with intentional root retention. The gingival attachment is incised, creating a small envelope flap. The tooth crown is amputated from the root with a cross-cut fissure bur attached to a high-speed handpiece under water irrigation. The resorbing root is further reduced with a round or pear-shaped bur to about 1–2 mm below the alveolar margin. The gingiva must be sutured tension-free over the defect, and a postoperative radiograph obtained.

This technique is not recommended if closed or open extractions are achievable and is contraindicated for teeth with periodontitis, endodontic disease and periapical pathology. Clients must be informed about the risks involved with this procedure (e.g. infection) and periodic monitoring of the surgical site must be performed by means of clinical and radiographic examinations (Reiter and Mendoza, 2002).

WARNING

Root pulverization

The practice of blindly pulverizing ('atomizing') fractured or retained roots using high-speed equipment is contrary to all principles of oral surgery and must be frowned upon and strongly discouraged. This amateurish technique can create considerable iatrogenic trauma, such as:

- Incomplete removal of the tooth root
- Overheating of hard and soft tissues, leading to bone necrosis and delayed healing
- Injury to inferior alveolar and infraorbital neurovascular bundles
- Possible repulsion of root fragments into the nasal cavity, the infraorbital canal or the mandibular canal
- Transection of salivary gland ducts in sublingual tissues
- Submucosal and subcutaneous emphysema
- Emphysema and air embolism.

Retrieval of root fragments using this technique may result in more damage than leaving them in place. Roots are either removed *in toto*, or allowed to remain buried if judged to be harmless (Kertesz, 1993) – the latter being decided on radiographic evaluation.

Extraction of specific teeth

Deciduous teeth

If the clinician identifies a permanent tooth erupting, and the corresponding deciduous tooth has not yet exfoliated, it may be wise to wait for a week or two before hastily extracting the deciduous tooth. Compared with their permanent successors, the roots of deciduous teeth are longer and thinner and may be partly resorbed. They are therefore more likely to fracture during extraction. A preoperative radiograph should be obtained to determine the proximity of the deciduous tooth root to the permanent tooth and to evaluate to what extent the root of the deciduous tooth has undergone resorption. Deciduous teeth are removed with closed or open extraction techniques, taking great care not to damage underlying tooth buds or the erupting permanent teeth. The keys to success are gentle technique (no force) and patience.

Persistent deciduous canines are common candidates for extraction. The maxillary deciduous canine is always distal to the permanent canine, whereas the mandibular deciduous canine is labial to the permanent canine (Kertesz, 1993). The extraction technique is much the same as for single-rooted permanent teeth. The deciduous tooth is loosened using fine luxators and elevators between the root and bone. Luxation/elevation may also be accomplished with a 22 gauge needle as a wedge lever.

Despite extra care being taken by the veterinary surgeon, the client should always be informed about potential complications associated with extraction of deciduous teeth near (developing) permanent teeth. Depending on the developmental stage of permanent successors, iatrogenic trauma may result in discoloration, enamel hypomineralization and hypoplasia, and crown/root dilacerations (bending) of the permanent tooth. Most deciduous tooth extractions are carried out after the permanent successor has erupted and so damage in the formative stages is less likely. Instruments should not be inserted between a deciduous tooth and its developing permanent successor, and levering against the latter must be avoided. A dangerous consequence of blind elevation of a deciduous tooth is the accidental elevation of the permanent tooth or tooth bud. Rotational forces should not be employed with extraction forceps, because this will often result in deciduous tooth root fracture.

If open extraction is deemed necessary, one or two releasing incisions are made, ensuring that they diverge and do not lie over the deciduous tooth root. A flap is raised, alveolar bone carefully removed, the tooth extracted and the flap sutured closed. A radiograph is taken if any doubt exists that the entire root was not extracted. Removal of a fractured root tip must be achieved, as it could affect eruption of the permanent successor.

Maxillary canine

This large, single-rooted tooth is, unless severely affected by periodontitis, difficult to extract using closed extraction techniques. Its root courses in a dorsal and caudal direction with its apex projected above the mesial root of the maxillary second premolar. Various flap designs with one or two releasing incisions have been described (Figure 11.11).

1. The gingival attachment around the tooth is incised. A horizontal gingival incision is extended rostrally to the midpoint between the canine and third incisor, another is extended caudally to the midpoint between the canine and first premolar. A vertical releasing incision begins three-quarters of the length of the canine root in the alveolar mucosa caudal to the rim of the nasal aperture, connecting to the rostral end of the gingival incision.
2. The flap outline is completed with a releasing incision that is made in the alveolar mucosa over the maxillary second premolar, sloping toward the mesiobuccal line angle of the first premolar. A mucoperiosteal flap is raised and alveolar bone removed.
3. A slot is burred in the alveolar bone along the mesial root surface for better elevator purchase (consider proximity of the first premolar root when burring a slot along the canine's distal root surface).
4. The canine tooth is elevated, the alveolus debrided and lavaged and the flap sutured closed.

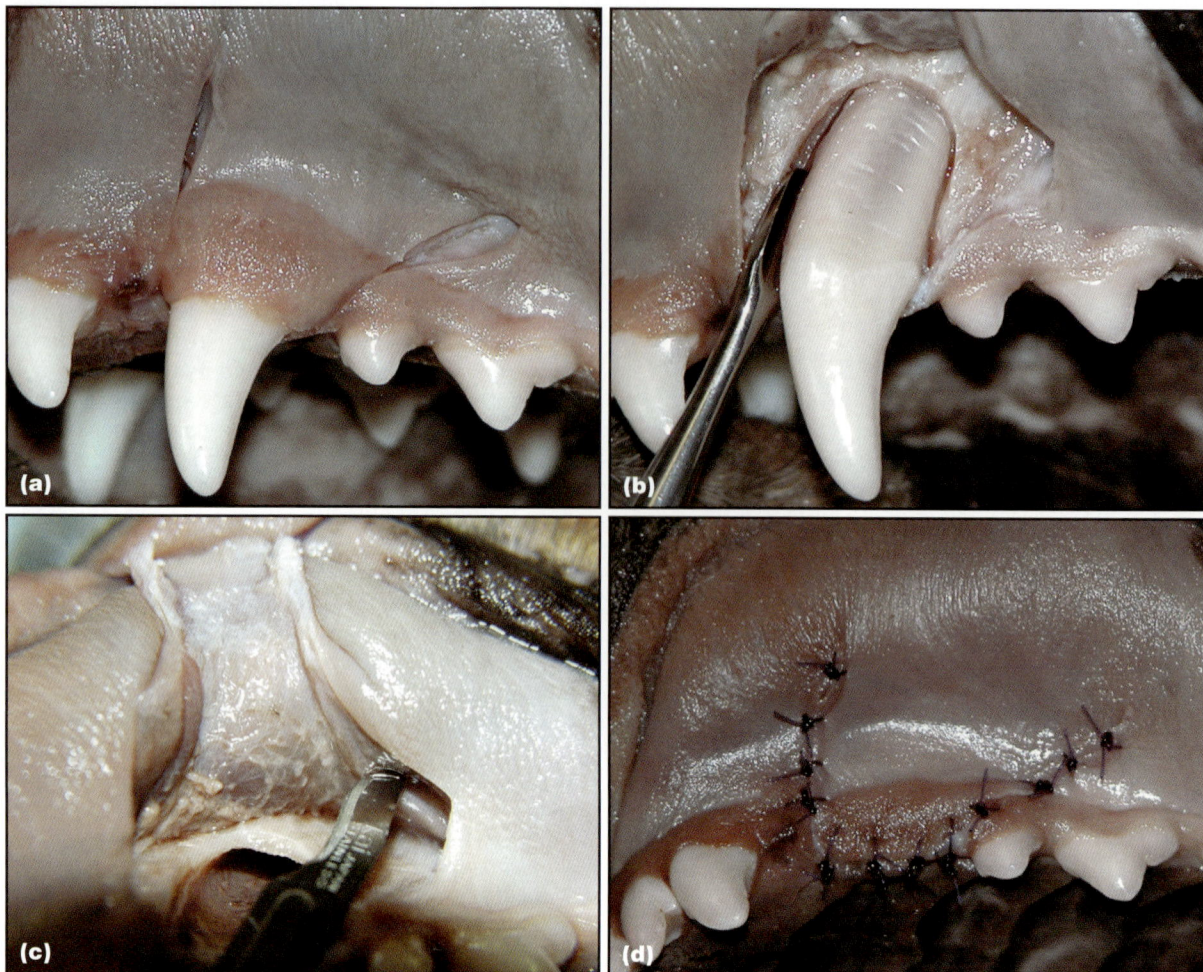

11.11 Open extraction of the upper canine in a dog. **(a)** Releasing incisions are apically divergent. **(b)** The tooth is elevated following removal of buccal alveolar bone. **(c)** The periosteum is incised at the base of the flap. **(d)** The flap is sutured to palatal gingiva.

During extraction, the apex of the root must not be tipped nasally, as this would perforate the thin plate of bone separating the alveolus from the nasal cavity, producing an acute oronasal communication. The elevator must also never be inserted palatally between the canine tooth and the alveolar bone. If fracture of the bony plate occurs and results in perforation, haemorrhage or emergence of flushing solution may be noted from the ipsilateral nostril. An acute oronasal communication is treated by suturing the mucoperiosteal flap over the alveolus, as one would routinely close the flap raised for the extraction procedure (Smith, 1998).

Mandibular canine

Unless the periodontal tissues are severely compromised, this tooth is difficult to extract using closed extraction techniques. Various flap designs with one or two releasing incisions have been described (Figure 11.12).

1. The gingival attachment around the tooth is incised. A horizontal gingival incision is extended caudally to the midpoint between the canine and first premolar. A vertical releasing incision begins three-quarters of the length of the canine root in the alveolar mucosa, connecting to the rostral

end of the gingival incision at the distolabial line angle of the third incisor tooth.
2. The flap outline is completed with a releasing incision that is made over the second premolar dorsal to the labial frenulum attachment, sloping toward the caudal end of the gingival incision. A mucoperiosteal flap is raised short of neurovascular structures emerging at the middle mental foramen and buccal alveolar bone is removed.
3. Slots may be burred in the alveolar bone along the mesial and distal root surfaces for better elevator purchase (consider proximity of the third incisor and first premolar roots when burring slots).
4. The canine tooth is elevated, the alveolus debrided and lavaged, and the flap sutured closed.

A lingual approach for surgical extraction of the mandibular canine has also been described (Smith, 1998). The mandibular canine root contributes considerably to the strength of the rostral mandible, which may be weakened after extraction. Osteopromotive materials may be packed into the alveolus prior to closing the extraction site.

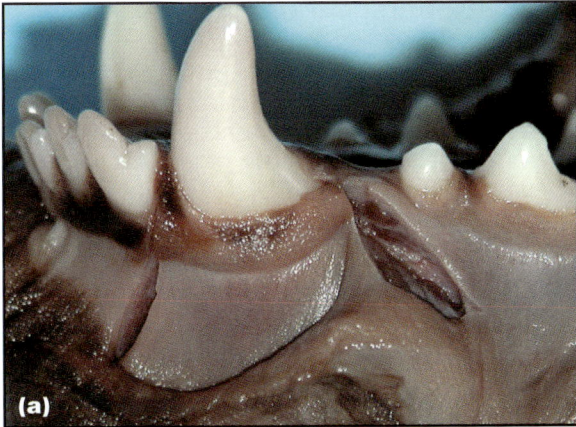

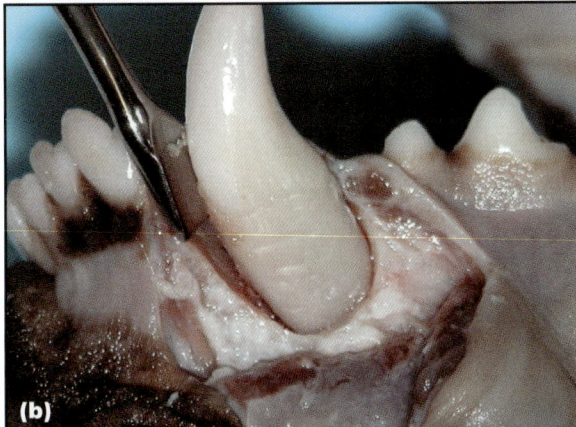

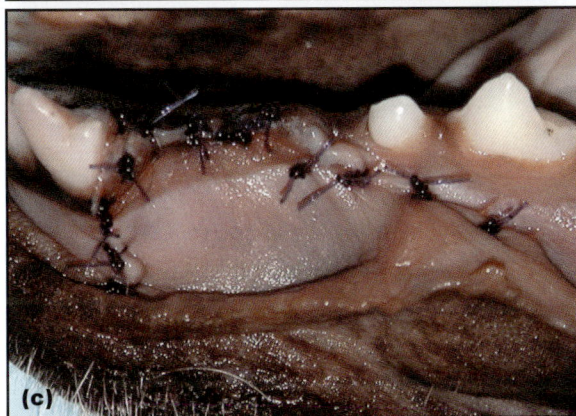

11.12 Open extraction of the lower canine in a dog. **(a)** Flap outline is created. **(b)** The tooth is elevated following removal of buccal alveolar bone. **(c)** The flap is sutured closed.

11.13 Open extraction of upper fourth premolar in a dog. **(a)** An elevator is inserted between the mesiobuccal and distal root. **(b)** Palatal view of the sectioned tooth crown. **(c)** The flap is sutured closed.

Maxillary fourth premolar

This three-rooted tooth has a large distal root and two mesial roots (mesiobuccal and mesiopalatal) emanating from a common root trunk. Various flap designs with one or two releasing incisions have been described (Figure 11.13).

1. The gingival attachment around the tooth is incised. The flap outline is completed with apically divergent rostral and caudal releasing incisions that begin three-quarters of the length of the roots in the alveolar mucosa, connecting the rostral and caudal ends of the buccal gingival incision. When making the rostral releasing

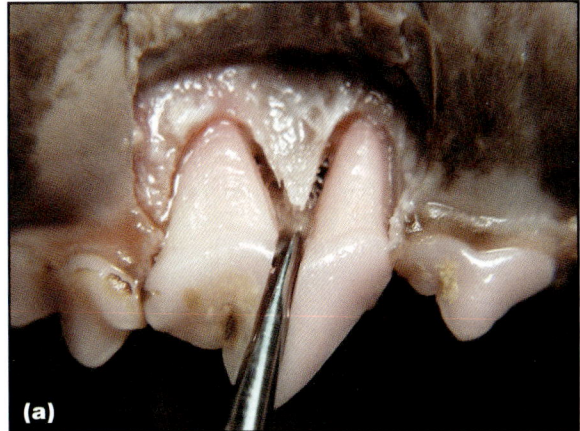

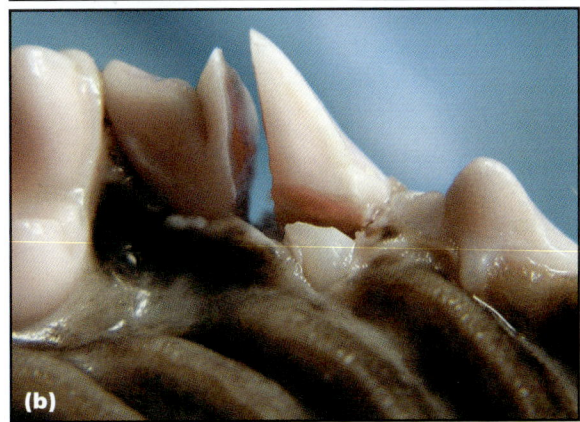

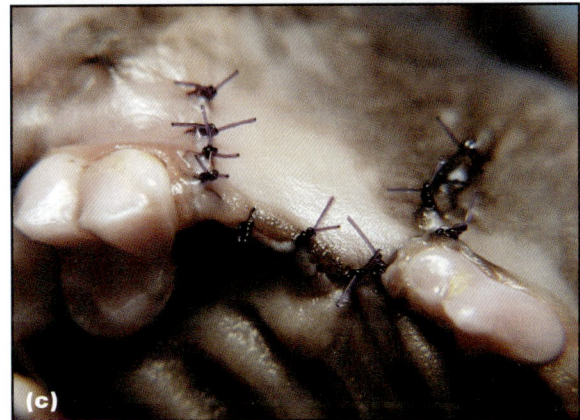

incision, the infraorbital neurovascular bundle emerging at the infraorbital foramen is to be avoided (particularly in brachycephalic breeds) (Emily and Penman, 1994). When making the caudal releasing incision, the duct openings of the parotid and zygomatic salivary glands are to be avoided.

2. After raising a mucoperiosteal flap, crown sectioning into single-rooted segments is performed, beginning at buccal and mesial furcation areas. The mesial and distal roots are separated by cutting between the two large cusps in a straight line from the furcation. The mesiopalatal root is separated by cutting in the

fissure created by the base of the main cusp and the palatine cusp. Alveolar bone is removed overlying the mesiobuccal and distal roots. Septal bone in the furcation area may also be reduced.

3. Slots may be burred in the alveolar bone along the mesial and distal root surfaces for better elevator purchase (consider proximity of adjacent tooth roots when burring slots). The mesiobuccal and distal roots are luxated, elevated and extracted.
4. Alveolar bone around the mesiopalatal root is removed, until it can be elevated and extracted. Care must be exercised to avoid driving the mesiobuccal root into the infraorbital canal or the mesiopalatal root into the nasal cavity.
5. The alveoli are debrided and lavaged, and the flap is replaced and sutured.

Maxillary first and second molars (in the dog)

These three-rooted teeth have one large palatal root and two buccal roots (mesiobuccal and distobuccal). They can often be extracted using the closed extraction technique. Excessive force must be avoided, as it can result in iatrogenic trauma to the eye and periorbital tissues due to the proximity of the ventral floor of the orbit. If crown-root segments resist elevation or root fractures have occurred, an open extraction approach must be considered.

1. The gingival attachment around the teeth is incised. The flap outline is completed with one vertical releasing incision that begins three-quarters of the length of the mesial root in the alveolar mucosa, connecting to the rostral end of the gingival incision. Care must be taken to avoid injury to the duct openings of the parotid and zygomatic salivary glands when the releasing incision is made.
2. After raising a mucoperiosteal flap, crown sectioning into single-rooted segments is performed, beginning at buccal and mesial/distal furcation areas. The palatal root is separated from the rest of the tooth by cutting in the fissure created by the two buccal cusps and the palatine cusp. The mesio- and distobuccal roots are separated by cutting through the fissure formed by the two buccal cusps.
3. Alveolectomy and root segment elevation is performed as described for the maxillary fourth premolar. The palatal root segment can often be elevated and extracted without further alveolar bone removal.
4. The alveoli are debrided and lavaged, and the flap is replaced and sutured.

Tension-free closure may not always be easily achieved at this site. Avoiding injury to the ducts of the parotid and zygomatic salivary glands, the skilful veterinary dentist will make a caudal releasing incision and/or free further mucosa to fully close the extraction site(s).

Mandibular first molar

This is a two-rooted tooth. In the dog, the mesial root is slightly larger than the distal root. In the cat, the mesial root is much larger and stronger, compared with the short and delicate distal root. Various flap designs with one or two releasing incisions have been described (Figure 11.14).

1. The gingival attachment around the tooth is incised. The flap outline is completed with two apically divergent releasing incisions that begin three-quarters of the length of the roots in the alveolar mucosa, connecting to the rostral and caudal ends of the gingival incisions.

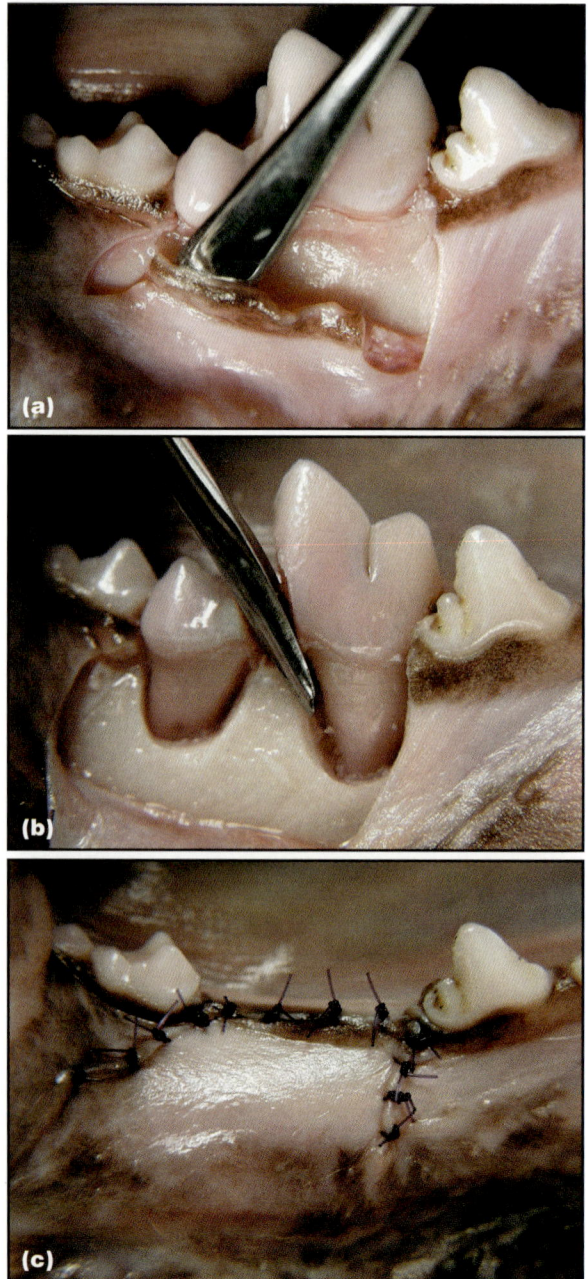

11.14 Open extraction of lower first molar in a dog. **(a)** A periosteal elevator is used to raise a mucoperiosteal flap. **(b)** An elevator is inserted between the mesial and distal roots. **(c)** The flap is sutured closed.

2. After raising a mucoperiosteal flap, crown sectioning begins at the buccal furcation point and continues via the shortest path through the crown in a distoocclusal direction.
3. Alveolectomy and elevation of the root segments as previously described, is performed. Good visualization of the roots and controlled root elevation decrease the incidence of iatrogenic mandibular fracture.
4. The alveoli are debrided and lavaged, and the flap replaced and sutured.

In small-breed dogs and some cats, the apical portion of the roots of mandibular cheek teeth may reach into the mandibular canal. Injury to the mandibular artery can result in haemorrhage that may significantly impair visualization of the surgical field. The extraction procedure is greatly complicated when root fragments are accidentally intruded into the mandibular canal.

Tooth extraction in cats
Tooth extraction in cats is performed in similar fashion as for dogs, but the following points should be borne in mind.

- The cat's skull is smaller and more fragile than that of the dog.
- The teeth of cats are narrower and smaller than those of a dog of similar body weight.
- The furcation point of the mandibular first molar in the cat is further distal than in the dog's mandibular first molar.

Feline teeth tend to fracture if extraction forceps are applied with force, and root fragments remaining in the alveolar sockets are a common complication, especially when the teeth are brittle due to tooth resorption (Reiter and Mendoza, 2002). Single-rooted segments after crown sectioning are more likely to fracture during leverage unless the force is applied very gradually. Traditional dental elevators are often too large for convenient use in cats, and smaller luxators, elevators and root tip picks/forceps should be used. It is imperative for successful extraction that root remnants are not retained, particularly in the presence of gingivostomatitis.

Multiple extractions in one quadrant
When extracting multiple teeth in sequence, it is important to consider which of the involved teeth is likely to be the most difficult to extract and use adjacent teeth to aid its extraction. The crown of one tooth may serve as a lever fulcrum for the dental elevator in extraction of an adjacent tooth. In dogs with severe generalized periodontitis and in cats with gingivostomatitis and tooth resorption, several teeth and even the entire quadrant may be included in a single mucoperiosteal flap (Figure 11.15). When performed properly, this technique is faster and less traumatic than prolonged use of luxators, elevators or forceps in a closed extraction technique. Releasing incisions are made with local neurovascular supply and effective closure in mind (Smith, 1998).

Fractured and retained roots
Extraction of the entire tooth and its root(s) is recommended. Exceptions to this rule include retained roots identified on radiographs that are completely buried under intact and healthy gingiva and show no signs of endodontic or periapical disease. However, retained roots with oral communication (sinus tracts through the gingiva) or associated with periodontal, endodontic or periapical disease must be removed (Reiter and Mendoza, 2002).

Narrow-bladed luxators and elevators are worked circumferentially around the root. A trough can be cut adjacent to the root fragment to allow insertion of even finer instruments. Special root tip (apical) elevators, picks and forceps are used to free and lift out very small root fragments. An oversized endodontic file can be used to retrieve the root fragment by inserting the file into the root canal and twisting to lock the file in place. With the aid of a root tip elevator or pick, the root may then be luxated, elevated and retrieved by pulling on the endodontic file. An alternative is to raise a mucoperiosteal flap and remove alveolar bone to outline the root fragment and facilitate its elevation and extraction. A radiograph should be taken to verify complete removal of the root.

Every reasonable effort must be made to retrieve fractured roots, but the risks associated with prolonged anaesthesia and increased removal of alveolar bone, especially in a weak mandible, must be weighed against the potential danger posed by a retained root. If the risk of complications from anaesthesia and tissue damage is greater than the advantage gained by extraction, leaving a root fragment in place after thorough lavage and closure of the surgical site may be an acceptable (though not ideal) treatment plan. Fractured and retained roots should be noted on the dental record/chart. Diligent monitoring for clinical signs associated with infection is required, supported by follow-up radiographic examination. The owner should be informed about the presence of fractured or retained roots, as they are usually the first to recognize a change in their pet's behaviour that may be as a result of pain and discomfort.

Unerupted and intruded teeth
Unerupted or intruded teeth in animals with a permanent dentition should be extracted. A consequence of leaving an unerupted tooth in place is the formation of a dentigerous (tooth-containing) cyst, whose epithelial lining may in some cases undergo neoplastic metaplasia.

1. A mucoperiosteal flap with one or two releasing incisions is raised.
2. Alveolar bone is removed over the tooth and its root(s), and the tooth is elevated and extracted. A multi-rooted tooth may be sectioned for a stepwise removal of crown-root segments. In the case of a dentigerous cyst, the epithelial lining of the cyst must be removed completely and submitted for histopathological examination.
3. The flap is replaced and sutured.

A clinically missing upper permanent tooth may have been intruded into the nasal cavity as a result of previous trauma. Patients can present with chronic

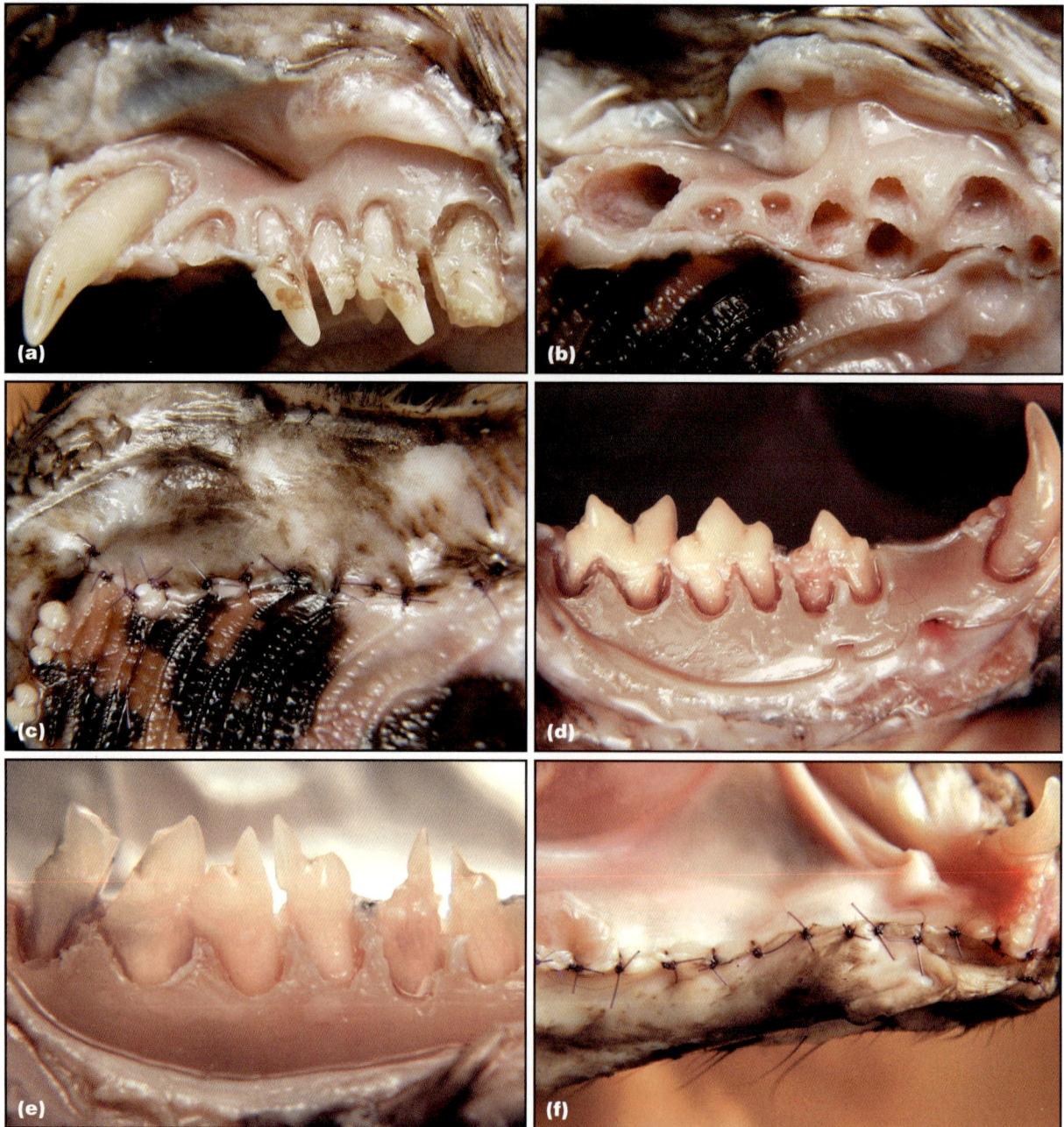

11.15 Multiple extractions in one upper and lower quadrant in a cat. **(a)** A mucoperiosteal flap is raised in the left upper quadrant, alveolar bone is removed, and the teeth are sectioned. **(b)** Coronal view of the debrided and lavaged alveoli. **(c)** The flap is sutured closed. **(d)** A mucoperiosteal flap is raised in the right lower quadrant and alveolar bone is removed; note unequal size of mesial and distal roots of the lower first molar in the cat. **(e)** Close-up of sectioned lower cheek teeth. **(f)** The flap is sutured closed.

rhinitis and epistaxis with owners unaware of the in-truded tooth. Radiographic identification and evalua-tion of the tooth position is required. Surgical removal of such teeth may be accompanied by severe haemor-rhage from the inflamed and infected nasal mucosa.

Perioperative management

Pain control
Topical anaesthetic gels may provide temporary relief from superficial pain, but their effects are extremely short-lived. Nerve blocks and field/infiltration blocks are performed intraoperatively with longer-lasting local an-aesthetics. Postoperative pain control is achieved with oxymorphone, hydromorphone, butorphanol, buprenor-phine and transdermal fentanyl patches. Non-steroidal anti-inflammatory drugs may be used for pain control in extractions and to reduce tissue swelling associated with open extractions (see Chapter 3).

Antimicrobial therapy
Bacteraemia is inevitable when procedures are per-formed in a mouth with plaque and calculus accumula-tion, inflamed mucosa and periodontal pockets. It has been described in cats and dogs during and after

ultrasonic tooth cleaning and extractions in healthy animals and usually lasts less than an hour. In rare cases, septicaemia may develop after poorly performed dental extractions are carried out in an immunocompromised patient (Reiter *et al.*, 2004).

There is a tendency to use antibiotics as part of the management of any animal with oral disease, but there is no justification for this. Bacteraemia can be prevented or reduced in severity by rinsing the oral cavity with dilute chlorhexidine gluconate (0.12 %) prior to commencing the surgical procedure. Antibiotic treatment is usually not required for single or multiple tooth extraction in an otherwise healthy patient. Unless there is a well founded positive reason for antibiotic administration, they should not be used.

Nutritional support

Oral intake may not be practical for the first few hours after anaesthesia. Hydration may be maintained with intravenous fluids. Water is offered once the animal has recovered sufficiently from anaesthesia. Soft food is offered 8–24 hours after anaesthesia and maintained for about 2 weeks. Most dogs and cats will eat and drink after multiple or even full-mouth dental extractions, and feeding tubes are rarely needed to bypass the oral cavity. However, some animals may refuse oral intake, and the owner is then instructed in syringe feeding of a liquid high-calorie diet. Hard treats and chew toys are withheld while the oral tissues heal.

Wound management

A water-based commercial mouthwash, dilute chlorhexidine gluconate solution (0.12%) or a chlorhexidine-containing gel is administered into the mouth once or twice daily for 2 weeks. Wound dehiscence is usually the result of tension on suture lines or compromised vascular support of flaps. Restraining devices (Elizabethan collar) may be used in some animals to prevent disruption of extraction sites. Re-examination is performed after 2 weeks to evaluate whether healing is normal or if further treatment is indicated.

Complications

Fractured roots

Fractured roots are a result of dental or mandibular/maxillofacial trauma, improper extraction technique or pre-existing root pathology (endodontic and periapical disease, dentoalveolar ankylosis and root replacement resorption). If the tooth being extracted has an inflamed pulp and an infected root canal, contains necrotic pulp or is affected by periapical disease, every part of the root must be removed to prevent further infection and inhibition of healing. Crown sectioning must be complete and leverage forces applied for elevation of root segments need to be directed as parallel to the roots as feasible and as far apical as possible, to prevent root fracture. The use of extraction forceps applied too far coronally on a tooth or root segment or applied with too much force is also likely to result in root tip fracture. An audible crack can often be

heard. A sharp-edged defect is visible and palpable at the end of the root. Dental radiography is an invaluable tool in determining the position and size of the retained root fragment, aiding in its complete removal. If a root fragment cannot be retrieved and is left in place, the patient must be evaluated by means of periodic clinical and radiographic follow-up. This allows for monitoring of healing of the surgical site and identification of sequestration of the root fragment should that occur.

Root intrusion into the nasal cavity, infraorbital or mandibular canal is a serious complication: retrieval of root fragments from these spaces is difficult. Access through soft tissue and bone away from the extraction site may be required, and the operator should be prepared for possible haemorrhage to occur. Referral of these cases to an experienced surgeon is desirable.

Haemorrhage

In the majority of extractions, haemostasis is easily effected. Cotton-tip applicators and suction using fine tips greatly assist in cases where bleeding impairs visualization and removal of a tooth or root fragment. Packing the empty alveolus with gauze for a few minutes is sufficient to arrest bleeding in most cases. Application of cold compresses made from shredded ice wrapped in a gauze sponge can reduce blood flow sufficiently to allow a clot to form and, at the same time, retard postoperative swelling after flap surgery.

In rare cases of excessive alveolar haemorrhage, the alveolus may be irrigated with thrombin solution or packed with materials to aid haemostasis. The gingiva must be sutured over the packs without tension. Vasoconstrictors are not recommended and should generally not be used in patients with cardiac problems, thyroid disorders or when halothane is used for inhalant anaesthesia.

Trauma to adjacent teeth, permanent tooth buds and soft tissue

Leverage against adjacent teeth must be avoided to prevent unwanted elevation and crown fractures of teeth not to be extracted. Complications of deciduous tooth extraction include damage to the underlying tooth buds of permanent successors. Instruments must not be inserted between a deciduous tooth and its developing permanent successor. Minor levering against the latter could result in accidental elevation of the permanent tooth.

Minor lacerations of adjacent gingiva commonly occur during the extraction process. More severe lacerations of soft tissues result from excessive elevation technique and slippage of sharp instruments. Gingival and alveolar mucosal defects thus created must be sutured appropriately. The use of a diamond disc for sectioning teeth is not recommended.

Sublingual oedema and salivary mucocele

Tongue manipulation, excessive elevation of the alveolar mucosa on the lingual aspects of the mandibles and other iatrogenic trauma can result in oedematous swelling of the sublingual tissues. The sublingual oedema may be severe enough that breathing could be compromised during recovery from anaesthesia, and such patients may benefit from a single injection of intravenous dexamethasone.

Excessive force and lack of instrument control can also cause injury to the ducts of the sublingual and mandibular salivary glands, causing extravasation of saliva into the sublingual tissues (sublingual salivary mucocele or ranula). If breathing and masticatory function are not significantly compromised, it is better to postpone surgical treatment (marsupialization; resection of sublingual and mandibular gland-duct complex), as the ranula often resolves on its own in a few weeks or months.

Orbital trauma

Iatrogenic trauma to the orbit may occur during extraction of caudal maxillary teeth. The cause of such trauma is related to the thin alveolar bone and proximity of the tooth roots to the ventral floor of the orbit. Orbital structures may be perforated by a pointed instrument, particularly in patients with severe periodontitis. Panophthalmitis may result. If antimicrobial and anti-inflammatory treatment fails, enucleation is an unfortunate result (Smith, 1998). Flushing of alveoli using a needle on a syringe may result in injection of non-sterile or tissue-damaging agents into the globe and is to be discouraged.

Fracture of the alveolus or jaw

A fractured alveolus occurs when excessive force is used during extraction, or when the bone overlying the root(s) has not been adequately removed. Unstable small bone fragments are removed before the extraction site is closed. Owners of animals with severe periodontal disease should be warned about an increased possibility of jaw fracture. The mandible may be prone to fracture during relatively routine pre- and intraoperative manoeuvres (when opening the mouth for intubation, placing a mouth prop, and during tooth extraction). Iatrogenic jaw fracture is most commonly associated with extraction of the mandibular first molar or canine and usually occurs when closed extraction techniques are used in areas weakened by extensive severe bone loss. This emphasizes the importance of preoperative dental radiography. A diseased and fractured mandible may never heal. Treatment includes extraction of diseased teeth in fracture lines, debridement of extraction sites and suturing of soft tissue to cover exposed bone, followed by orthopaedic repair.

A leather, nylon, plastic or in-clinic fabricated tape muzzle can be used to support the jaw while a fibrous union is formed. The muzzle is applied snugly enough to maintain the canine dental interlock, but loosely enough to permit the tongue to protrude and lap water and semi-liquid food. An initial layer of tape is formed into a loop, encircling the muzzle and mandibles with the sticky side of the adhesive tape outermost. A second layer is then added, with the sticky side facing inward, directly on top of the first layer. A loop around the neck is added (sticky side out for the first layer, then sticky side in). For cats and short-nosed dogs, an additional middle piece is placed from the loop over the muzzle extending over the forehead to the neck loop. Care should be exercised when using tape muzzles in

brachycephalic breeds as this may interfere with temperature homeostasis. Partial mandibulectomy is a last resort for pathological jaw fracture if other methods of repair are not successful or possible.

Oronasal communication

Causes of oronasal communications involving the maxillary alveoli include severe periodontitis, periapical disease and iatrogenic trauma. If the nasal cavity has been penetrated during the extraction process (acute oronasal communication), a flap should be raised to close the extraction site. History of a chronic oronasal fistula typically reveals that a maxillary canine tooth has been lost or was previously extracted. Periodontitis results in resorption of the thin alveolar bone separating the root and nasal cavity. A deep periodontal pocket may be present on the palatal aspect of a maxillary canine tooth, causing communication between the oral and nasal cavities even though the tooth is still in place. A chronic oronasal fistula results in rhinitis, sneezing, ipsilateral nasal discharge and difficulty in eating and drinking, and a defect may be seen in the rostral palate, with oral epithelium confluent with nasal epithelium.

A single-layer buccal-based flap procedure is usually sufficient to repair a chronic oronasal fistula. Epithelium lining the fistula on the palatal side is resected, and apically diverging incisions are created into the alveolar and buccal mucosa using a No. 15 scalpel blade. A full-thickness mucoperiosteal flap is raised with a periosteal elevator. The periosteum is incised at the base of the flap (as described earlier in this chapter to improve flap advancement). The flap is mobilized by blunt submucosal dissection using small Metzenbaum scissors, advanced to cover the defect, and sutured to hard palate mucosa without tension in a simple interrupted pattern. Alternatively, a two-layer flap technique may be used: the first flap provides an epithelial surface for the nasal cavity and a connective tissue surface facing the oral cavity; the second flap is designed to cover the connective tissue surface of the first flap and also provides an epithelial surface for the oral cavity (see *BSAVA Manual of Canine and Feline Head, Neck and Thoracic Surgery*).

Trauma from opposing teeth

This may occur, particularly in cats, when a maxillary canine tooth is extracted. Normally this tooth and supporting structures (gingiva and bone) keep the lip out of the way of the lower canine when the cat closes its mouth. After extraction of the maxillary canine the upper lip is not held out of the path of the opposing mandibular canine, with the result that it may be pinched, punctured or lacerated. The opposing tooth can be treated by several means: (i) coronal reduction; (ii) orthodontics; or (iii) extraction.

Tongue hanging out of mouth

The rostral mandibular teeth serve as a basket to contain the tongue when it is at rest. When mandibular canine teeth are extracted, the tongue may not be held in the mouth at all times, particularly in dogs. Commissuroplasty can be performed in cases of excessive drooling and lip dermatitis, though this procedure is most commonly indicated after partial or complete mandibulectomy procedures.

Emphysema and air embolism

Emphysema may occur after tooth sectioning or removal of alveolar bone using pneumatic high-speed equipment. It may also result from blowing air or air/water spray into submucosal tissues, particularly after deep submucosal dissection of large mucoperiosteal flaps. Emphysema can be effectively reduced or prevented with gentle digital pressure applied to the sutured flap for a few minutes to evacuate air bubbles and provide a seal between soft tissue and bone. Blowing air or air/water spray into alveolar sockets or on to bleeding tissues is contraindicated and risks causing air emboli.

Local and systemic infection

Wound dehiscence is usually a result of tension on suture lines. The extraction site is treated by means of resuturing, or left to granulate and epithelialize (healing by secondary intention). Infection and necrosis of alveolar bone occasionally occurs, particularly if the extraction procedure was excessively traumatic or caused loss of vascular supply to a segment of alveolar bone. Excessive heat generated during alveolectomy or alveoloplasty may also result in bone necrosis. Treatment consists of removal of sequestered bone, curettage until healthy bleeding bone is reached and a blood clot formed, and closure of the site with a healthy soft tissue flap. The rare condition of alveolitis (dry socket) in cats and dogs (more common in humans) is best prevented by allowing a blood clot to form in the debrided and lavaged alveolus after extraction and before suturing of the extraction site. An extraction site that seems to be non-healing for 7 days or longer following surgery should be considered for biopsy to rule out the possibility of neoplasia.

Bacteraemia has been described in cats and dogs during and after ultrasonic teeth cleaning and tooth extraction. Systemic infection as a direct result of tooth extraction is anecdotally reported.

References and further reading

Buffa EA, Lubbe AM, Verstraete FJ and Swaim SF (1997) The effects of wound lavage solutions on canine fibroblasts: an in vitro study. *Veterinary Surgery* **26,** 460–466

Emily P and Penman S (1994) Extraction and oronasal fistula closure. In: *Handbook of Small Animal Dentistry, 2nd edn*, eds. P Emily and S Penman, pp. 95–105. Pergamon Press, Oxford

Gorrel C and Robinson J (1995) Periodontal therapy and extraction technique. In: *BSAVA Manual of Small Animal Dentistry, 2nd edn*, eds DA Crossley and S Penman, pp. 139–149. BSAVA, Cheltenham

Harvey CE (1990) Basic techniques – extraction and antibiotic treatment. In: *BSAVA Manual of Small Animal Dentistry*, eds CE Harvey and H Orr, pp. 29–35. BSAVA, Cheltenham

Harvey CE and Emily PP (1993) Oral surgery. In: *Small Animal Dentistry*, eds. CE Harvey and PP Emily, pp. 312–377. Mosby-Year Book, Inc, St. Louis, Missouri

Holmstrom SE (2000) Exodontics (extractions). In: *Veterinary Dentistry for the Technician and Office Staff*, ed. SE Holmstrom, pp. 205–222. WB Saunders, Philadelphia

Holmstrom SE, Frost P and Eisner ER (1998) Exodontics. In: *Veterinary Dental Techniques for the Small Animal Practitioner, 2nd edn*, eds. SE Holmstrom, P Frost and ER Eisner, pp. 215–254. WB Saunders, Philadelphia

Kertesz P (1993) Oral surgery: I. Extractions. In: *A Colour Atlas of Veterinary Dentistry and Oral Surgery*, ed. P Kertesz, pp. 149–164. Wolfe Publishing, Aylesbury

Reiter AM, Brady CA and Harvey CE (2004) Local and systemic complications in a cat after poorly performed dental extractions. *Journal of Veterinary Dentistry* **21**, 215–221

Reiter AM, Lewis JR, Rawlinson JE and Gracis M (2005) Hemisection and partial retention of carnassial teeth in client-owned dogs. *Journal of Veterinary Dentistry* **22**, 216–226

Reiter AM and Mendoza K (2002) Feline odontoclastic resorptive lesions – an unsolved enigma in veterinary dentistry. *The Veterinary Clinics of North America: Small Animal Practice* **32**, 791–837

Smith MM (1998) Exodontics. *The Veterinary Clinics of North America: Small Animal Practice* **28**, 1297–1319

Verstraete FJM (1999) *Self-Assessment Color Review of Veterinary Dentistry*. Manson Publishing, London

Appendix

Conversion tables

Haematology and biochemistry

	SI unit	Conversion factor	Conventional unit
Haematology			
Red blood cell count	10^{12} / l	1	10^6 / µl
Haemoglobin	g / l	0.1	g / dl
MCH	pg / cell	1	pg / cell
MCHC	g / l	0.1	g / dl
MCV	fl	1	$µm^3$
Platelet count	10^9 / l	1	10^3 / µl
White blood cell count	10^9 / l	1	10^3 / µl
Biochemistry			
Alanine transferase	IU / l	1	IU / l
Albumin	g / l	0.1	g / dl
Alkaline phosphatase	IU / l	1	IU / l
Aspartate transaminase	IU / l	1	IU / l
Bilirubin	µmol / l	0.0584	mg / dl
BUN	mmol / l	2.8	mg / dl
Calcium	mmol / l	4	mg / dl
Carbon dioxide (total)	mmol / l	1	mEq / l
Cholesterol	mmol / l	38.61	mg / dl
Chloride	mmol / l	1	mEq / l
Cortisol	nmol / l	0.362	ng / ml
Creatine kinase	IU / l	1	IU / l
Creatinine	µmol / l	0.0113	mg / dl
Glucose	mmol / l	18.02	mg / dl
Insulin	pmol / l	0.1394	µIU / ml
Iron	µmol / l	5.587	µg / dl
Magnesium	mmol / l	2	mEq / l
Phosphorus	mmol / l	3.1	mg / dl
Potassium	mmol / l	1	mEq / l
Sodium	mmol / l	1	mEq / l
Total protein	g / l	0.1	g / dl
Thyroxine (T4) (free)	pmol / l	0.0775	ng / dl
Thyroxine (T4) (total)	nmol / l	0.0775	µg / dl
Tri-iodothyronine (T3)	nmol / l	65.1	ng / dl
Triglycerides	mmol / l	88.5	mg / dl

AP1 SI and conventional units. Measurements in SI units are multiplied by the conversion factor to give concentrations in conventional units.

Hypodermic needles

		Metric	Non-metric
Needle gauge		0.8 mm	21 G
		0.6 mm	23 G
		0.5 mm	25 G
		0.4 mm	27 G
Needle length		12 mm	$^1/_2$ inch
		16 mm	$^5/_8$ inch
		25 mm	1 inch
		30 mm	1.25 inch
		40 mm	1.5 inch

Suture material sizes

Metric (Ph. Eur.)	USP
0.4	8/0
0.5	7/0
0.7	6/0
1	5/0
1.5	4/0
2	3/0
3	2/0
3.5	0
4	1
5	2
6	3

Index

Numbers in *italics* indicate figures

Abrasion *26,* 153
Abscess
    malar *25*
    periapical 151, 152
    periodontal, in dogs 115
Acanthomatous ameloblastoma 167–8
Acepromazine maleate (ACP) 46
Actinomyces 129
    hordeovulneris 122
    viscosus 122
Actinomycosis in dogs 122
Acute gingivitis in cats 129
Acute necrotizing ulcerative gingivitis *126*
Acute periapical abscess 151
Acute periapical periodontitis 150–1, 152
Air embolism 195
Airway maintenance 44–6
Alcohol-based hand-rubs 63
Alendronate 175
Alpha$_2$ adrenergic agonists 46, 52
Alveolar bone
    loss in dogs 100, 101
    radiology 19
Alveolar mucosa *16*
Alveolar process 17
Alveolitis 195
Alveolus, fracture *157,* 194
Amalgam, health and safety considerations 65
Ameloblastoma
    acanthomatous 167–8
    central 168
Amelogenesis imperfecta 87
Amoxicillin 116
Amoxicillin–clavulanate 113, 116, *141,* 145
Amyloid-producing odontogonic tumour 168
Anaesthesia
    for extraction 192
    gas scavenging 62
    induction
        inhalational agents 48
        injectable agents 47–8
    local/regional 52–5
    maintenance 48–9
    monitoring 49
    patient evaluation 41–2
    patient preparation
        endotracheal intubation 44–5
        fasting 42–3
        fluid therapy 43–4
        pharyngostomy intubation 45
        premedication 46–7
        tracheostomy 46
    recovery 49–50
    risk classification *42*

Analgesia 50–2
    after extraction 192
    in feline chronic gingivostomatitis *142*
    for gingivectomy 164
    pre-emptive 46
Ankylosis 112, 193
Anodontia 84, 85
Anterior cross bite 79–80, 83
Anticholinergics 46
Antimicrobials
    after extraction 192–3
    in feline chronic gingivostomatitis 141
    in periodontal disease in dogs 109, 113–14
Apexification 155
Apexogenesis 20
Apically repositioned flap in dogs 111, *112*
Arkansas sharpening stone 70
Attached gingiva *16*
Attachment loss (periodontal) 100–1, *132*
Attrition 152–3
Autoclaves, safety 64
Avulsion 156–7

Bacteria, role in plaque development
    in cats 128–9
    in dogs 98–9
Bacterial aerosol 59, 62
Benzodiazepines 46
Biofilms in dogs 99
Bi-pedicle advancement technique 92
Bisecting-angle technique of radiography 39–40
Bone loss 133
Brachycephalic skull 10, 77, 78
Brachygnathia 77
Bullous pemphigoid in dogs 119–20
Bupivacaine 54, 55
Buprenorphine *142,* 192
Burns
    chemical *158*
    electrical *157*
Burs 72, 75–6
Butorphanol *142,* 192

Calcification disorders 87, 89
Calcium hydroxide pulp-capping agents 149–50, 155
Calculus 33
    forceps 68
    formation
        in cats 129
        in dogs 102
    index *34, 132*
    removal, in dogs 106–9
Candidiasis in dogs 122
Canine distemper 123
Canine odontoclastic resorptive lesion (CORL) *165,* 176

Index

Index

Index

Index

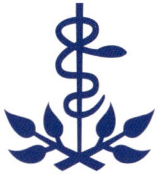

BSAVA Manuals

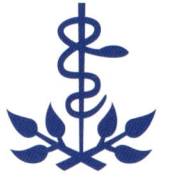

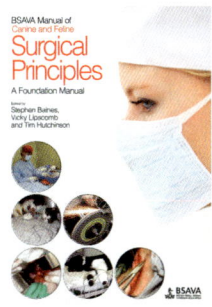

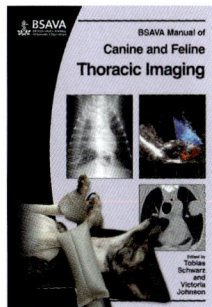

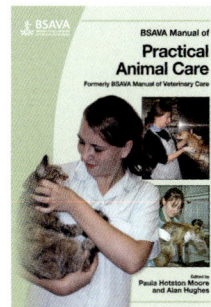

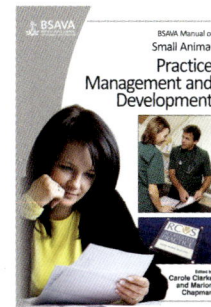

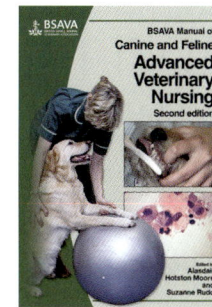

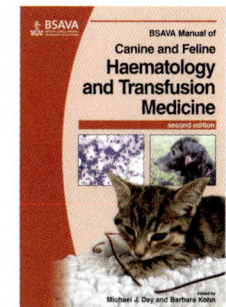

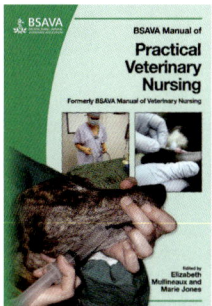

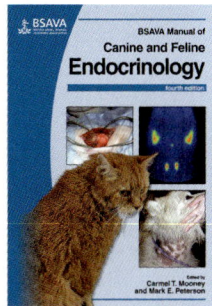

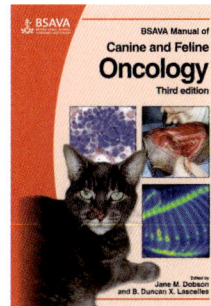

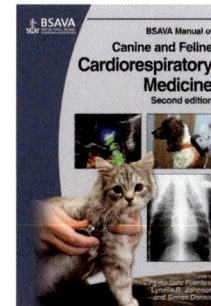

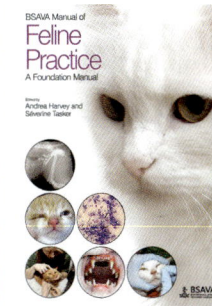

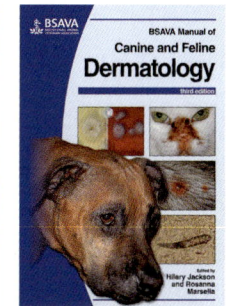

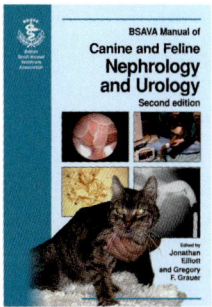

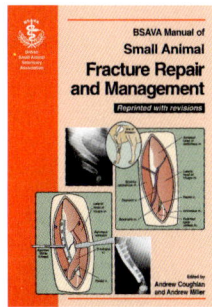

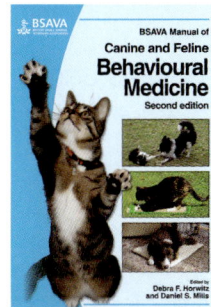

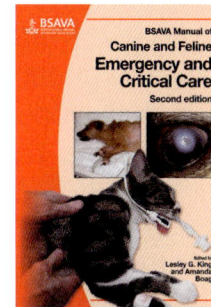

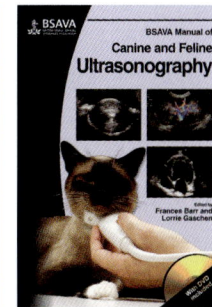

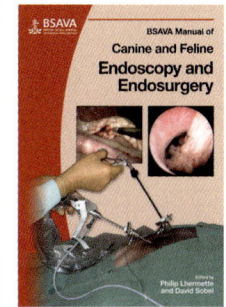

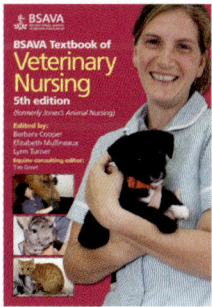

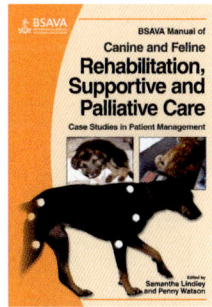

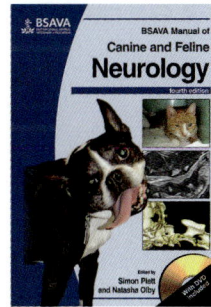

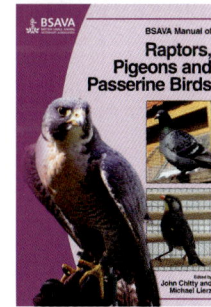

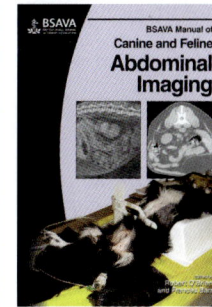

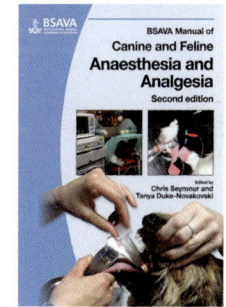

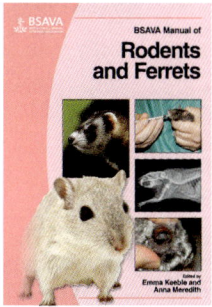

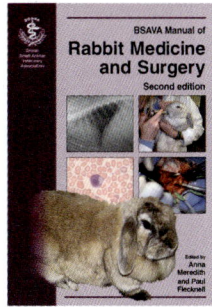

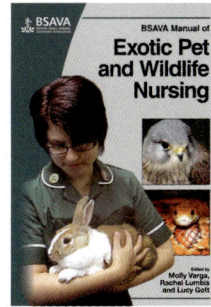

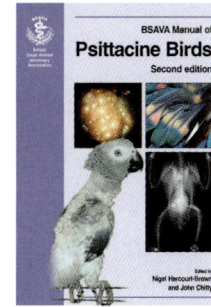

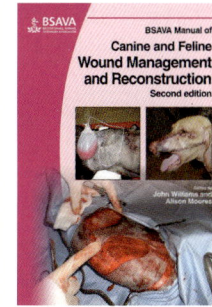

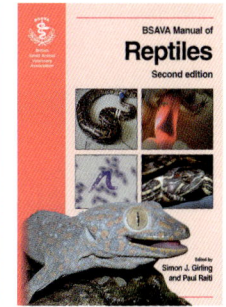

BSAVA Manual of Canine and Feline **Surgical Principles** — A Foundation Manual — Edited by Stephen Baines, Vicky Lipscomb and Tim Hutchinson

BSAVA Manual of **Canine and Feline Thoracic Imaging** — Edited by Tobias Schwarz and Victoria Johnson

BSAVA Manual of **Practical Animal Care** — Formerly BSAVA Manual of Veterinary Care — Paula Hotston Moore and Alan Hughes

BSAVA Manual of Small Animal **Practice Management and Development** — Edited by Carole Clarke and Marion Chapman

BSAVA Manual of Canine and Feline **Advanced Veterinary Nursing** — Second edition — Edited by Alasdair Hotston Moore and Suzanne Rudd

BSAVA Manual of Canine and Feline **Haematology and Transfusion Medicine** — second edition — Edited by Michael J. Day and Barbara Kohn

BSAVA Manual of **Practical Veterinary Nursing** — Formerly BSAVA Manual of Veterinary Nursing — Edited by Elizabeth Mullineaux and Marie Jones

BSAVA Manual of Canine and Feline **Endocrinology** — fourth edition — Carmel T. Mooney and Mark E. Peterson

BSAVA Manual of Canine and Feline **Oncology** — Third edition — Jane M. Dobson and B. Duncan X. Lascelles

BSAVA Manual of Canine and Feline **Cardiorespiratory Medicine** — Second edition — Edited by Virginia Luis Fuentes, Lynelle R. Johnson and Simon Dennis

BSAVA Manual of **Feline Practice** — A Foundation Manual — Andrea Harvey and Séverine Tasker

BSAVA Manual of Canine and Feline **Dermatology** — third edition — Edited by Hilary Jackson and Rosanna Marsella

BSAVA Manual of Canine and Feline **Nephrology and Urology** — Second edition — Edited by Jonathan Elliott and Gregory F. Grauer

BSAVA Manual of Small Animal **Fracture Repair and Management** — Reprinted with revisions — Andrew Coughlan and Andrew Miller

BSAVA Manual of Canine and Feline **Behavioural Medicine** — Second edition — Edited by Debra F. Horwitz and Daniel S. Mills

BSAVA Manual of Canine and Feline **Emergency and Critical Care** — Second edition — Edited by Lesley G. King and Amanda Boag

BSAVA Manual of Canine and Feline **Ultrasonography** — Edited by Frances Barr and Lorrie Gaschen

BSAVA Manual of Canine and Feline **Endoscopy and Endosurgery** — Edited by Philip Lhermette and David Sobel

BSAVA Textbook of **Veterinary Nursing** — 5th edition — (formerly Jones's Animal Nursing) — Edited by: Barbara Cooper, Elizabeth Mullineaux, Lynn Turner

BSAVA Manual of Canine and Feline **Rehabilitation, Supportive and Palliative Care** — Case Studies in Patient Management — Edited by Samantha Lindley and Penny Watson

BSAVA Manual of Canine and Feline **Neurology** — fourth edition — Edited by Simon Platt and Natasha Olby

BSAVA Manual of **Raptors, Pigeons and Passerine Birds** — Edited by John Chitty and Michael Lierz

BSAVA Manual of Canine and Feline **Abdominal Imaging** — Edited by Robert O'Brien and Frances Barr

BSAVA Manual of Canine and Feline **Anaesthesia and Analgesia** — Second edition — Edited by Chris Seymour and Tanya Duke-Novakovski

BSAVA Manual of **Rodents and Ferrets** — Edited by Emma Keeble and Anna Meredith

BSAVA Manual of **Rabbit Medicine and Surgery** — Second edition — Anna Meredith and Paul Flecknell

BSAVA Manual of **Exotic Pet and Wildlife Nursing** — Edited by Molly Varga, Rachel Lumbis and Lucy Gott

BSAVA Manual of **Psittacine Birds** — Second edition — Edited by Nigel Harcourt-Brown and John Chitty

BSAVA Manual of Canine and Feline **Wound Management and Reconstruction** — Second edition — Edited by John Williams and Alison Moores

BSAVA Manual of **Reptiles** — Second edition — Edited by Simon J. Girling and Paul Raiti

Tel: 01452 726700   Fax: 01452 726701
Email: administration@bsava.com   Web: www.bsava.com

BSAVA Manual of
Canine and Feline
Neurology
4th edition

Edited by
Simon Platt and Natasha Olby

This new edition of the best-selling *BSAVA Manual of Canine and Feline Neurology* has been expanded and updated to reflect the many developments in this field. The Manual covers diagnostic procedures and the clinical presentations and therapeutics of neurological diseases, with new chapters on genetic aspects and the science behind the traditional Chinese approach to adjunctive medicine, including information on acupuncture. The advances made in the use of MRI are also fully reflected.

A major addition for this fourth edition is the accompanying DVD, which contains over 100 video clips both of neurological examination and lesion localization. Further reading lists are also included on the DVD.

Contributors:
T James Anderson (UK); Sònia Añor (Spain); Rodney S Bagley (USA); Cheryl Chrisman (USA); Joan R Coates (USA); Peter Dickinson (USA); A Courtenay Freeman (USA); Laurent Garosi (UK); Carley Giovanella (USA); Nicolas Granger (UK); Krista Halling (USA); Nick Jeffery (USA); Sam Long (Australia); Mark Lowrie (UK); Karen Muñana (USA); Gabby Musk (Australia); Dennis O'Brien (USA); Natasha Olby (USA); Mark Papich (USA); Jacques Penderis (UK); Simon Platt (USA); Michael Podell (USA); Roberto Poma[†]; Luc Poncelet (Belgium); Amy Pruitt (USA); Anthea Raisis (Australia); Diane Shelton (USA); Korin Saker (USA); Diane Shelton (USA); John Sherman[†]; Beverley Sturges (USA); Donald E Thrall (St Kitts); Heather Wamsley (USA)

ORDERING DETAILS

British Small Animal Veterinary Association
Woodrow House, 1 Telford Way, Waterwells Business Park, Quedgeley, Gloucester GL2 2AB

Tel: 01452 726700
Fax: 01452 726701
Email: administration@bsava.com
Web: www.bsava.com

BSAVA reserves the right to change these prices at any time
2006PUBS12

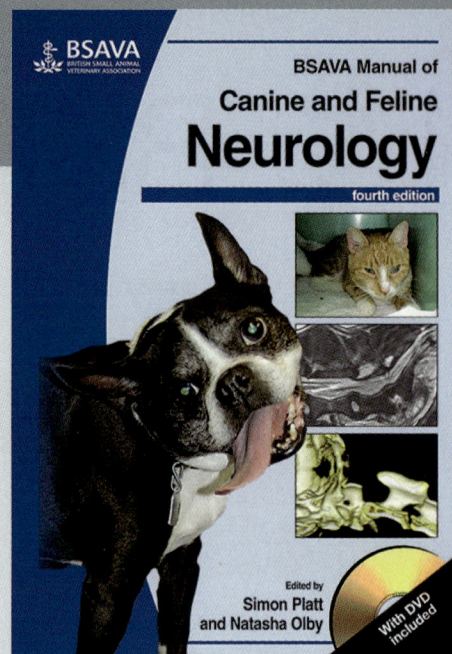

Contents:
The neurological examination; Lesion localization and differential diagnosis; Clinical pathology; Electrophysiology; Neuroimaging; Tissue biopsy; Genetic diseases; Seizures; Coma, stupor and mentation change; Disorders of eyes and vision; Head tilt and nystagmus; Neurological abnormalities of the head and face; Tremors, involuntary movements and paroxysmal disorders; Neck and back pain; Tetraparesis; Paraparesis; Monoparesis; Exercise intolerance and collapse; Tail, anal and bladder dysfunction; Neurological emergencies; Anaesthesia and analgesia; Principles of neurosurgery; Drug therapy for diseases of the central nervous system; Radiation therapy of the nervous system; Rehabilitation of the neurological patient; Treatment of neurological disorders with traditional Chinese veterinary medicine; Appendix 1 – Neurological disorders associated with cat and dog breeds; Appendix 2 – DAMNITV classification of diseases; Appendix 3 – Conversion tables; Index

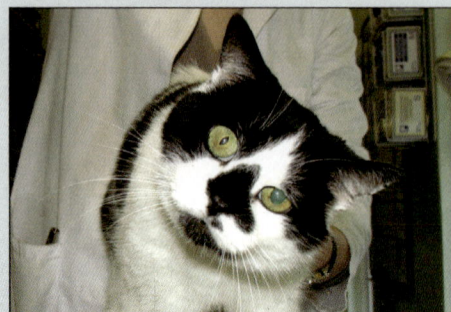

Published 2013
552 pages plus DVD
ISBN   978 1 905319 34 3

Price to non-members: £89.00
MEMBER PRICE: £55.00

BSAVA Manual of

Canine and Feline

Surgical Principles

A Foundation Manual

Edited by

Stephen Baines, Vicky Lipscomb and Tim Hutchinson

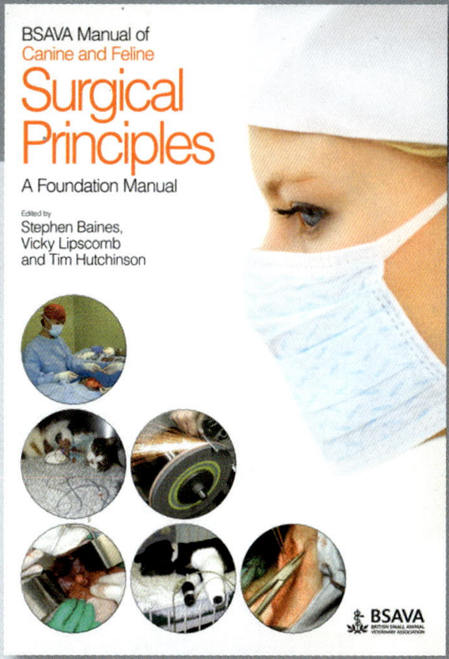

Meticulous attention to the basic principles of surgery is critical if a good surgical outcome is to be achieved. Good surgeons are not those who are simply skilled at surgery, but those who ensure that every aspect of patient care is performed at the highest standard. Complications that arise following surgery are often attributable to a lack of understanding or appreciation of the importance of these basic principles.

The *BSAVA Manual of Canine and Feline Surgical Principles* provides a solid grounding in best practice for the basic principles of veterinary surgery, which will be particularly helpful for veterinary students, new graduates and veterinary nurses as well as any veterinary surgeon wishing to update their knowledge.

- Surgical facilities and equipment
- Perioperative considerations for the surgical patient
- Surgical biology and techniques

WHAT THEY SAY

"...a well-crafted, well-balanced, well-organized new surgery textbook...a good source of information for veterinary students, surgical residents and general practitioners..."
Journal of Small Animal Practice

ORDERING DETAILS

British Small Animal Veterinary Association
Woodrow House, 1 Telford Way, Waterwells Business Park, Quedgeley, Gloucester GL2 2AB

Tel: 01452 726700
Fax: 01452 726701
Email: administration@bsava.com
Web: www.bsava.com

BSAVA reserves the right to change these prices at any time
2005PUBS12

Contents:
Surgical facilities – design, management, equipment and personnel; Sterilization and disinfection; Surgical instruments – materials, manufacture and care; Surgical instruments – types and usage; Suture materials; Surgical staplers; Surgical lasers; Preoperative assessment; Preoperative stabilization; Fluid therapy, and electrolyte and acid-base abnormalities; Shock, sepsis and SIRS; The immune and inflammatory response to anaesthesia; Postoperative management; Principles and practice of analgesia; Principles of nutritional support; Aseptic technique; Healing of elective surgical wounds; Surgical wound infection and antimicrobial prophylaxis; Hospital-acquired infection; Haemostasis and blood component therapy; Principles of operative technique; Suture patterns and surgical knots; Index.

Contributors:
Sophie Adamantos (UK), Davina Anderson (UK), Nick Bacon (USA), Stephen Baines (UK), Noel Berger (USA), Andy Brown (USA), Dan Chan (UK), Liz Chan (UK), Terry Emmerson (UK), Peter Eeg (USA), Gillian Gibson (UK), Rob Goggs (UK), Mike Hamilton (UK), David Holt (USA), Arthur House (Australia), Karen Humm (UK), Geraldine Hunt (USA), Tim Hutchinson (UK), John Lapish (UK), Liz Leece (UK), Vicky Lipscomb (UK), Anette Loefler (UK), Kathryn Pratschke (UK), Veronica Salazar (UK), Chris Shales (UK), Tom Sissener (Canada), Jeffrey Wilson (USA)

Published 2012
312 pages
ISBN   978 1 905319 25 1

Price to non-members: £75.00

MEMBER PRICE: £49.00

**Order online at
www.bsava.com
to save on P&P**

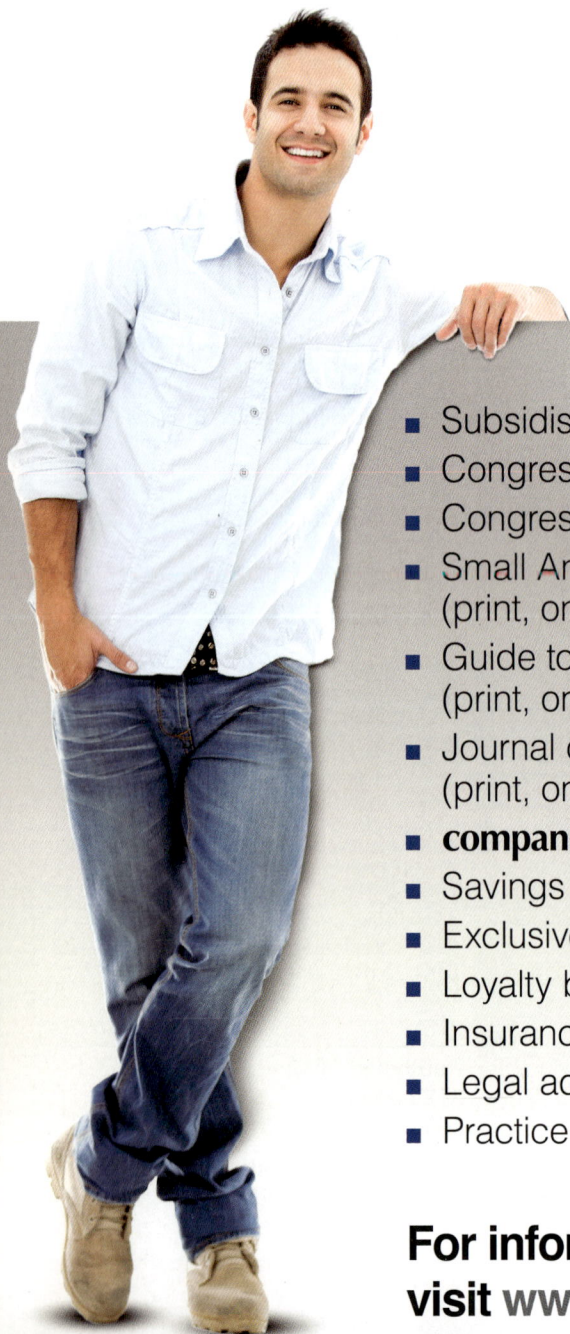

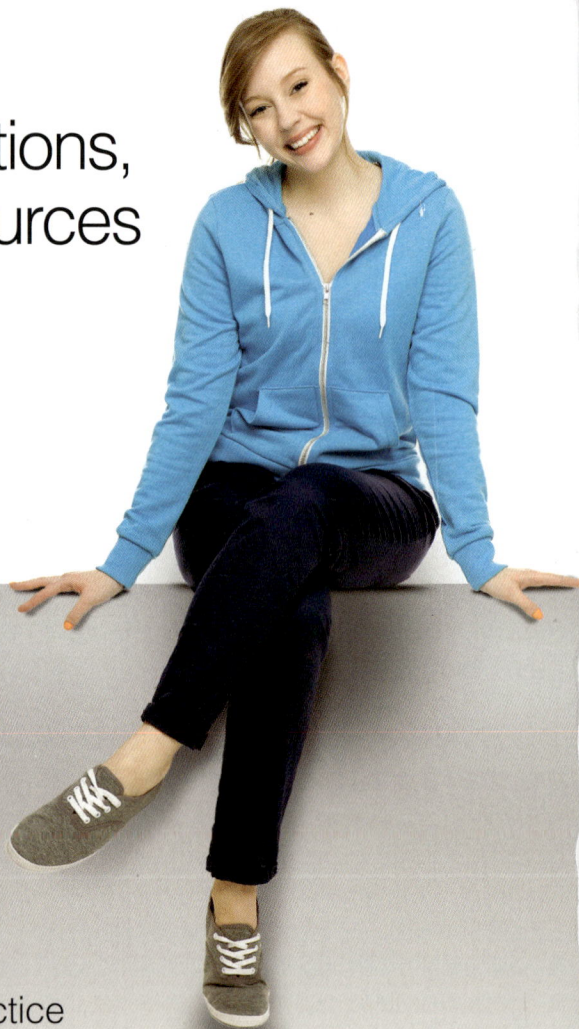